The Healer's Tale

Life Course Studies

David L. Featherman
David I. Kertzer
General Editors

Nancy W. Denney
Thomas J. Espenshade
Dennis P. Hogan
Jennie Keith
Maris A. Vinovskis
Associate General Editors

The
HEALER'S
TALE

*Transforming Medicine
and Culture*

Sharon R. Kaufman

THE UNIVERSITY OF WISCONSIN PRESS

The University of Wisconsin Press
114 North Murray Street
Madison, Wisconsin 53715

3 Henrietta Street
London WC2E 8LU, England

3   4   5   6   7   8   9   10

Printed in the United States of America

Library of Congress Cataloging-in-Publication Data
Kaufman, Sharon R.
The healer's tale : transforming medicine and culture /
Sharon R. Kaufman.
368 p.   cm.—(Life course studies)
Includes bibliographical references and index.
ISBN 0-299-13550-0
ISBN 0-299-13554-3 (pbk.)
1. Physicians—United States—Biography.   I. Title.
II. Series.
R153.K24   1993
610'.973'0922—dc20
[B]   92-34798

For Seth, Sarah, and Jacob

CONTENTS

PART III *Generalists, Scientists, and Curers:*
 1930s and 1940s

PART IV *Power and Influence: 1946–1970s*

ACKNOWLEDGMENTS

I AM DEEPLY indebted to the seven physicians whose lives are portrayed in the following pages. Neither they nor I knew how long this project would take when I began the first interview in 1987. Listening to their stories has deepened my understanding of medicine's transformation during the twentieth century. Getting to know these doctors has enriched my own life tremendously. They each spent three days with me, talking about their lives and patiently and graciously answering my questions. Over the next few years, by letter and telephone, they responded to my requests for more information. I asked them to read both the original interview transcripts and the edited, final version of the narratives for accuracy. They read and commented on a first draft of the entire manuscript. And they found and sent me most of the photographs included here.

In the pages that follow, it is obvious that they are timeless role models in medicine. They are also role models for a good old age. As I write this, they are well into their eighties and remain actively engaged in making the world a better place through their scholarship and their ongoing contributions to their universities, medical and nonmedical organizations, and local and national communities. It has been a great privilege to know them.

During the years of this project, two of the doctors still had demanding schedules, traveled extensively, and went to their offices daily. I wish to thank Jeannie Shapin, secretary to Dr. Jonathan Rhoads at the Department of Surgery, University of Pennsylvania, and Rosalie Feinen, secretary to Dr. John Romano at the Department of Psychiatry, University of Rochester. They have been especially helpful to me over the past four years.

I spoke with many people around the United States in my search for appropriate physicians to include in this project. I am grateful to them all for their help. Paul Beeson, J. Andrew Fantl, Joseph Kushner, Michel Mandel, Ann Morris, Marcia Ory, Hamilton Putnam, and Guenter Risse suggested the participating doctors.

I owe a special debt to Karol Ortiz, who read the manuscript in its early stages and challenged and enriched my thinking about medicine's changes, means, and ends. She encouraged me to think deeply about medicine's evolution and the physicians' careers and urged me to ponder carefully the relationship of life history research to contemporary problems in medicine. I cannot thank her enough. David Plath read the entire manuscript and helped me refine my ideas and clarify my writing. Adele Clarke and Margaret Clark read portions of the manuscript and offered valuable suggestions. Amy Einsohn's astute editorial suggestions contributed to the book's final form, as did the comments of Eric Cassell, Jennie Keith, and David Kertzer.

Guenter Risse, chairman of the History of Health Sciences Department, UCSF, introduced me to the field of the history of medicine. I thank him for his early guidance and encouragement. Gay Becker, my invaluable colleague and friend at the Institute for Health and Aging, UCSF, gave me moral and practical support throughout this project. I thank the institute staff, especially Sue Churka-Hyde, Edwina Newsom, and Norton Twite, for their assistance over the years with tape transcription and word processing. I am grateful to all my colleagues at the Institute for Health and Aging, the Department of Social and Behavioral Sciences, and the Medical Anthropology Program, UCSF, for their support in facing the challenges of being a "soft" social scientist on a health-sciences campus.

Finally, I wish to thank Allen Fitchen, for his confidence in my work, and the staff at the University of Wisconsin Press, for their fine attention to all the details that turn a manuscript into a book.

This project was supported in part by a grant from the Academic Senate, University of California, San Francisco.

San Francisco
June 1992

The Healer's Tale

PROLOGUE

Public Consciousness and Confusion

CONTEMPORARY Western medicine stands between culture and nature and manipulates both. Medicine has traditionally manipulated nature in its attempt to prevent or intervene in the ravages of disease. We continue to expect it to do so. More recently medicine has also begun to transform culture with its increasing power to manipulate natural processes. Such profound transformation makes us uneasy. Our ideas about the beginning of life, the finality of death, and the process and role of motherhood, for example, are deeply held cultural beliefs about human nature itself. The emergence of a baby into the world, the visible and palpable cessation of respiration and heart beat, a woman who conceives, bears, and raises a child—these fundamental matters of life, death, and motherhood are now changing. What we have always considered "natural" is now reconsidered in light of the results of medical technology: "live" twenty-four-week-old fetuses; "brain dead" individuals enabled to breathe through respirators; women who contribute an egg toward or gestate a baby or who nurture one from someone else's egg/gestation. Yet our long-held cultural conceptions of a natural birth, natural death, and natural mother have not been ultimately replaced or superseded by clear, acceptable definitions created by medical possibility. On the contrary, medical advances have forced us to reconsider the boundaries of life and death and have made it unclear when life begins, when death occurs, and what a mother is. The confusion generated by the blurring of traditional boundaries between culture and nature permeates national consciousness. Consider the following news stories.

HOW DO WE DEFINE
THE ORIGINS OF LIFE?

San Francisco Chronicle, August 8, 1989 (Associated Press)
Husband vs. Wife
1st Day of Trial in Embryo Dispute
Maryville, Tennessee—Trial began yesterday in a divorce case in which the judge must decide whether seven frozen embryos should go to a husband who does not want children now or to a wife who cannot conceive naturally.

Junior Lewis Davis, 30, sued for divorce from Mary Sue Davis in February and asked that Mrs. Davis, 28, be barred from ever using any of the seven fertilized eggs without his consent. Mrs. Davis contends that she should be able to have the eggs implanted without his consent because the implantation procedure might be her best chance of having a child.

"The question of how we classify these embryos is vital," Jay Christenberry, Mrs. Davis' attorney, said in his opening statement. "While the couple's rights are important, there are other rights we must consider." . . .

The case is thought to be the first of its type in the United States.
Not a Person
A medical ethics expert testified yesterday that the embryos deserve special respect but should not be given the same rights as a person . . .

New York Times, May 27, 1990
New Turn in Couple's Fight over Frozen Embryos
Knoxville, Tennessee, May 26 (Associated Press)—A woman who won custody of seven embryos last September in a widely publicized court ruling now says she plans to donate them to a fertility clinic so that they can be used by a childless couple.

But her former husband, who fertilized the embryos and is her opponent in the continuing legal fight over them, says her decision has no bearing on his appeal . . .

San Francisco Chronicle, September 14, 1990
Tennessee Ruling Grants Joint Custody of Embryos
Judges Overturn Ex-Wife's Lower-court Win
Knoxville, Tenn.—The Tennessee Court of Appeals yesterday granted joint custody of seven frozen embryos to a divorced couple, overturning a landmark ruling that had granted custody to the woman . . .

The three appeals court judges made it clear during oral arguments that they wanted to avoid the ethical and philosophical questions of the case—such as whether the embryos are alive and deserving of legal protection—and stick to the issue of what to do with them.

WHAT IS A MOTHER?

New York Times, August 12, 1990 (Carol Lawson)
Couple's Own Embryos Used in Birth Surrogacy
. . . Four years after the Baby M case, which provoked calls for strict regulation of surrogate motherhood, if not an outright ban, surrogacy is not only actively practiced but expanding in a new direction, bringing new hope to some families and, at the same time, highlighting a host of ethical and legal concerns.
Wife's Eggs and Husband's Sperm
The Baby M case involved what physicians now call traditional surrogacy, in which the surrogate mother is impregnated through artifical insemination with the sperm of the husband from the couple who have hired her. The surrogate is thus the genetic mother of the baby.
In contrast, the Venezuelan couple are beneficiaries of what medical and legal experts call gestational surrogacy. The wife's eggs and the husband's sperm were brought together in a petri-dish in a hospital laboratory in Pasadena in the process known as in vitro fertilization . . .

Los Angeles Times, October 25, 1990 (Robert Steinbrook)
Menopausal Pregnancy Becoming a Reality
5 Women with Nonfunctioning Ovaries Give Birth in Researcher's Embryo Implant Study
Physicians using advanced reproductive technologies have enabled some menopausal women in their 40s to bear children, according to a report in today's New England Journal of Medicine.
The achievement, which involves eggs transferred from another woman, hormonal supplements and test-tube fertilization, is the latest in a fast-moving field that has pushed back the limits of pregnancy. It opens up the possibility of childbearing well into middle age but also promises to raise legal questions and debate about the ethics of giving birth late in life.
"The limits on the childbearing years are now anyone's guess," said Dr. Marcia Angell, executive editor of the New England Journal . . .

New York Times, November 4, 1990 (Seth Mydans)
Science and the Courts Take a New Look at Motherhood
　　As advances in technology bring into question basic assumptions about life and death, medical and legal scholars are suggesting that motherhood may in the future be defined less in terms of biology than in terms of intent.

　　The biological definition of motherhood lost a good deal of its certainty late last month with a court decision and the announcement of a medical advance that presented contrasting new versions of this elemental concept.

　　In the court case, a judge in California denied parental rights to a surrogate mother who had carried and given birth to an implanted fetus with which she had no genetic connection. Comparing her with a foster parent, he ruled that her womb was little more than a home in which she had sheltered and fed the legal offspring of the genetic parents.

　　A few days later, an advance in fertility research put the priorities in the opposite order, making it possible for a woman past the age of menopause to carry, give birth to, and claim as her own an implanted embryo that was a genetic stranger to her.

　　"In these two instances we have exactly the same biological situation, yet we want different legal results," said Lori B. Andrews, the author of two books on surrogate motherhood. "The law has always looked at parenthood in terms of biology. Now it needs to be more creative. You need to move to something like pre-conception intent. It has always been the legal presumption that the mother who gives birth is the legal mother. It made sense. It was the only way, the one certainty. But it's not certain anymore." . . .

　　Measures addressing surrogacy were introduced in every state legislature after the highly publicized Baby M case in 1987 and 1988, but few were adopted. Two states, Michigan and Florida, now forbid paid surrogacy arrangements and five other states, while not banning them, have deemed surrogacy contracts legally unenforceable.

　　None of the states has yet answered, for legal purposes, the newly complicated question: What is a mother? . . .

WHO CONTROLS DEATH?

New York Times, January 10, 1991 (Lisa Belkin)
Reverse Right-to-Die Case in Minnesota
　　Minneapolis—In a case that medical ethicists and legal experts say is apparently a first, a Minneapolis hospital plans to go to court for permis-

sion to turn off a patient's life support system against her family's wishes.

For eight months, 87-year-old Helga Wanglie has lain in Hennepin County Medical Center dependent on a ventilator for oxygen and a feeding tube for nutrition, unaware of and unresponsive to her surroundings. Her doctors say that she will never recover and that they do not want to give medical care that they describe as futile.

But Mrs. Wanglie's husband and two children describe her as an extremely religious woman who would prefer even this life to death.

"This is the opposite of Cruzan," said Arthur Caplan, director of the Center for Biomedical Ethics at the University of Minnesota, referring to Nancy Cruzan, the Missouri woman whose family fought for years to remove her from the feeding tube that was keeping her alive . . .

New York Times, July 19, 1989 (Martin Tolchin)
When Long Life Is Too Much: Suicide Rises among Elderly
Washington, July 18—Reversing a half-century trend, the suicide rate among elderly Americans steadily increased in the 1980's, according to Government records.

The 25 percent increase from 1981 to 1986, the last year for which the Government has records, brought the suicide rate among those 65 and older to 21.6 per 100,000 people, as against an overall national rate of 12.8. The trend perplexes health care experts, who note that the elderly are generally more financially secure and healthier, and they live longer than their forebears . . .

But some experts speculate that the technological advances extending the lives of the elderly sometimes bring a quality of life that they cannot accept . . .

New York Times, May 23, 1989 (Lisa Belkin)
Doctors Debate Helping Terminally Ill Die
Houston, May 23—With medicine preoccupied by AIDS, a question that doctors once only whispered has emerged as a subject of open medical debate: should doctors be allowed to help their patients kill themselves?

Leading medical journals give space to advocates of doctor-assisted suicide for terminally ill patients and to others who argue against what is also being called voluntary euthanasia. And efforts are under way in four states to put the question to the voters.
Doctors Willing to Help
"The discussion has shifted," said Earl E. Shelp, a Southern Baptist minister in Houston who is teaching a seminar on AIDS and a course

on medical ethics at Dartmouth College this semester. "It is being discussed now not as an absolute prohibition, but as a question of under what circumstances should it be allowed," he said.

The issue is not merely theoretical. Terminally ill patients often ask their doctors to help them die. And though such help is illegal, there are doctors who agree to assist their patients . . .

New York Times, December 3, 1990 (Isabel Wilkerson)
Murder Charge Filed against 'Suicide Doctor'
Women Died after Using Physician's Death Machine
Chicago—A Michigan doctor who connected a woman suffering from Alzheimer's disease to a homemade suicide device and watched as she pushed a button and died was charged yesterday with first degree murder.

The case is being closely watched as a watershed in the debate over whether physicians should be allowed to assist terminally ill patients who want to take their own lives . . .

New York Times, December 14, 1990 (Tamar Lewin)
Judge Clears Doctor of Murdering Woman with a Suicide Machine
A Michigan judge threw out murder charges yesterday against Dr. Jack Kevorkian, who touched off a bitter nationwide debate over euthanasia in June when he connected a 54-year-old woman with Alzheimer's disease to his homemade suicide machine, then watched as she pushed a button and died.

After a two-day preliminary hearing on the case in Clarkston, Mich., Judge Gerald McNally of Oakland County District Court ruled that the prosecutors had failed to prove that Dr. Kevorkian, 62, had planned and carried out the death of the woman, Janet Adkins. Judge McNally said it was Mrs. Adkins and not Dr. Kevorkian who had caused her death . . .

Dr. Kevorkian said yesterday that while he was convinced that he had done the right thing, he had been taken aback by the magnitude of the response to Mrs. Adkins' death and was pleasantly surprised by the judge's decision.

His lawyers praised the ruling, and said they were heartened by the debate the case had inspired . . .

San Francisco Chronicle, August 9, 1991
Book with Advice on Suicide Hits Top of a Best-Seller List
New York—A new book that advises terminally ill people on how to

take their own lives has surged to No. 1 on the hard-cover advice category on the New York Times best-seller list . . .

The book is "Final Exit" by Derek Humphry, executive director of
the Hemlock Society, an organization in Eugene, Ore., that advises on
how to commit suicide . . .

Humphry said in a telephone interview yesterday that people are
"tired of ethical debate among theologians and philosophers."

"There's tremendous desire for personal control and choice over
one's dying."

INTRODUCTION

Medicine, Nature, Culture

THE ETHICAL DEBATE, court decisions, and cultural confusion generated by new medical technologies and practices have permeated much of contemporary life. Modern medical research and practice have given us many innovations: organ transplants, artificial organs, implanted devices, and infusion systems; gene splicing and genetic engineering; laboratory fertilization and embryo transfer; prenatal diagnosis of genetic defects and gender selection of children; sperm banks; artificial insemination; in utero surgery; genetically engineered vaccines; and the prolongation of life by artificial means. In doing so, medicine has produced a paradox. Though medicine has accelerated our sense of power and control over our destinies, it has, at the same time, also shaken the foundations of our definitions of life, death, and the natural life span. It has confused us.

Because advances in medical knowledge and application have so altered our knowledge of ourselves, our limitations, and our possibilities, medicine plays an evocative role in contemporary society. Each new discovery in the laboratory, each new groundbreaking surgical procedure or experimental drug therapy forces us to reconsider the limits of medicine's ability to cure, to expand our notions of the viable body and self. Each new medical development confronts us with existential questions about our humanity. What, in fact, is it to be a human being if we can replace organs with plastic and still survive? Where does our autonomy end and our dependence begin when we come to rely on technology to keep us alive? What does dependence mean when a cardiac pacemaker enables us to be independent? What is a "quality" life? Is it a life free of pain, or a life enabled to persist despite pain? Medicine draws attention to questions about our identity and our limits as human beings

11

while its discoveries and practices provoke a reconsideration of the forms and possibilities of human existence.[1]

Medicine has always played a dominant role in defining the human being. For example, ancient civilizations posited that four substances constitute the human body: black bile, yellow bile, phlegm, and blood. These substances were thought to function in a specific relationship to the seasons, the planets, and an entire cosmological system. For hundreds of years, in many parts of the world, conceptions of the body based on these substances and their relationship to nature guided medical diagnosis and treatment and shaped people's understanding of themselves and their place in the natural world. Galen, the famous Greek physician who lived around A.D. 130, conceived of "vital spirits," "natural spirits," and "animal spirits" to describe physiological processes. His ideas shaped medical thinking for centuries. Fifteen hundred years later, the roots of modern biological theories began to replace earlier conceptions of human functioning when observation, experimentation, and what we now call the scientific method came into use. For example, after William Harvey conducted his experiments on blood flow and circulation (published in 1628), the heart was discovered to be a pump, and current theories of the relationship between circulation and respiration could begin to develop.

Contemporary medicine, too, has given us frameworks for understanding how we function and how we may better function. Thus it has given us better knowledge of who we are as biological organisms. It has also given us at least a partial vocabulary for describing ourselves as psychological and cultural beings. But unlike its precursors, contemporary medicine has not clarified our relationship with the natural world. In fact, developments in modern medicine have forced our reconsideration of the meaning of "nature" and "natural." And as our biological knowledge becomes more precise, our psychological and cultural understanding becomes more obscure.

Assumptions about the origins and limits of life and finality of death are the anchors of existential awareness. Doubting those assumptions is highly unsettling. One reason the field of bioethics has emerged with great fanfare in the last decade is that we desperately want, need, and are searching for experts to take responsibility for defining life and death with clarity and sureness, and to create order, consistency, and predictability from the new chaos into which the application of medical knowledge has plunged us. Professionals in health care as well as the public are turning to bioethics for resolution of the many existential ambiguities medical advances have created. Such ambiguities are rooted in two larger subjects: the separation and opposition of nature and culture, and the relationship between technology and morality.

NATURE AND CULTURE:
BLURRED BOUNDARIES

Medicine has blurred our once firmly established boundaries between nature and culture and, by doing so, has challenged their very definitions. This fact is of fundamental importance when we consider the idea, proposed by the anthropologist Claude Lévi-Strauss, that the greatest distinction in human thought is the separation of nature and culture.[2] In the Western world, and particularly in America, we can begin with the cultural assumption that nature and culture are independent entities, autonomous of one another.[3] It is widely believed that nature was here first; culture was superimposed when human beings evolved relatively recently—a few million years ago. One of humankind's primary activities has been to tame, control, and remake nature to suit our cultural purposes, first of all, for the procurement of food, clothing, and shelter, and then for the acquisition of wealth and the production of material comfort.

Separation and opposition of nature and culture is maintained in popular thought by at least two of our broadest cultural institutions—science and religion. In our everyday view of science, nature is potentially knowable and predictable if we can, by rational means, discover its own laws and order through observation, measurement, and dissection.[4] Religion, on the other hand, confronts phenomena that are natural—including birth, death, and disease—by looking at them as unknowable, in some essential way, to humankind. Religion's aim is not to know nature, but rather to make our coexistence with the unpredictability of nature palatable through the creation of prayer, faith, and ritual.

Developments in modern medicine undermine the culturally produced autonomy of nature from culture so fundamental to the modern Western ethos. Examples of their new and uncertain relationship abound. Notions of motherhood and family are obsolete, because reproductive technologies create the options of surrogate (as opposed to natural/biological) motherhood and test tube (to be distinguished from natural) babies. Traditional (natural) ways of dying can be supplanted by technologically or pharmaceutically controlled death. Identical twins have always been thought to be a phenomenon of nature. Now, multiple embryos, brought into existence at the same moment, containing similar genetic material, can be frozen, only to be grown separately, at different times in a woman's womb.[5] The resulting children look alike but are different ages. What now are twins? The human body, itself the result of nature and the evolutionary process, can exist (more and more often for prolonged periods of time) with some of its natural organs aided by artifical devices or replaced by artifical organs. Medicine gives us new possibilities and options for considering the relationship between nature and culture. At the same time, medicine is weakening traditional cultural definitions about the work of nature and the natural world of the human organism without replacing these definitions. In doing so, medicine creates existential dilemmas. The work that needs to be done by society to resolve those dilemmas is only just beginning.

TECHNOLOGY AND MORALITY

Many have observed that medicine is driven by means, not ends. More refined technological devices and procedures, more powerful diagnostic tools, more sophisticated interventions capture the attention of both the medical community and public and move medicine irrevocably onward at ever greater speed. The devices, tools, and procedures dominate our thinking. Their use is not informed by a shared cultural mandate which considers their long-term social worth or their ability to alter the meaning of nature and culture. The very speed with which innovations are produced and the authority with which they are employed makes society powerless to intervene: by the time we have considered some of the implications of the new technologies, it is too late to stop either their use or their integration into the biomedical enterprise and medicine's self-definition.[6]

Because medical innovations force us to reconsider culture and nature, definitions of morality—what constitutes correct, appropriate behavior—become obscured: Is the laboratory creation of babies still human reproduction? Is it ethical? Should parents-to-be have the right to screen their progeny genetically for intelligence or athletic ability? to choose the sex of their baby? Should comatose or frail and demented individuals be kept alive by artificial means? and for how long? Should terminally ill people be able to choose the time and method of their death? The questions are endless.

We live in an age in which individual rights, personal preference, and immediate gratification are valued more strongly than are notions of community, social responsibility, and long-term goals. This is evident in the low priority our national policy places on a clean environment, public education, and access to health services, for example. In the realm of health care, lack of shared values about the worth or potential of actual medical interventions troubles our decision-making after the fact. We employ the technology and then are forced to ponder and evaluate the ramifications of what we have done. Decisions in medicine about an appropriate course of action are determined by the immediacy of solving particular problems in specific situations with the best technology available. The "technological imperative,"[7] not some firm set of beliefs and goals, is shaping medicine.[8]

The technological imperative—the means—is paired with medicine's moral imperative—its ends: to save lives and manage the course of disease. The moral imperative guides and rationalizes medicine's specific practices, especially reliance on and commitment to uses of technology. These means and ends exist as basic assumptions and give meaning to medical practitioners' actions. Yet they are taken for granted by most of us and thus have been largely unexamined. Medicine's ends are particularly problematic. They are not based on a consideration of what, or how much, or when, or for whom technological intervention and the saving and managing of lives is appropriate. How and why did this problem arise? Why do physicians and patients alike have so much difficulty articulating shared values about medicine's means and ends?

THE LIFE IN MEDICINE

This book grew out of my awareness of the evocative nature of contemporary medical research and practice. I wanted to explore the development of medicine's means and ends by examining how these were experienced in the individual careers of significant contributors to twentieth-century medicine. I have centered my inquiry on the life history, rather than on other kinds of historical material, because of my conviction that subjective reflections on individual choices and practices in medicine are valuable sources for understanding medicine's current dilemmas. Examination of the personal narrative is one method for knowing how we moved from the past to the present and how we have formed our conceptions of the future. Such narratives serve both as sources for identifying and examining the development of means, ends, values, and practices and as documentation of medicine's twentieth-century transformation and its impact on cultural forms.

Life histories of selected physicians who have "seen it all" can illuminate some of the ways in which medicine has come to have such a profound impact on nature, culture, and thus ourselves. Doctors who were trained before antibiotics and the world of high-tech and who have practiced since the 1930s have seen medicine change drastically, from an honorable and duty-bound occupation of comfort and care, to a powerful profession of creating and administering cures, to the currently God-like and unsettling pursuit of re-creating human life. Physicians who were leaders in their particular fields have contributed to those changes. Their life histories can offer individual, subjective perspectives on medicine's transformation.

During the lifetimes of the seven physicians whose stories follow, medicine's very definition changed dramatically. When they entered the profession, its primary activities were diagnosis and care; medicine could cure relatively few diseases. During their careers, care was superseded by cure, and the long-held values of consolation and empathy came to be informed by the standardized and quantifiable methods of laboratory science. Gradually, medicine's traditional goals of diagnosis and support of the patient were overshadowed by the emergence of a seductive, powerful, scientific, and operational way of understanding disease and human suffering and of valuing human life. Medicine's transformation was not planned or anticipated by individual physicians or, in fact, by anyone. It has evolved in pragmatic response both to specific, localized challenges in patient care and disease management and to the availability of new technologies. As physicians have become able to save more lives, they have not, by and large, stopped to ponder the implications of their day-to-day activities for medicine's identity or for its impact on the meaning of life, death, nature, and culture.

I wanted to examine how medicine's transformation occurred by looking at the lives of individuals who participated actively in that transformation. I wanted to know how social values, expectations, and attitudes, as well as scientific ideas, diseases, and treatments, shaped their careers and changed over decades. I specifically asked the doctors to ponder the effects of medicine's changing values on their lives and their specialties and to discuss how the values of the 1920s and 1930s were transformed over the course of their careers.

Much attention has been paid in recent years to the politics and institutions that have shaped post–World War II American medicine and the rise and decline in medical authority and power vis-à-vis other American institutions. The stories of the seven lives which follow represent a more intimate portrait of developments in medicine, because they consider those larger forces only as background. I gathered life histories because I wanted to uncover what it was like to become and practice as a physician in America during the middle of the twentieth century. One of my goals was to have doctors describe their lives in medicine in order to illustrate how the profession made them and how, given the opportunities they encountered and the constraints they faced, they created the profession while making themselves. Another goal was to examine those narratives as examples of medical culture, tradition, and changing values and as reference points for our current social and ethical debates. Excursions into the structure and details of a life give us a picture of the self in culture, a picture neglected by studies of politics and institutions. Physicians' life histories provide one basis, one perspective, for understanding medicine's dominant role in simultaneously defining human potential and obscuring the nature of the human being.

The midlife years of the doctors portrayed here coincided with the growing prestige, power, and authority of medicine in the United States. They were at the height of their careers during medicine's "Golden Age," that brief, unprecedented height of prosperity, autonomy, and influence (1945–1965).[9] Indeed, their lives in medicine contributed to the Golden Age. Yet, their stories do not dwell on medicine's scientific advances, or on its political or social prestige. Indeed, their accounts present some of medicine's shortcomings and failings. The doctors did not promote a view of a profession dominant in the larger world. Instead, they described their personal development—and medicine's transformation—through the day-to-day routine of practicing medicine.

American medicine can be conceived as a cultural system. Within that conception, the book is structured to move between two conversations and two tasks. One conversation is held between myself and each doctor in the form of the life history narratives which follow. The corresponding task is to portray developments in medicine from the varied viewpoints of seven of its distinguished practitioners. The doctors' accounts reveal "insider" understandings of the evolving goals, frustrations, and ideals of twentieth-century American medicine.

The second conversation ponders the implications of the narratives for understanding medicine's transformation. The task is both to place the doctors' accounts in a historical and social perspective and to examine some of the taken-for-granted, inevitable features of the culture the doctors describe. The goal of presenting these two conversations is to make explicit some of the tacit rules, values, developments, and definitions in the culture of medicine that have contributed to our current state of moral confusion.

While we look to the future and try to sort out and resolve the ethical dilemmas and confusion created by contemporary medical knowledge and practices, the traditions of medical science and activity are ever present. Our understanding of medicine's means, ends, ambiguities, and evocative nature will be richer if we pay attention to its immediate past.

SEVEN DOCTORS

THE WORK OF the individuals whose life histories I collected was, according to their colleagues, highly respected during their entire careers. The career paths of these doctors were not so unusual that they were known as mavericks, yet their work, in one way or another, extended or challenged the dominant ideas and practices of their time.[1]

I looked for researchers and clinicians, university-based physicians and private practitioners. Of the seven doctors whose stories are included here, four were university-based, three of them full-time. It was easier for me to locate appropriate academic physicians for this project, because the academic world is small. I asked university-based physicians, "Who are the outstanding doctors in your field trained during the 1920s and 1930s?" It was much more difficult to locate appropriate solo practitioners in other parts of the country without the connecting networks of the university world, because those people do not usually have national reputations. But there is another reason for the emphasis here on academic physicians. During most of this century, definitions of what constitutes medical knowledge and practice—in research, in patient care, in defining the specialties, and in the education of the next generation of physicians—were created and re-created primarily by doctors who had university careers. Thus it seemed appropriate to emphasize their voices.

I specifically chose doctors whose range of work was broadly rather than narrowly defined, because a broad practice in medicine was most typical of the period during which these doctors were trained and were establishing their careers. The specialties included here are internal medicine, general surgery, general psychiatry, obstetrics and gynecology, and pediatrics. Though ophthalmology, otolaryngology, and dermatology were established specialty fields before the 1930s, I decided not to interview doctors in those fields for two reasons. First, I concentrated on the branches of medicine that affect the greatest number of people. Second, I examined the broad fields of medicine in existence between the First and Second world wars that have had the greatest impact on our thinking about medicine's relationship to culture and nature and medicine's ability to define the human being. The subspecialties that came into existence after these seven doctors had established their careers—cardiac surgery, oncology, neonatology, reproductive endocrinology, for example—have more dramatically than ever drawn attention to cultural, biological, and ethical questions about our identity and to questions about medicine's purpose. But those subspecialties are recent innovations; they did not exist before the Second World War. The broad fields discussed by these physicians foreshadowed those developments.

Women were minorities in medicine before the Second World War. For the most part, they went into pediatrics, psychiatry, and public health, because those were the fields most frequently open to them. I interviewed one woman, a pediatrician, as representative of a pathway available to women of that era. Jews were also minorities in medicine before the war. I interviewed one Jew in order to learn more about discrimination during the years between the wars. I chose a Jew rather than a member of a different religious or ethnic minority because it was common for Jews of that period to aspire to independent, medical careers. Following the Second World War, many Jews who had chosen medical careers in the 1920s and 1930s became very prominent in all fields of American medicine.[2]

Sons of doctors were favored by medical school admission committees and made up approximately one-quarter of medical school classes between the wars.[3] Four of these seven doctors followed in their fathers' footsteps. They came from middle-class families. The three whose fathers were not doctors had to work their way through medical school. Two of those were from poor families.

It also seemed important to seek both geographic and educational variety among the interviewees. I wanted to collect stories of growing up in different regions of America. And I wanted to know the ways in which medical education in both great and not-great institutions had an impact on the career path. Finally, the seven interviewed are doctors about the same age. They were born in 1906, 1907, and 1908, and were all between the ages of eighty and eighty-three during the period of the interviews, 1987–1989.

These individuals shared two remarkable traits at the time the interviews were conducted. They each possessed a physical vitality unusual for their years, and they each had a keen, penetrating intellect. Without exception, they engaged me and my questions with a clear, direct gaze, and they worked very hard to reflect on, remember, and evaluate their long lives. Telling the story of one's life from the perspective of eighty years is a challenging task and requires much energy. I was acutely aware of that fact during the three days I spent with each person. All these doctors accepted the challenge with grace, seriousness, humor, and a desire to represent themselves and their careers as accurately as possible. Watching them and listening to them, I suspected that they created the life history with the same intelligence, directness, and commitment as they had engaged the practice of medicine.

J. DUNBAR SHIELDS

Through inquiries made to academic physicians, private practitioners, and medical societies in the New England states, I searched for an appropriate physician from a smaller town who was not affiliated with a major university. I discovered J. Dunbar Shields of Concord, New Hampshire. He has a distinguished statewide reputation and had just been honored with the Laureate Award given by the American College of Physicians (1989). He was instrumental in establishing internal medicine as a specialty in the state. Warm, friendly, and enthusiastic, Dr. Shields greeted me in the new, small home he and his wife "were still getting used to" in Concord, after moving from the large home they had lived in for fifty-three years. Photographs of his three children, grandchildren, and great-grandchildren fill the walls of his home, and he talked about them fondly during my visits. A large and complex drawing of his family tree hangs in his small study. Dr. Shields is a man embedded in caring family relationships. He told me repeatedly that his family has greatly enriched his life, his understanding of people, and his ability to interact well with colleagues and patients. He made me feel at ease as we walked to his study, and while we talked, he struck me as a man genuinely interested in people and their problems. Not wanting to represent his life in medicine through rose-colored glasses, he candidly discussed the limitations, frustrations, and false starts of medicine which had an impact on his ability to help people. Through a pursuit of new and appropriate treatments

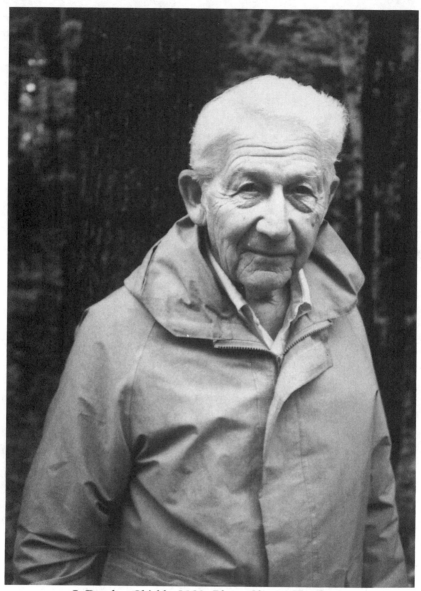

J. Dunbar Shields, 1989. Photo: Sharon Kaufman.

which could ease suffering and prolong the lives of his patients, he dedicated much of his career to overcoming medicine's limitations.

The son and grandson of general practitioners in the rural South, J. Dunbar Shields, Jr., fought becoming a doctor during his youth. But by the time he graduated from Mississippi Agricultural and Mechanical College (now Mississippi State College) in chemical engineering, he realized he had wanted to be a doctor all along. He was raised on a gracious plantation in Natchez, Mississippi, and from a young age was keenly aware of the devastating, long-term impact that the Civil War had on the economy of the South and the personal lives of its citizens. His grandfather treated the wounded soldiers of the North and South. His father treated and educated the residents around Natchez, white and African American alike. Dr. Shields grew up wanting to serve the community.

He attended Tulane University School of Medicine in New Orleans and interned at St. Luke's Hospital (now St. Luke's–Roosevelt Hospital Center) in New York City. Desperate for a job in 1933, Shields answered an ad for a doctor in Concord, New Hampshire. He thought he would stay there for about a year, just long enough to save money for returning to the South. But his general practice was so successful that he decided to remain in Concord. Over the years, he directed his efforts to clinical medicine and developed a wide range of interests.

Like the majority of doctors of his era, Shields worked as a general practitioner before the Second World War, though his goal was to specialize in internal medicine. He was one of the first doctors in New Hampshire to take the internal medicine board exams in 1947, which qualified and licensed him as a specialist.

Throughout his career, Shields was an innovator. He had the first electrocardiogram machine in Concord. His specialization in the treatment of polio and tuberculosis, led him to an interest in respiratory therapy. Before professional therapists existed he trained a nurse in the techniques of respiratory therapy. He also founded the Respiratory Therapy Department at Concord Hospital.

Later in his career when he became increasingly concerned with medicine's relationship with, and impact on, a wider society, his horizons expanded. He served as governor of the New Hampshire chapter of the American College of Physicians from 1968 to 1974. Also in 1968, after having worked his way through the executive positions in the New Hampshire Medical Society, he became its president. He was active in state legislative affairs as well.

Though his activities expanded to areas of administration and leadership, he remained a clinician, grounded by the primacy of the physician-patient relationship. While we were preparing for our first interview session together, Dr. Shields said to me: "This is a role reversal; I am usually the one to take the history. This will be new for me. The history is one of the most important things in medicine. The other important thing is listening to the patient. Those have always been the most important things, and they still are."

SAUL JARCHO

Two colleagues suggested I interview Saul Jarcho of New York City, who became widely known as a fine clinician through his many years of government service. His publications in the field of medical history earned him a national reputation.

The modest apartment in New York City that Dr. Jarcho has shared with his wife for more than forty years is a library. The walls of every room are lined, floor to ceiling, with books written in many languages. Many are older volumes that he began acquiring sixty years ago. During the course of our conversations he fondly pulled some of them from their shelves to show me. Dr. Jarcho is a scholar to the core. Detailed observations and fastidious, comprehensive research have characterized all his pursuits, from patient care and the understanding of disease patterns to his prolific historical studies. In fact, he characterizes himself as "probably excessively conscientious."

Dressed impeccably in a suit and tie during our interviews, he had a formal, reserved appearance. However, while we talked his kindness, thoroughness, deep sense of responsibility, and compassion for the human condition shined through. He is greatly distressed both by the encroachment of federal regulations on the ability of the physician to provide optimal medical care and by the growing litigiousness of American society, and he spoke about those developments passionately. He is also deeply concerned about the narrow education most physicians receive, both in medical school and during the undergraduate years, and the negative ramifications of narrow-mindedness for patient care and for the well-being of the physician.

As a young man, Saul Jarcho was torn between being a scholar of classics, history, and literature and becoming a doctor. He was educated

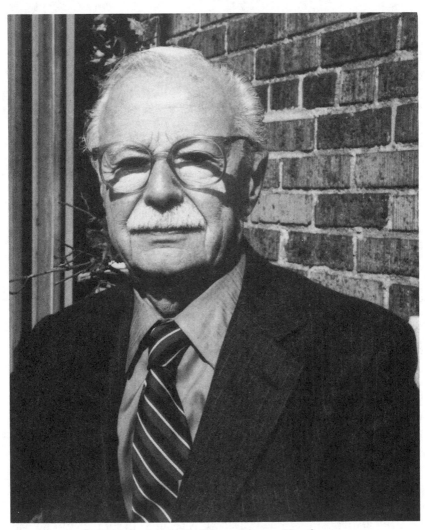

Saul Jarcho, 1989. Photo: Sharon Kaufman

at Harvard College and received a master of arts degree in Roman literature from Columbia University. Jarcho grew up in New York City, the son of middle-class Russian-Jewish immigrants. Jarcho's father, a successful physician, would not let him consider any career other than medicine. He felt that Jews needed to remain independent and that medicine was one of the very few professions in which Jews could both excel and remain in control of their destinies. The president of Harvard, Abbott Lawrence Lowell, on learning that Jarcho intended to be a doctor, advised him to study anything but premedical subjects during his undergraduate years. So Jarcho was able to follow his scholarly inclinations while preparing for a career in medicine.

Throughout his professional life, he pursued his scholarly studies while practicing medicine. At several junctures, his scholarship was part of his career: During the Second World War, he conducted research for, and later became director of, the Medical Intelligence and Health Education Division of the Office of the Surgeon General. After the war, he conducted research projects on the distribution of certain diseases and explored problems in pathology, publishing several case studies on his research. His interest in the history of medicine began to develop during the 1930s, and from then on he studied and published widely, especially on the history of Italian medicine.

He taught pathology at Johns Hopkins University School of Medicine for two years (1934–1936) and at Columbia University before the Second World War. Later, as an attending physician at Mount Sinai Hospital in New York, he conducted bedside teaching. These teaching activities were an extremely gratifying part of his career.

He developed an early interest in tropical diseases and studied and practiced in Puerto Rico during his training years. That interest and experience, coupled with his fluency in Spanish, enabled him to treat Hispanic patients quite successfully. His reputation spread, and he was frequently called in New York to treat Spanish-speaking patients who had acquired their diseases in the tropics. Because he also spoke several languages besides Spanish, he served as a consultant for other non-English-speaking patients.

Jarcho's primary interest was always to understand the patient in his or her cultural context, which included language, behavior, migration patterns, family heritage, and religion. He understood that those factors all played a part in disease acquisition, in the patient's understanding and conception of illness, and in the patient's response to treatment. He firmly believes that wide-ranging conversation with the patient, though time consuming, is always valuable, because "it helps to disclose the patient's character and problems."

PAUL BRUCE BEESON

All roads led to Paul Beeson. Physicians in academic medicine, community hospitals, and private practice suggested that I interview him, as did a few colleagues in the academic world who are not doctors. His research and academic career and the fact that he edited a major textbook of medicine for many years[4] have made him one of the most distinguished living American internists.

Dr. Beeson greeted me in a plaid flannel shirt and corduroy slacks at the door of the spacious home he and his wife had just built in a town near Seattle. Although he was recovering from hip replacement surgery, he walked around easily and told me that since he had retired he was enjoying some of the rough chores around the property, such as chopping wood. He reminded me of a modern-day country squire. Our conversations took place in his study—the walls lined with photographs of classmates, colleagues, and doctors he had trained over the years as well as diplomas, honors, and awards. He spoke articulately about the ethics of medical experimentation, the training of doctors, and the changing bedside manner of physicians—all issues he has pondered carefully over the years.[5] Deeply considerate of student, colleague, and patient needs and how those needs have changed over time, Beeson has always had a strong conviction about being fair-minded. His grasp of teaching principles, relationships with patients and their families, and research over a fifty-year period is enormous. His love of and excitement about practicing medicine, in the past and the present, is overflowing.

Born in Montana, raised in Alaska, Paul Beeson is the son of a physician and surgeon. His father went to Anchorage to heal the sick and treat the wounds of pioneers, adventurers, and laborers who came to work on the railroad and live in America's last frontier. Beeson attended the University of Washington in Seattle. From there he went to McGill University medical school in Montreal and interned in Philadelphia at the University of Pennsylvania. He thought he would be a general practitioner and spent two years in general practice with his father and brother in Ohio. Residency training began in New York, in the then not very

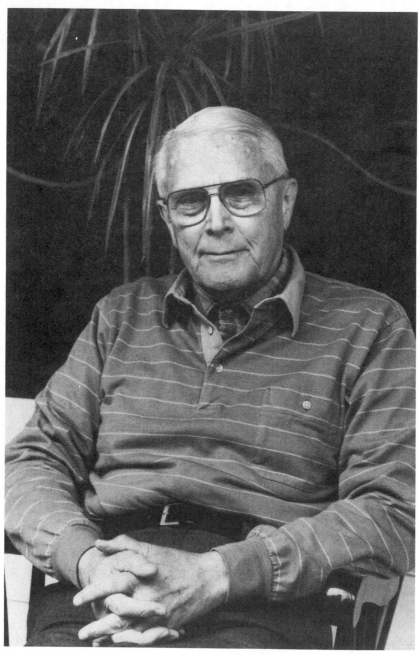

Paul Beeson, 1980s.

prestigious private service of the New York Hospital. The opportunity to continue his residency and become a researcher at the Rockefeller Institute, the premier institute for medical research in the United States, proved to be his intellectual awakening. That experience opened his eyes to the worlds of research and academic medicine.

Beeson began his research career at the Rockefeller Institute under the direction of Oswald Avery, who, at the time Beeson was there, was working on what would be the discovery that DNA is the basic genetic material of the cell. From Rockefeller, Beeson went to the Peter Bent Brigham Hospital, Boston, where he was chief medical resident to Soma Weiss. Weiss trained him in the art and science of physical diagnosis and the conduct of bedside teaching. After the war Beeson taught and practiced at the medical school of Emory University in Atlanta and became chief of the Department of Medicine there (1946–1952). His pioneering in research, most specifically into the mechanisms of fever and infectious disease, earned him a worldwide reputation. From Emory, he went on to chair the Department of Medicine at Yale (1952–1965). He also edited successive editions of a major textbook of medicine for many years.

Sir George Pickering chose Beeson to be the second Nuffield professor at Oxford, England, where he worked for nine years (1965–1974). That experience culminated in his being made an honorary knight commander of the British Empire (1973). When he retired to the United States, he became a Veterans Administration distinguished physician at the Veterans Administration hospital in Seattle, Washington. Beeson's career path and comprehensive approach to medicine as a science, practice, and philosophy have been compared with those of Sir William Osler (1849–1919), the most distinguished and admired North American physician of the preceding era.

"I didn't have much of any clear idea of what I wanted to do throughout my general practice in Wooster, Ohio, with my father and brother. At Rockefeller, a combination of events got me started. I found that I enjoyed reading and got great satisfaction from it. I realized I did want to be a good internist. I don't think I was sure that I wanted to stay in academic medicine, but the chance to go to the Brigham as chief medical resident was just a marvelous opportunity. I had found out what a great teacher Soma Weiss was, so I jumped at that. After four years at Emory in the department of Eugene Stead, I knew I did want to stay in academic medicine and I did want to become chairman of a department.

"I want to make it abundantly clear that I just feel the luckiest person in the world to have been propelled into medicine. I have thoroughly enjoyed it. I can't imagine myself having done anything else; I can't picture a life in business or politics."

MARY B. OLNEY

A pediatrician in San Francisco suggested I interview Mary Olney, whose outstanding reputation as one of the most respected women doctors in northern California was widely known. She was the protégée of Francis Scott Smyth, known as one of the founders of modern pediatrics in California. Olney's work in pediatric cardiology and diabetology earned her a national reputation.

I met with Dr. Olney in her office near the University of California in San Francisco. Though she had recently retired, her private office was so crammed full of papers from current projects that we held our conversations in an examining room. Dr. Olney has never married; her life has been one of total commitment to medicine and the care of thousands of children. As a practitioner, she was highly regarded and in great demand because of her combined clinical skills, all-pervasive compassion, and insights into the role of the family in the child's health and welfare. She has always been tremendously excited about the role basic scientific discoveries can play in improving the quality of life for disabled children and their families.

As we talked, her astute mind and selfless character were evident. Service to children was her highest priority throughout her career, and it is through the value of service that she defines pediatrics and, indeed, the scope of medicine. Traveling six thousand miles to look for an appropriate camp site when her diabetic youth camp was forced to move, educating families about the cause, control, and treatment of diabetes and other diseases, working with the psychological problems and emotional vulnerabilities of children were all part of her vision of complete medical care and were ways in which she served children, their families, and the community. At the end of our interviews, Olney spoke about Mother Theresa's dedication to children and how useful it would be if our society could learn from her methods of care. Mother Theresa stands out as her model of devoted service.

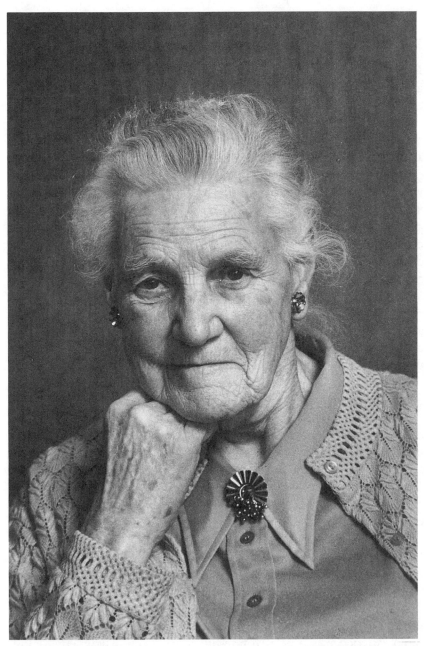

Mary B. Olney, 1988. Photo: Randolf Falk. Courtesy Alumni Faculty Association, University of California, San Francisco.

Mary Olney wanted to be a doctor from the time she was a young child growing up in Richmond, California. Her father owned a dry goods store; her mother owned and managed a ranch on the Sacramento River delta. Olney spent her youth working in the store in the winter after school and harvesting fruit from the ranch during the summer. She attended the University of California for both her undergraduate and medical training. She worked as a librarian and editor to support herself during the first two years of medical school. By the end of her internship at the University of California, San Francisco, Olney wanted to go into orthopedics, but she was told that no residency program in orthopedics would allow a woman "to put her hands on a patient." She was also informed that she would need a ten thousand dollar reserve to start practice, because orthopedics cases were handled mostly by insurance companies, which paid very slowly. Facing those two impediments, she decided she could not pursue her first choice in medicine. Her biggest turning point was the decision to take a residency in pediatrics at UCSF.

After a year of further training at the University of Chicago, Olney returned to UCSF's Department of Pediatrics as an instructor and then as an assistant professor. Early in her career, she felt that the greatest challenges would be in the university setting, so she decided to limit her private practice to half-time. She taught medical students and nurses throughout her career, and she worked in the university hospital clinics, where she specialized in cardiology and diabetology.

During her residency and early instructor years Olney was deeply influenced by her department chairman, Francis Scott Smyth, who was a pioneer in the holistic approach to children's health. Inspired by Smyth's approach, Olney had a desire to take pediatrics beyond the hospital and clinic setting—to do more for the child. In 1938, she started a summer camp for diabetic children. It was an instant success. Over the past half century, the camp has grown, flourished, and enriched the lives of countless children and their families under Olney's leadership.

"I do not see a cure for diabetes within the immediate future. There will always be psychological problems that accompany it. We still have to teach that ability, not disability, is what counts. Until there is a cure for diabetes, there is a need for camp, for its psychological contributions, social contributions, and medical contributions. To get all three in one camp experience is pretty wonderful. It has been a wonderful, most gratifying experience."

JONATHAN EVANS RHOADS

Dr. Beeson suggested I interview Jonathan Rhoads, whose great commitment to patient care, the scientific understanding of the patient's surgical needs, and university and community service (both local and national) is widely known and respected.

Dr. Rhoads met me in the waiting room of the Department of Surgery at the University of Pennsylvania. Our interviews were conducted in his office there. He is a tall man with a clear and steady gaze. He had stopped performing surgery only months before I interviewed him, and I noticed that his hands are as steady as his gaze. He is perhaps the most physically agile of the seven physicians. A slender man with a powerful presence, he strides down the halls easily; I had to run after him when he raced to hold open an elevator door. In contrast with his energetic physical appearance, he speaks softly and slowly, considering every thought carefully. During our interviews, he reflected on innovations in surgery during this century and on his roles in surgical research and training, in public education, and in the governance of the university. His greatest pride is in two areas: first, the benefits to postsurgical care resulting from the long-term research carried out in his laboratory, and second, the many surgeons he trained over the years who have gone on to become either leaders in academic medicine or well-known and highly regarded community surgeons.

The son of a general practitioner, Jonathan Rhoads was born into a prominent Quaker family that had lived in the Philadelphia region for generations. Following the pattern of many Quakers from that area, Rhoads was educated at the Friends School in Germantown, and then attended Haverford College. He did not firmly decide on medicine as a career until his senior year at Haverford. He attended Johns Hopkins University School of Medicine and returned to Philadelphia for his internship at the Hospital of the University of Pennsylvania. He remained there for the rest of his career, first as a surgical resident, then as assistant and associate professor, and later as chairman of the Department of Surgery. He chose surgery as his specialty toward the end of his internship after his exposure to a charismatic surgeon, I. S. Ravdin. Under Ravdin's direction during a five-year residency, Rhoads devoted his efforts to experimental research in addition to general surgery. Along with his colleagues at the surgical research laboratory, he studied the

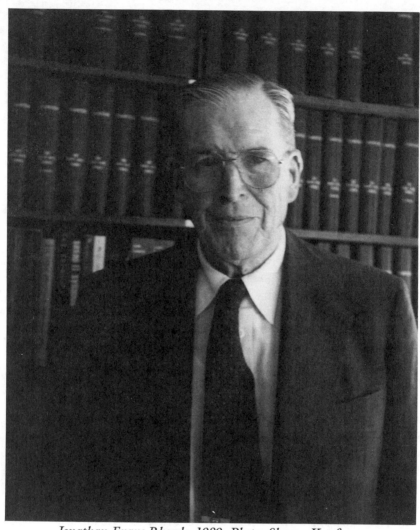

Jonathan Evans Rhoads, 1989. Photo: Sharon Kaufman.

problems of nutritional deficiencies following surgery and pioneered in treating those problems. He carried on the nutritional research throughout his years at the University of Pennsylvania.

During the height of his career, he was deeply involved with broad educational matters beyond the medical school. He served on the Philadelphia Board of Education and as provost of the University of Pennsylvania. Later in his career, he was president of the American Cancer Society and a member of the federal government's National Cancer Advisory Board.

Of his hospital and research career, he said: "Many of the cases I was involved with suffered from nutritional deficits. Our central research project was how to resolve these, particularly among patients who could not eat and had to be fed intravenously. In my earlier years at the university, there was no way of giving those patients sufficient food, and we concentrated on methods to do this. We were successful in finding two ways to accomplish it, one of which has been widely adopted. In retrospect, contributions to the nutrition of surgical patients, and the success of many doctors completing our residency program have been the most satisfying accomplishments of my time at the University of Pennsylvania."

C. PAUL HODGKINSON

C. Paul Hodgkinson became one of my seven interviewees at the suggestion of an academic obstetrician/gynecologist and former trainee of his. Known as one of the pillars of clinical research in gynecology, Dr. Hodgkinson established the basic groundwork for an important area of clinical investigation—lower urinary tract infections in women. He devoted many years to help establish and then guide his specialty as an organized field of medicine. He volunteered his time for the American College of Obstetricians and Gynecologists from the time of its inception and became its president in 1960.

Dr. Hodgkinson greeted me warmly in the comfortable home he shares with his wife in a suburb of Detroit. It was the end of winter and our interviews were conducted in the sun room adjacent to the living room. He told me right away that he very much misses practicing medicine and that almost every night he dreams about some aspect of his medical career. Throughout our discussions, he became animated and

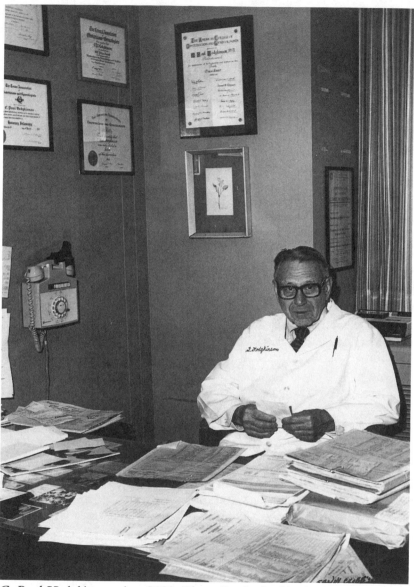

C. Paul Hodgkinson, circa 1983. Photo: Sandy Crabb. Courtesy Department of Gynecology and Obstetrics, Henry Ford Hospital.

lively when he related a story, an experience he had had, which illustrated a point he was trying to make or an answer to one of my questions. An exceptionally hard worker throughout his life, Dr. Hodgkinson struggled at various points in his career to expand his horizons, to become the kind of doctor he wanted to be. He recalls his weakness in English grammar and composition; when he wanted to begin writing scientific papers, he bought grammar books and studied them for hours. Later, on a tour through South America as president of the American College of Obstetricians and Gynecologists, he learned to give speeches in Spanish.

At the time of our interviews, he was deeply troubled by the high cost of malpractice insurance for doctors in his field, battles among doctors and hospital departments over money, and the tendency in recent years for doctors in his specialty to practice "defensive medicine." Yet he remains idealistic about the role the individual doctor can play in medical research and practice and about medicine's prospects and promise in general.

The son of a merchant tailor in New Castle, Pennsylvania, C. Paul Hodgkinson began to earn a living at the age of fifteen, working in drugstores. At the age of twenty-two, after he had completed pharmacy school and was working as a pharmacist, he decided to become a doctor. He was married and had a child when he began medical school at the University of Buffalo, where he spent his first year. He transferred to Temple University School of Medicine in Philadelphia in his second year and graduated from there, having worked his way through medical school as a druggist.

Hodgkinson chose Henry Ford Hospital in Detroit for his internship because of the salary that institution offered—one hundred dollars a month. Salaries for interns were highly unusual at the time, and with a wife and child to support, he needed an income. Hodgkinson thought he would be a general practitioner until he saw how specialization worked at Henry Ford Hospital. After a three-year general surgical residency, he switched to obstetrics and gynecology because of the influence of Dr. Jean Paul Pratt, then chief of the division of gynecology and obstetrics at Ford. Aside from several years in military service during the Second World War, Hodgkinson spent his entire professional life at Henry Ford Hospital. He was chief of the Department of Gynecology and Obstetrics for twenty-four years and had a large obstetrical practice as well. He specialized in the early diagnosis of breast cancer and conducted research into stress urinary incontinence for many years.

"I don't think there is anything I wanted to do that I couldn't do in medicine and research. A lot of things in research experiments I started, I either devised or made myself. I didn't ask somebody else to make it and I didn't ask for money. I just gathered the things up for the project I wanted and did it. I think that has happened to me almost all my life. I knew what I wanted to do and I went out and found a way of doing it. I don't think I was ever held back. I think you make your own opportunities."

JOHN ROMANO

A psychiatrist in San Francisco suggested I interview John Romano, a pivotal figure in the specialty's development, an outstanding and inno- vative teacher, and an extremely articulate and colorful speaker. He was responsible for integrating psychiatry into the medical school curricu- lum at Rochester, a reform that was widely accepted across America. He has also written extensively, reflecting on psychiatry's relationship to other medical fields and to society at large.[6] Romano's affiliations and commitments have been perhaps the broadest among this group, spanning psychiatric research, patient care, teaching, university service, and a myriad of community activities. Along with a handful of others of his generation, he was responsible for shaping modern psychiatry in America.

We talked in his large office/library at the University of Rochester. The table between us was stacked with newspapers, an eclectic display of journals, and recently published books that he was in the midst of read- ing. He has both wide and penetrating interests. He became a psychia- trist because he felt it was the broadest and most humane of the medical specialties and because he was intrigued by the unanswered questions about relationships between mind and brain and among mind, brain, and disease.

Dr. Romano devoted much of his career to the care, treatment, and understanding of the mentally ill, and he speaks compassionately about the dimensions of anguish and suffering he has seen over the years. His knowledge of and experience with so much pain—and with medicine's relative impotence to ameliorate it—has not weighed heavily on him, for he possesses a sense of humor that has served him well over the years and has pervaded his reflections.

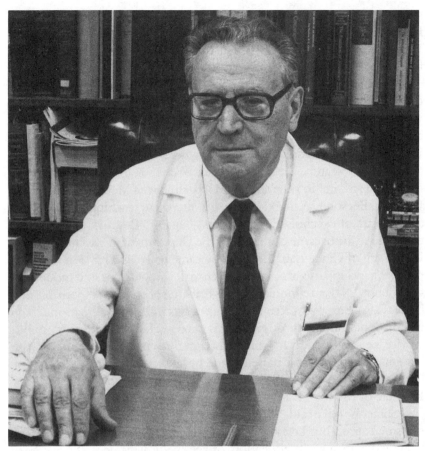

John Romano, 1983, on the occasion of Dr. Romano's 75th birthday. Courtesy Edward G. Miner Library, University of Rochester Medical Center.

John Romano grew up in Milwaukee, the son of poor Italian immigrants. His father was a music teacher. His grandfather was a stonecutter and builder. At the conclusion of our interview sessions, Romano took me for a walk around the outside of Wing R at Strong Memorial Hospital, the wing for the Department of Psychiatry that was built when he came to Rochester to chair the department in 1946. While we stood outside, he told me: "My grandfather was a stonemason. And I guess I have a part of that in me. Working with the architects and builders over a two-year period was a great achievement for me. I have so much pride in this building." His pleasure at having followed in his grandfather's footsteps is evident, glowing. His comment is an expression of continuity of family ties and outright pride in his heritage. The tangible edifice of Wing R has given him as much satisfaction over the years as the ideas he has created and instituted and the knowledge he has fostered within it.

Romano worked his way through Marquette University and School of Medicine. His interest in psychiatry began to develop during his last year of medical school and during his internship. His career as a psychiatrist officially began with his residencies and fellowships at Yale, the University of Colorado, and Harvard, where, with no mentor, he began to conduct research. He joined Soma Weiss's staff at the Peter Bent Brigham Hospital to start the new Department of Medicine—the same year Paul Beeson was there. There, his interest in teaching doctors to be more aware of psychological problems began to flourish. At the age of thirty-three, he became chairman of the Department of Psychiatry at the University of Cincinnati. In 1946 he came to Rochester. His teaching program and inpatient unit for psychiatric patients became models for the country. Never relinquishing his teaching or patient responsibilities, he was also extremely active in university, city, regional, national, and international affairs throughout his career. His dedication to public service is exemplifed by his ten-year struggle to procure adequate health insurance for psychiatric patients, and by his serving as a founding member and first chairman of the Research Study Section of the National Institute of Mental Health.

"Someone once said, 'A man has but one song to sing in his life.' I am not sure I agree, but I do know a major theme of my professional life has been and remains the education of the medical student. I have been privileged to participate in the teaching of medical students for fifty-two years. My goal was to assist the physician of today and tomorrow, whatever may be his discipline, to become aware of man in human as well as in infrahuman mammalian terms. I learned that in order to point to this objective, it was necessary to participate actively in clinical research; in the education of special professionals such as psychiatrists, social workers, psychologists, nurses, and others; to care for the sick and their families directly; to participate actively in the government of the medical school and the university of which I was a member; to participate in establishing and furthering patient care facilities throughout the community in which we lived and in which we served; and to take part in several national and international ventures in my field."

Although their characters are as distinct as their specialties, these doctors have several strong personality traits in common. They share a deep compassion and kindness for their patients and an absolute devotion to their profession. For the most part, they dedicated their careers to all three pillars of medicine: research, teaching, and patient care. Each, in his or her own way, has demonstrated an insatiable curiosity about problems in medical science and an ongoing enthusiasm for medicine's promise to ameliorate suffering and contribute to knowledge of disease.

The physicians are extremely modest about their remarkable achievements. In retrospect, the doctors speak of luck, opportunity, and support when describing their growing responsibilities and authority in their fields. They sought and accepted the greatest challenges their fields had to offer. Yet they talk only of hard work, a sense of responsibility, the desire to solve compelling medical problems, and their commitment to what they were doing.

An understanding of the whole of medicine pervades their discussions, and they are able to articulate the evolving relationships between their own specialties and other medical fields. They began their careers as generalists in long internships and/or private practice, during which time they came to appreciate the scope of general medical practice and the varieties of illness. The knowledge and perspectives of their generalist years became deeply ingrained and were not supplanted by specialist knowledge acquired later. Perhaps these seven doctors are among the only generation of American physicians to be generalists as well as specialists. That dual perspective has both shaped their discussions of the nature of medicine and their roles in it and contributes to the ways in which they describe and characterize themselves. Their dual perspective also creates a moral stance unique to their era: They emphasize compassion and the need to put the good of the individual patient above all other concerns and simultaneously stress personal investment in the emerging sciences of medicine. Furthermore, the doctors look beyond the needs of the individual patient and the press of scientific discovery to the community; they conceive medicine to be a civic duty and a social responsibility.

PART I

Becoming a Doctor: 1920s and 1930s

Guerir quelquefois,
Soulager souvent,
Consoler toujours.

(To cure sometimes,
To help often,
To comfort and console always.)

*—French motto made famous by
Edward Livingston Trudeau, M.D., 1848–1915*

MEDICAL MORALITY

Past and Present

THE SCOPE of medicine has changed dramatically since these seven physicians' training years. Medicine's very definition, in fact, has been transformed in ways that no one could anticipate. Since the mid-1960s at least, contemporary medicine has considered the rights of the individual patient—to autonomy in decision-making, to other medical opinions, to choice of treatments, to education, for example—as valuable and central to medical practice. Such an emphasis is based on individualism as the primary value in Western society.[1] In its ideal and most extreme form, particularly in North America, this individualism stresses the autonomy of a distinct, deep, natural self which aims to exist within, yet be free from the constraints of, society and culture.[2] This form of individualism, which began to emerge in the Western world following the Second World War, has contributed to the current confusion we feel about medical advances. Within medicine, individualism is expressed in a morality that emphasizes the rights of beings whose very existence is sustained or created by modern medical technology: frozen embryos, twenty-week-old fetuses, comatose persons, surrogate mothers, "brain dead" organ donors, persons with organ transplants, the extremely frail elderly. Contemporary morality, both within and outside of medicine, pays attention to the priority and sacred value of the individual, even if an individual's life is extended or maintained solely by technological means.

In contrast, family, community, or society's rights—if thought to exist at all—are not expressed, highly valued, or asserted in contemporary social life. Acts of social responsibility (such as the obstruction of nuclear weapons plant construction or toxic waste dumping) are rarely publicly rewarded and, in fact, are frequently punished. The word "duty" is rarely used in conversation, for it connotes obligation, outside the self, to a broader social good. Duty has little meaning in a culture where individualism is emphasized. Within medical moral debate, no-

45

tions of social good or community needs are poorly defined and articulated, and they represent a lesser priority than that of individual rights.

Recent expressions of morality are to be contrasted with a morality of generalized social responsibility which pervaded medicine in the 1920s and 1930s. During that period, when these doctors were being trained, medicine could be characterized by its sense of duty, charity, and social obligation, though it was an obligation based on social inequality. Medicine entailed service to the sick in the broader interests of society. The object of medicine was the social good. Similarly, moral behavior was not only a quality expressed by the individual physician acting as an autonomous agent; ideally, morality was thought to be inherent in the practice of medicine itself. For these doctors, morality evolved from a sense of duty coupled with a sense of empathy and caring.

These individuals first observed the duty and caring in their family role models, their parents. The four whose fathers were doctors absorbed what a doctor did and how a doctor was supposed to act. What stands out many years later in their descriptions of their parents' activities are the moral attributes of their fathers' doctoring expressed in public and social terms. Shields's father became a doctor to assist his own father and to relieve pain. He "took care of" the entire community by starting schools and educating African American children in addition to practicing medicine. Jarcho remembers his father's strong ethical principles. He abolished the practice of fee-splitting at the hospital where he was chief of staff and worked successfully to have African American physicians appointed there. Beeson's father, a general practitioner who had expertise in trauma, made it possible to survive and thrive while taming America's last frontier, Alaska. And Rhoads's father served his community through disease prevention, primary health care, and working as the school physician.

Olney's and Hodgkinson's parents, not doctors, were active in lodge and church work, respectively. Romano's mother, a welfare worker, had the ability to calm hysterical people and bring order to dysfunctional families. She organized and prepared food, clothing, and shelter for the sick and impoverished in her community. All seven of the doctors remember their parents acting, above all, in the public interest.

These doctors, while growing up, absorbed their parents' sense of duty and need to serve the community. They emphasize parental values as critical to their character development and to the ways in which they came to practice medicine. Descriptions of their own youths show an emerging sense of awareness, understanding, empathy, and desire to serve the people around them. Shields and Rhoads, who both fought becoming doctors, finally decided they wanted to do something "socially useful" and that being a physician was the best way to accomplish that goal. Jarcho's early love of languages served him well from the start of his medical career. He realized he could understand and thus work to solve patients' problems by communicating with them in their own languages. Beeson got to know the uneducated working class during his summer jobs and felt that that knowledge would make him a better doctor. Romano, through the jobs that supported his medical education, developed empathy for marginal people of all kinds—alcoholics, vagabonds, homeless, mentally ill. Olney worked among the gypsies, migrant farm laborers, and other downtrodden individuals when she was a child; those early contacts made lasting impressions. Later, when as doctors they met socially and economically marginal people in medical environments, they had a broader knowledge of what these people's lives were like and, thus, what care for them would specifically entail.

PERCEPTIONS OF MEDICINE'S LIMITS

Doctors of the 1920s and 1930s did what doctors have always done. They offered their patients a variety of treatments and worked toward understanding the mechanisms of disease and causes of suffering. They could not do very much to intervene in the biological processes of disease in the way these processes have subsequently come to be understood and treated. The list of effective drugs in use during the 1920s and 1930s is very short. For example, opium and its synthetically isolated derivatives—morphine, codeine, and heroin—were used to relieve pain. Acetamenophen was used for fever and pain. Aspirin relieved pain, fever, and the inflammation of arthritis and rheumatism. Chloral hydrate was used as a sedative to relieve anxiety and insomnia. The barbiturates, most commonly phenobarbitol, were popular sedatives. Quinine was used to treat malaria. Diphtheria antitoxin had been in use since 1891 and was saving lives. Digitalis and the organic nitrates—amyl nitrate and nitroglycerin—were used for short-term relief of heart disease. Salvarsan stopped the progress of syphilis, though it did not cure the disease. The discovery of insulin in 1922 saved and prolonged the lives of diabetics. And liver extract was found to be a cure for pernicious anemia in 1926.[3] Shields spoke in great detail about the dearth of treatments and what that meant to the practicing physician. The therapeutic role of the doctor was clear-cut: attempt to cure, devise ways of caring for the sick, relieve pain and suffering, be at the bedside.

I asked the doctors to describe for me their understanding of the powers and limits to medical and biological science at the time they entered medical school. Beeson responded:

> At the time, my concept of medical practice was that of a general practitioner, like my father. I knew there were specialists. But by today's standards, they were very rare birds. When I entered premedical studies, I vaguely saw myself doing medicine, pediatrics, obstetrics, and general surgery. As for my concept of biological science, it seemed pretty static. I appreciated that I would need to know anatomy, pathology, and physiology. But what we learned at that time was all in textbooks, and comparatively little new knowledge in such fields was being produced. I suppose I accepted the need to learn what was known about such preclinical subjects, then learn to be a doctor in the apprentice role. I thought my improvement would come along naturally, with practice and observation of the existing body of knowledge. I am confident that nobody foresaw the explosion in basic understanding that would result from the new funding of medical research that came along after World War II. The tidal wave of American doctors going into specialty practice was a direct result of the massive infusion of money into medical research. That led to undreamed-of complexities in diagnostic and therapeutic practices.

Rhoads told me:

> When I started out, the sense of medicine's limits, held by the community, were perhaps more realistic then they are now. Patients knew that to enter a hospital was to become a member of a group of persons, many of whom died. They had strong reservations about going to surgeons and often insisted on meeting their surgeons at home before they would submit to admission. I think the public was as optimistic about science then as it is now but were more cognizant of the limitations of what medical care could provide.

In spite of their relatively limited ability to cure diseases, doctors were respected and revered. Their diagnostic, treatment, and caring skills were sought after. They represented solace, comfort, benevolent authority, and most important, the relief of pain and suffering. The few dramatic cures in existence—for rabies and diphtheria, for example—did not affect very many individuals, but they did affect public opinion. The physician was viewed as someone with great potential to be a healer.[4] The seven individuals participating in this project had a highly optimstic faith in medicine's future and a specific trust in the ability of science to solve medical problems. Their faith reflected the new prestige of science during that era. Scientists were heroes. The ideas that scientific discoveries could solve social problems and that science could accomplish almost anything were widely held.[5]

FEATURES OF MEDICAL TRAINING

It is ironic that, while medicine's identity has changed so fundamentally over the past sixty years, methods of training physicians have hardly changed at all. Observers of medical education have noted that, although the content of medical education is ever-changing to keep abreast of new discoveries, techniques, and procedures in the biomedical sciences, the structure of medical education has remained nearly as it was sixty years ago.[6] That fact has made numerous educators ponder whether or not emerging doctors are being trained adequately to evaluate the relevance and appropriateness of the highly technical skills they are learning, or to make sense of medicine's changing goals and responsibilities in the context of their own practices.

In this section, the physicians reflect on the dominant features of medicine that shaped their education during the 1920s and 1930s. All seven physicians describe four features of medicine that were central to the training experience. First, the primacy of using one's own senses to learn the art of physical diagnosis stands out as essential to being a doctor. Touching a patient and listening for certain sounds were critical for making an accurate diagnosis, a skill needed for becoming a respectable and respected physician.

Second, although certain teachers during the medical school years are remembered positively for their specific knowledge and teaching ability, senior physicians or professors from that period are rarely singled out as role models, as persons whose specific influence these individuals can recall. (Hodgkinson's experience is an exception.) Beeson and Jarcho stress this most decisively. In fact, Jarcho talks about the profound influence his father had on the way he learned to make therapeutic decisions, rather than the influence of any particular teacher. Beeson and Olney note that their actual teachers of the procedures and techniques of medicine were the interns and residents, those doctors only one, two, or three years ahead in their training. This feature of medical training has not changed over the past decades.[7] Olney and Romano mention the contribution of nurses to their basic medical training as well. Yet ward rounds were conducted by senior physicians who volunteered their time to teach medical students. From those men the doctors learned the style and standards of bedside medical practice.

Third, they recall that the most commonly seen diseases at the time were syphilis, rheumatic fever and rheumatic heart disease, typhoid, tuberculosis, and the pneumonias. Syphilis, rheumatic fever and rheumatic heart disease, and many of the pneumonias could not be cured. Hodgkinson remembers ministering to patients who were "doomed to die." Jarcho recalls graduating from medical school perplexed and worried that he could not actually do anything for sick people. The doctors were not learning to cure diseases; this fact both troubled them and anchored them to medicine's ultimate limitation.

Fourth, medicine was learned by observing and treating poor patients in large charity hospitals. All the doctors recall their clinical training in those hospitals during their third and fourth years as excellent. They recall the care given to those patients as excellent also. The doctor-patient relationship was characterized by inequality and social distance. The role that relationship played in shaping physicians' morality is discussed following the narratives.

Medical students of that era traditionally were upper- and middle-class white males who did not need to pay for their educations. Olney, Hodgkinson, and Romano were exceptions to the norm. They each speak a great deal about the work they had to do to earn a living while in medical school. There were simply no institutional mechanisms for paying for a medical education at the time. Moreover, working was frowned upon; medicine was supposed to be all-consuming. Olney recalls the University of California's strong sanctions against working: "They would flunk out anyone they caught working," she said. Yet one-third of her classmates held jobs.

Contrasting qualities of the internship are recalled by the physicians. Shields remembers most vividly the physician's powerlessness to cure diseases and the hours spent devising and implementing treatments that could, at best, prolong a patient's life but not save it. Beeson, like others of his generation,[8] recalls the tightly knit men's club feeling among his fellow interns. No one was married. No one had money for entertainment outside the hospital. There was no salary. They did not leave the hospital often. Yet they shared an intense, exclusive experience, and there was time for fun, talk, and camaraderie. Jarcho remembers the absence of marriage, money, and freedom as well, but recalls it as a monastic experience rather than having the feeling of a men's club. Romano paints a picture of an internship not nearly as exclusive, clublike, or enjoyable as Beeson's. What stands out most in his accounts is the range of physician competence he encountered. He recalls how indiscriminate surgery, fads in medicine, morally reprehensible behavior, and poor teachers shaped his attitudes about how a doctor should behave, what a doctor should be. Hodgkinson remembers the varied chores—doing blood work, giving intravenous injections, and changing patients' dressings—and the fact that his one-year internship helped him mature. Jarcho and Rhoads stress the relatively great responsibility interns had for patients because there were few residencies at that time. The medical hierarchy was not as long or complex as it became later, and interns were able to communicate directly with the chiefs, thereby having (or seeming to have) more autonomy and control. Olney focuses on what she learned from patients during the internship. She chose to work in a county hospital setting where she met a variety of indigent patients. She began to understand the meaning of serious illness to all families—deprivation. That fact had an enormous impact on her and focused her concern later when she became a pediatrician.

The importance of using one's own senses in physical diagnosis, the lack of senior professors as role models, the responsibility of interns, the dominance of infectious, lethal diseases that they were powerless to cure, and the fact that they were trained on poor patients who did not pay for their care were the major features of medicine that shaped the nature of the profession and the moral outlook of physicians who were trained in the late 1920s and the 1930s. The doctors' narratives invite us to ponder how those features of medical education have changed, and why. As examples of medicine's transformation, the narratives serve as guideposts to changes in medicine's morality. It is hoped that they can also serve as reference points in contemporary conversations about the goals and purposes of medical training in the future.

THE NARRATIVES:
DOCUMENTS OF TRANSFORMATION

We now turn to the doctors' narratives themselves, as cultural and historical documents with which to understand better medicine's transformation from an occupation of help, comfort, and consolation to a profession of cure and a pursuit of extending, enhancing, and re-creating
human life. Medicine's remarkable and profound evolution was unplanned and, with the exception of a handful of astute observers, unanticipated. The rapidity with which this transformation took place and the
fact that it was largely unpredictable and unexamined have made more
urgent and unsettling the widespread moral and social dilemmas it has
produced. The fact that the entire transformation occurred in *these physicians' lifetimes* makes their narratives, and those of others of their generation, of special historical significance. For the following narratives are
specific examples of the ways in which medicine has been an agent of
cultural change. My hope is that they can serve as a stimulus for discussion about medicine's ever-growing impact on society and about the
evolving relationship between medicine and culture.

SHIELDS

Care and Ignorance in New Orleans and New York

"MY FATHER was a doctor. His father was a doctor. My father was a country doctor practicing in a terribly depressed area of the South—the area around Natchez, Mississippi. I'm absolutely sure he never liked to practice medicine. He was a good doctor and an excellent obstetrician, driving a buggy and staying there all night, delivering breech births and so forth. But he never made any money practicing medicine. That was in the early 1900s. Seventy-five percent of his practice was with poor blacks. If those people lived on a plantation, the plantation owners would pay him a certain amount of money every year. That's the only way he made any money. I felt that he would much rather have been a farmer. But he became a doctor to help out his father with his practice. He was devoted to helping family members and he was devoted to public affairs, particularly education. I always admired him tremendously, but I didn't look up to him as a role model. I tried not to be a doctor and I don't think he wanted me to be a doctor. He didn't want to push me into being a doctor.

"I think I picked Tulane medical school mainly because it was in New Orleans. I loved New Orleans. I certainly thought I would practice in the South. Tulane was an excellent medical school and one of the top ones in the country. And it was only 150 miles from home. I started in the fall of 1927; I was twenty years old. It was such a contrast to the cow college I had attended in Mississippi.

"I went to medical school with a good friend from Natchez. We lived in the top of a house near the medical school. We studied together. In medical school in those days, we studied as a team. It was helpful to study that way. It was hard because I had poor training. We worked like dogs, each trying to outdo the other. All we did was study, morning, noon, and night. As a matter of fact, my mother and father came down to see me and they were worried about me because I couldn't talk or think about anything else.

"After I got out of that horrible first year, I enjoyed medical school. It

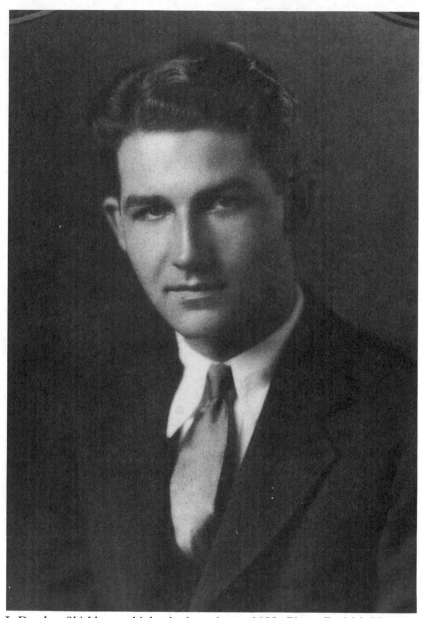

J. Dunbar Shields as a high school graduate, 1922. Photo: Earl M. Norman.

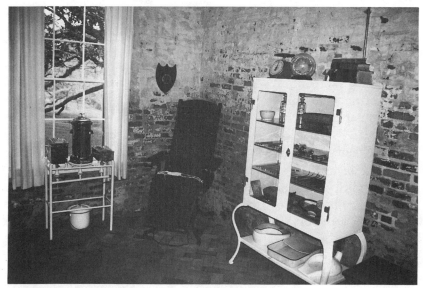

The treatment room of Dr. Shields' father, circa 1920s. Now part of the Mount Repose Medical Museum, Natchez, Mississippi.

was fun. Back in those days, medicine was very poorly taught. There was much too much memorization. We had to practically memorize *Gray's Anatomy.* That was poor teaching and we wasted a lot of time on that.

"After the second year, it was learning medicine. The last two years were excellent. I had some excellent teachers. They taught us basic medicine. For instance, they showed us how to examine patients. We learned from them how to recognize the signs of infection. We learned the importance of using our senses to come to conclusions. They encouraged curiosity and they tried to instill in us a thirst for medical facts. Above all, they stressed the necessity of learning and reading medicine for the rest of our lives.

"Tulane was one of the first places which had a special building for clinical medical training. In the junior year, we had our own little offices where we actually saw patients. We were connected with Charity Hospital, a tremendous institution. And we saw patients there. The patients were underprivileged, poor people. Their care was paid for by the state. Rich people went to Touro Infirmary and Baptist Hospital. There were no private facilities at all in Charity Hospital. Patients were housed in very, very big wards—maybe forty or fifty people in a ward—with no curtains around the bed. The wards were segregated, black and white. I saw mostly black patients. It was a well-respected institution where good medicine was practiced.

"We saw a lot of malaria. The venereal diseases. Syphilis and its effects were rampant. We saw the pelvic inflammatory diseases that resulted from venereal disease. We saw a great deal of rheumatic fever and rheumatic heart disease. Typhoid was still with us. And we saw the great disease, tuberculosis. We didn't have much tuberculosis at Charity Hospital, though, because it was treated in special institutions. We had some dengue fever, a mosquito-born fever. Pneumonia was a killer then, and appendicitis was a killer. And we saw a lot of pellagra. Tulane people saw quite a bit of leprosy, because we went up to Carville, the leper colony. But we could do nothing for leprosy then. The only thing we could cure was malaria.

"While I was in medical school, I wanted to take care of people as some of the great clinicians did. But in addition, I had a great desire to be a leader in academic medicine. That was a different goal than most of my classmates had. I think I worked harder than most of them. I graduated second in my class of about 140, in 1931.

"There were two women in my class. They were pioneers and there must have been some antagonism toward them from some of the people in the class. But they did all right. We lost a lot of the class in the freshman and sophomore years. But the two women graduated. The class was all white. There were a few Hispanics.

"When I look back, I was in medical school in an era of very little light. We could do so very little. We felt this more when we were interns, when we had more prolonged contact with patients. We had just so little to work with. But I had the feeling very early that there were going to be tremendous advances, and that was another reason to be a doctor. We were going to be able to do so much more. I wanted to be able to do something for these people. I had faith in the researchers. I was very much interested in the chemistry of medicine and the whole biological process. I was very interested in basic science involving medicine.

"I remember a young girl I saw in the first part of my internship. She had subacute bacterial endocarditis. We knew that the individual with SBE was going to die. And this girl was perfectly beautiful, probably eighteen years old. She had four beautiful-looking brothers. At that time, we had no medication. I had to watch her die by degrees. I remember racking my brain to death trying to figure out some way to do something for that girl. We tried all kinds of things. This was early in our knowledge of bacteriophages, which were the product of bacterial growth. We thought we could inject them into the body and perhaps kill the infection. Bacterial endocarditis was a streptococci infection that grafted onto a heart valve previously damaged from rheumatic fever. It was associated with destruction of red blood cells, and there was a lot of anemia. At that time we could give streptococcal vaccine to donors. We injected her four brothers with the killed strep veridans bug. And those boys ate huge quantities of raw beef. They lived on raw beef. We took their blood very, very frequently, and gave it to their sister in direct transfusions to treat the anemia. At the same time, we hoped we were giving her antibodies that would help. We wouldn't mix the blood with any kind of anticoagulant. We had a machine that had two syringes. One person would take the blood from the donor and pass the syringe to the recipient before it had a chance to clot. That was the early start of immunology, and I was fascinated by immunology. And it was nothing, just nothing, compared to today. It was an illustration of what we couldn't do. It was an illustration of what we were trying so desperately to do. And it was an illustration of how ineffective we were. We kept that particular girl alive for months by giving her a lot of blood and by supporting her. She stayed on the ward for nearly a year. We just couldn't do anything really.

"Well, medicine had done some things. We had taken care of yellow fever. We had taken care of malaria. Two scourges. And we were doing some things for tuberculosis. We were doing pneumothoraces and crushing the phrenic nerve. We could treat pellagra, and we could treat pernicious anemia, a vitamin deficiency as well. We treated them by feeding the patient whole liver. We could give quinine and relieve pain. My father's reason to be a doctor was mainly to relieve pain. We had morphine, thank God, and some of its derivatives. We had aspirin and we had phenobarbital. We used sodium bromide. For syphilis we were giving arsenicals—we called it 606—by intravenous injection. And we were rubbing the patients with mercury. We also gave potassium iodide. We treated syphilis for long periods of time. We were curing people, but the cure was almost as bad as the disease. People were made terribly ill and their veins were always giving out. We were not too skillful in the use of IVs. If syphilis got into the brain or the spinal fluid, there was nothing we could do at all. Even intravenous feedings were very new. We couldn't give anything but glucose or saline. We were making progress, although it was minimal. I didn't by any means expect the great explosion that happened after the war, with penicillin and with research. But I thought medicine was going to improve.

"We not only couldn't and didn't do things, we did horrible things. We had no cure for typhoid fever. One of the medical treatments for typhoid fever at that time was starvation. The story was that you fed a cold and starved a fever. There was quite a bit of typhoid around Natchez, and those patients were given nothing to eat. My father was an influence on me in this regard. He was a therapeutic nihilist really. Necessarily so. The typhoid bacillus had not been isolated in his time. But he noticed that the cases of typhoid occurred along the creeks, the water sources. He felt that the disease came from food and water in some way. He saw people with typhoid starve and get weak and die. But he also saw some people get well. He felt that if he could keep up their strength long enough, they would get well. So he fed his typhoid patients. He had quite a reputation in that area at the time for his treatment of typhoid fever: 'If you need to be treated for typhoid fever, you'd better go see Dr. Shields.'

"What did we do for colitis? I was terribly guilty in that regard. I gave a low residue diet. Irritable colon was a scourge in those days. As a matter of fact, I wrote a paper on it. I gave a paper on my handling of the irritable colon with a low residue diet at the state medical society meeting. I was doing just the opposite of what they do now—high fiber.

"How about ulcer? When I was in my internship, one of my relatives had an ulcer. So I set out to cure him. I gave him a Sippy diet, which was all milk and cream, and I gave him antacids. We didn't have the aluminum compounds or the magnesium compounds in those days. We had to give them Sippy powders. Sippy was a doctor who invented this regimen. So I gave him that and all he did was get worse. Now of course we don't give them milk, because that stimulates the acid-forming glands in the stomach. We did so many things wrong because of our ignorance.

"I'm the only doctor I ever knew who got through medical school and the internship without doing any obstetrics. I just hated it. I guess that was my reaction to the fact that my father was such a good obstetrician. At Tulane, when I was on obstetrical duty, there was always an intern or resident there. I always found some nice guy who would do it for me, so I never did it. Twice during my years of practice, I almost got fouled up in having to deliver a baby. I went out on house calls and found the women right in the middle of a delivery. I called another doctor.

"I started the internship at St. Luke's Hospital in New York in 1931. It was called a one-year internship and a one-year residency, but it wasn't. It was a two-year internship. I never had a residency. That's where I made the decision not to go into academic medicine. I really wasn't terribly disappointed. St. Luke's was more of a clinical institution than Cornell and the College of Physicians and Surgeons.

"At Tulane, I hadn't been particularly affected by the Depression. The South was already depressed anyway. We didn't notice any difference. But in New York it certainly was felt. It was a time when people were jumping off of buildings. But I wasn't affected by the Depression. As interns, we were so isolated. At St. Luke's, we got our eight dollars a year and our food and uniform. We lived in intern quarters in the hospital. We had good rooms, but lousy food.

"The first six months we worked in the lab, and that was a bad deal in a way. The theory was that we would learn the basics. We did blood counts, blood chemistries, urinalyses. We did very basic things because we couldn't do many things then. We did have a flame photometer, so we could do fairly decent chemistries—blood types and cross matchings. We weren't doing any research. It was purely a clinical lab at St. Luke's. We also saved the hospital a lot of money, as they didn't have to pay technicians. During the last six months, I became the house officer in charge of two big medical wards and had interns under me. I really was responsible for the works. We worked hard, sometimes eighteen hours a day when we had a lot of sick patients. There are good parts about that. We learned and we contributed without pay. We worked hard and we weren't too involved in the mechanics of making money. It was a good existence. We learned a lot; no question about it.

"We treated heart disease with digitalis. The low sodium diet had not come in yet. We tried to treat it with some diuretics. We had caffeine derivatives. And we had mercury, which was a diuretic. We used injections of a mercurial salt, intramuscularly. But those didn't amount much to anything. We kept patients quiet, gave oxygen when they needed it, and gave digitalis. There was so much heart failure and accumulation of fluid that we had to do a lot of aspiration of the chest and abdomen.

"Pneumonia was a big disease, a big killer. We had nothing specific to treat it. Except we did have—and this took a lot of time—intravenous antitoxin serum. We could give it for Types 1, 2, and 4 pneumonia, but we couldn't give it for Type 3. At that time, Type 3 was the bad pneumonia, because the bacillus had a capsule on it that we couldn't penetrate with medication. We had to type the pneumonia right away, by getting a blood or sputum culture. If we could type it, we could give serum. But we had to watch very closely, because the individual might be allergic to the serum. But when it worked, it was a wonderful thing. We had this very, very ill patient who was probably going to die. We gave him this serum, and within an hour there was the so-called crisis when the fever just crashed down and all the toxemia went away. We were great, great heroes. It was just like giving penicillin today, except it acted more dramatically. That was for pneumococci pneumonia. But then we had primary atypical pneumonia, which we didn't know what to do with. But recognizing it and giving supportive treatment was important and was all we could do.

"People stayed in the hospital until they got well, felt well, and wanted to go home—sometimes for months or a year. There were no nursing homes or facilities to which to send them. And you had to have good care at home to send them home early. There was so little we could do that rest was a very important factor, particularly in heart disease. I remember Dr. Burch, the head of medicine at Tulane, was a great exponent of rest for heart failure. He had a service at the Veterans Marine Hospital. He took people who were suffering terribly from the horrors of New Orleans heat and put them in a room with air conditioning so they could be comfortable. So many people died there [in New Orleans] during the summer. He kept them at absolute rest. He prolonged their lives because of that.

"One of the few things we could do was make people rest. Their positions in bed were important too. We had to mobilize every conceivable resource to treat people at that time. It was harder then from that point of view. Now, doctors have so many more treatments. There are so many medications with such horrible side effects that are so dangerous that doctors have to know a lot more.

"I stayed at St. Luke's for a while after I finished my two-year internship there. I took a couple of months in radiology. I was interested in radiology and I wanted to round out my training. I did fluoroscopic exams and read pictures and so forth.

"I probably could have gone into academic medicine after the internship. I was offered a job associated with one of the clinicians on the staff of St. Luke's. But in 1933 they didn't have much money to offer, and it was a cutthroat business. During the Depression years everyone was competing for the few crumbs that fell. Medical positions in academia were built on a hierarchy system, and one needed to displace the person above in order to reach the top. We had to fight for a position on a hospital staff. When I finished the internship, I didn't have any money at all. I was flat broke with a seven-thousand-dollar debt, and I had to go and make some money for a while."

JARCHO

Scholar in Medicine

"I AM CERTAIN that at about the age of six, seven, up to ten, I very much wanted to be a physician. I used to see sick beggars in the street and wonder what I could do for them. That feeling was influenced by my father, who was a doctor. But after I had been through four years at Harvard and had spent one year in the Classics Department at Columbia, I wasn't at all certain that a physician was what I wanted to be. The reason I became a doctor may have been that my father didn't know any other way in which a young Jewish man could earn a living.

"At Harvard I was influenced by two professors, John L. Lowes, professor of English, and Edward K. Rand, professor of classics. Professor Rand took me aside one day about 1925 and said, 'If you want to become a professor of classics I will back you. But remember, you are Jewish, and the chances are against you. While I offer you my backing, I think you would be wiser to go into medical school.'

"So I never really made the choice to become a doctor. How could I have gone against my father and Professor Rand? Whether or not the decision was made by my father or me, there were not many professions in those days in which a man could be his own boss. And for Jews the opportunities were measurably smaller. The fact of being one's own boss has made medicine almost unique.

"In the autumn of 1926 I entered the College of Physicians and Surgeons [now Columbia University College of Physicians and Surgeons]. In my class of about a hundred students, there were four or five women. There were three Puerto Ricans. There were a few Italian-Americans from City College, and a few Jews from City College.

"Years later, in 1932 or 1933, the pathologist, Dr. Paul Klemperer, asked who in medical school influenced me. I said, 'Nobody,' and he was horrified. No one had. I had never spoken to the chief professor of medicine, Dr. Walter Palmer, or to the professor of physiology, except during the final examination. I never saw the professor of chemistry, Dr. Geis. I never spoke to the professor of surgery, Dr. Alan Whipple. I was living on the stimulus provided by the professors of English and classics at Harvard. One of the reasons I admired Professor John L. Lowes so much is that he insisted on observation—simple observation. That was observation of literary texts, poems, and novels, but it applies also to the observation of human beings.

"On a few occasions in the second year I had a good teacher named Herrick, a likable, admirable man. We had him when we were learning percussion. We stripped to the waist and everybody was percussing his neighbor. I did not find it easy to learn this art. Suddenly Herrick was behind me. Pointing me out to the whole class, he said, 'I see that there are still some among you who cannot percuss properly.' I went home broken in two. I had a very good teacher in medicine the fourth year, Dr. Dickinson Richards. But he didn't influence me as my Harvard professors had. The teaching of therapeutics was underemphasized by the Department of Medicine; hence I emerged from medical school somewhat troubled about what I could do for a sick person.

"Medicine in the third and fourth years was taught mainly on the wards of the hospitals, where we saw the serious cases. But how do you treat the ordinary cases which you see in practice? Nowadays, medical schools are becoming alert to this. I think that more of the teaching will be done in outpatient clinics, and even in the home. What they teach on the ward is in the literal sense an abstraction. It is drawn out, drawn away from the total body of knowledge.

"I graduated from Physicians and Surgeons in 1930 and obtained an internship in medicine, which was to start at Mount Sinai six months later, in January 1931. I had a free period of six months before the internship began. I decided to go to Puerto Rico to the School of Tropical Medicine. I obtained various letters of introduction and worked there for two months. I acquainted myelf with the leading endemic diseases, and I did laboratory work. I also traveled to almost every town and village in the island, met the physicians, learned about conditions, and began to speak Spanish. This proved to be extremely helpful later. At times I would sit in a laboratory at the school, look out the window, and see women walking right by in the street having the grotesquely swollen legs of elephantiasis. And I worked in the clinics, where I saw the malaria patients and people who had sprue [a diarrheal disease]. I paid a number of visits to the leper colony and to the tuberculosis sanitarium. I worked in one clinic in which each physician took fifty patients in a day, some of whom had walked all night to get to the clinic.

You can imagine how one trained by the conscientious teachers at the College of Physicians and Surgeons would react to finding himself with nothing more than a couple of minutes in which to make a diagnosis and prescribe treatment. This caused moral pangs, but I did what I could. The patients very often brought sacks of fruit or coconuts in lieu of payment.

"I also learned about the relation among the ecological and social conditions and the diseases. I became interested in schistosomiasis. This occurs in people who go into the water of mountain streams; the infected snails reside there. I would go and help collect snails in that water.

"After two months in Puerto Rico, I presented myself at the New York Lying-In Hospital on the last day of August 1930, where I had a four-month obstetrical internship waiting for me. I had selected this appointment because my father was by then an obstetrician and gynecologist and, second, I felt that in the event of some financial catastrophe, this would be some immediate way of earning a living.

"During the first three months I delivered women in their homes in the slums. There was no assistance from a nurse, no ambulance to carry the equipment. I had to look for the building—the number was often illegible or missing—climb the malodorous stairs, where there might be no illumination, and enter the apartment. I took everything off the kitchen table, covered it with newspaper, put the woman on it, shaved her, examined her, and many hours later (because we were too conscientious and came too soon) delivered her, tied the umbilical cord, delivered the placenta, washed and dressed the child, wrote the birth certificate, washed the instruments, packed them up, and dragged myself back to the hospital.

"One saw things. In one apartment, a small tenement, I found the woman but no one else. By that time I had some experience and knew that her being alone was a bad sign. If, at that moment of life, the patient is alone, there is something socially wrong and badly so. She was a Latin. I conducted the delivery in Spanish. She then said to me, 'Now that you have delivered the child, what are you going to dress him in?' My bag contained a belly band, which I wrapped around the child. I remembered that I had a large new and unused pocket handkerchief, which I then put around the baby's abdomen and chest. There was no sheet on the bed, but there was a pillowcase. I put that over the child, fearing that the totality of all this might not be enough. I looked around and saw that of the two windows, one had a window shade. I ripped it down and wrapped that around the child and went back to inform the hospital.

"In the last month of this four-month appointment, we delivered women in the hospital. In the deliveries, both those done in the patient's home and those done in the hospital, we were required to use the Gwathmey method of anesthesia. In medical school I had been taught by one of the greatest obstetricians in the United States and one of the best teachers, Dr. Benjamin Watson. He had been professor at Edinburgh and Glasgow. I had never heard of the Gwathmey method and was afraid of it. It consisted of administering an enema containing, I think, some ether in olive oil. I am by no means certain of this formula now. We also gave the woman an injection of magnesium sulfate intramuscularly. I had no confidence in this, and whenever I could find a reason for not giving it, I didn't give it. If I was obliged to give it, I gave it in a greatly reduced dose, and nothing bad happened.

"After leaving the Lying-In Hospital at the end of 1930, I started a two-and-a-half year internship at Mount Sinai. It was a rotating internship, ending with a year in medicine. It was a form of internship that has disappeared, greatly to the disadvantage of the profession and the public. We spent time in pediatrics, surgery, in all the other specialties. We worked some months in the laboratory, usually in bacteriology. It was very instructive for a doctor to have this as firsthand experience. When we went to the patient's bedside to take a blood culture, we were responsible for cultivating the bacteria, if any, and at the same time we acquainted ourselves with the clinical problem. It was an extremely valuable experience. We had very capable physicians. We had a large variety of difficult problems and we had a very high autopsy rate. The hospital was famous for its high proportion of autopsies. This was a great enrichment of one's educational opportunities. Moreover, I was able to work successfully among Latins who knew little or no English and was able to detect unobserved tropical diseases in some of them because of special training in Puerto Rico. There were many Puerto Rican patients on the wards of Mount Sinai. They were examples of tropical poverty and of wretched neglect by the federal government.

"We saw a great deal of vascular disease, heart disease, including rheumatic heart disease, which is primarily a disease of the heart valves. In the autumn we would see typhoid. We even saw typhus, Brill's disease. Brill's disease is a form of typhus in a patient who had had typhus years before. Brill observed this at Mount Sinai, where he was a physician. I saw a good deal of cancer of the gastrointestinal tract—stomach and colon. We sometimes saw chorea, but not often. Neoplastic disease and heart disease were common. We also had a lot of cases of bacterial endocarditis because the hospital was famous for that. The disease was close to 100 percent fatal. The diagnosis was sometimes extremely difficult; our hospital excelled in it. We also had Tay-Sachs disease and Gaucher's disease, diseases commonest among Jews—on the pediatric wards mainly. We were just before the age of antibiotics. Therefore, much of the treatment was nursing care, diet, encouragement.

"We also saw Graves' disease, exophthalmic goiter: the neck is swollen, the thyroid gland is enlarged, and the eyes protrude. In those days, we treated patients by thyroidectomy, which is a very difficult undertaking. The operation is not so difficult anatomically, but you have a patient with a heart rate that may be 120, who is at the height of nervousness, uncontrollable, and the problem is difficult to treat. Then radioactive iodine came into use, and other drugs, doing away with the need for much of the surgery.

"The hospital excelled in surgery in addition to medicine, particularly in surgery of the gastrointestinal tract. There were a good many cases of duodenal ulcer, bad cases requiring operation. Also, there were cases of cancer requiring excision of part or all of the stomach. A member of the staff had invented a treatment of tumors of the urinary bladder by burning them out electrically, that is, fulguration through the cystoscope. So there was a good deal of that.

"I don't have much to say about the Depression per se. We knew from taking clinical histories what trouble there was, but actually we were so overworked that I don't think the economic condition of the country impinged very strongly on us at that time. We had all we could do to do our work. Certain things were thrust upon us as obvious. I remember being called down to the front office at Mount Sinai one December day. There was a Puerto Rican whom nobody could speak to, a man with a little boy who was not even wearing a jacket, just a shirt, shuddering in the cold. I said to him, 'Where did you come from?' He had just come from Puerto Rico. They hadn't eaten. I asked, 'How did you get the money to come?' He used the Spanish expression '*juntando chavos*'—joining pennies together.

"I served certain nights in the reception ward. At one time, I served every other night for several months. On some weeks I was on duty two

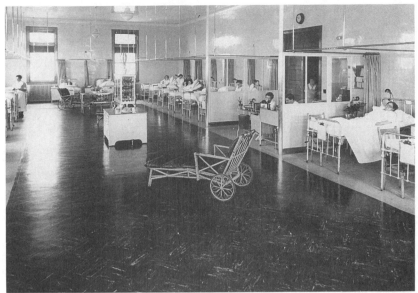

Medical ward, 1930s. The Mount Sinai Hospital. Courtesy of the Archives of the Mount Sinai Medical Center.

nights running, plus days. Many of the patients had had accidents. Occasionally, if I saw a man whose trouble I thought to be simply hunger, I would put a bandage on his head and keep him overnight; I thereby eluded the vigilance of the night supervisor and would slip the patient food during the night. The next day, we'd let him out. Diagnosis: Suspected Fracture of the Skull—Observation. We did that occasionally. The ones who saw the problems of the Depression were not the indoor physicians, but the physicians who worked in the outpatient clinic. They really saw it.

"At that time, Mount Sinai was not part of a medical school, but there was a large amount of valuable informal teaching plus innumerable staff meetings. Every day we made ward rounds with the older doctors. And we discussed each case with them or as many of the serious cases as time allowed; this took all afternoon and might last from 2:00 P.M. until dinner. On the medical wards the intern responsible was expected to know each case history by heart. He usually recited it during the rounds. Later on I was an attending physician at Mount Sinai and conducted ward rounds also. That was a voluntary effort; we were not paid.

"My father helped me financially throughout my college and medical education, including the internship. There was no salary for interns. You simply had your room and board and uniform and laundry. At the end of the internship, if all your charts were in order, the hospital gave you a lump sum of fifty dollars. We were not permitted to be married, and further, there was no question about disobeying any orders. Without knowing it, the hospital was repeating the medieval pattern of poverty, chastity, and obedience.

"One reason for the excellence of the attending staff at Mount Sinai was that promotion was 'through the laboratory.' That is, internship or work in the clinic was not considered enough. You also needed a foundation in some branch of laboratory science, usually pathology, which was then considered the principal basis of clinical medicine.

"There was no residency then at Mount Sinai. The internship lasted thirty months and ended with six months as house physician. During the last six months I was the person principally responsible for the health and survival of seventy of the toughest patients they had. That was the equivalent of a residency at that time.

"I think I learned most of what medicine was like from my father. He was extremely conscientious, extremely attentive. He was a strong man and worked very hard. Physical strength was important. One made house calls; I'm considered to be among the last who did. I learned therapeutic methods from my father. I learned to apply mustard plasters, which were valuable for pneumonia, since they helped with the pain. I learned about dosages of drugs. I learned how to prescribe; in those days that was important. My father was a master at prescribing. The writing of prescriptions was not taught adequately in medical school and not at all during internship. My father was also very strong against unnecessary operations, unnecessary procedures.

"My father was very strong on ethics, and ironbound about it. He was very strongly against fee-splitting: some doctors referred patients to other doctors who gave back part of the fee, instead of picking the best consultant for the patient's illness. He worked at the Sydenham Hospital in New York, which no longer exists. One of the first things he tried to do there was get rid of the doctors who split fees. He became chief of staff and hence was able to accomplish this. That was one of the main ethical problems he dealt with, and he talked about it on many occasions. He also struggled to have black physicians appointed to the staff at Sydenham Hospital. This was in the 1920s. He had seen plenty of racial persecution in hellish czarist Russia, where he was born. He recognized that the neighborhood would have a black majority, and that was an added reason why he felt that black physicians should be appointed. He was successful. It became an interracial hospital. Those were the main things that I learned from him—ethics and therapeutics."

BEESON

Quintessential Doctor from Alaska

"MY FATHER WAS a general practitioner and surgeon. I can remember the sign on his office door; it always read: Physician and Surgeon. I spent most of my childhood in Anchorage, Alaska, which had about two thousand people at the time. My father was the only doctor in Anchorage. I learned a great deal about being a doctor from watching what my father's life was like. His work consumed his life. He was surgeon for the Alaska railroad, which was a government project. The railroad was being built from Seward, an all-winter port, up to Fairbanks. The headquarters was in Anchorage, which was midway between them. There was a big construction operation going on up and down the railroad. My father handled all of the trauma, obstetrics, pediatrics, whatever, with almost no possibility of referral to anyone, because at that time it was a seven-day trip by steamship to Seattle. He was a very capable person. I think his special abilities were in surgery and in trauma rather than in medicine.

"I learned a lot about being a doctor from being essentially the only child. My brother was eight years older than me and was away at school all the time. I heard snatches of conversations between my father and my mother about what he was doing. I remember frequently hearing the telephone ring in the middle of the night. He gave some instruction to the nurse at the hospital nearby, or he often got up and went. So I did get some idea of what being a doctor was like.

"I think I knew as much about medicine as any young person does in deciding on a career in medicine. The fact is, you don't know what it is like until you actually get into it. It doesn't matter whether you are from a doctor's family or not. The idealism of helping mankind and the aura that surrounds the doctor in the doctor-patient relationship are what you think about in the beginning.

"I went to McGill medical school because my brother was there. I was twenty years old when I began. McGill was a five-year school and very rigid; they all were at that time. We had hours and hours of lectures and very formal, tough examinations. We sat and scribbled in lecture

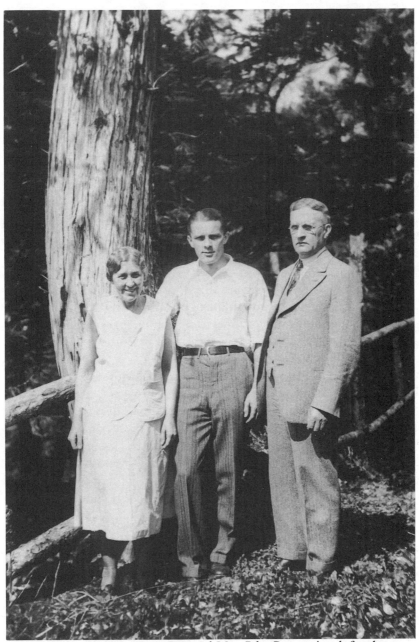

Paul Beeson with his parents, Dr. and Mrs. John Beeson, just before he entered medical school, 1928.

rooms and then memorized it and gave it back in examinations. I did well scholastically and I enjoyed studying what I was told to memorize. It wasn't until I was at the Rockefeller Institute years later that I really started to love learning. I never used a medical library throughout medical school or internship. Never. The great Osler Library is at McGill. Bibliophiles come there from all over the world. I went into that place once with another medical student, and William Francis, the curator, was there. He was delighted to see a couple of medical students. He came out of his office and greeted us so warmly and started to show us around. Meanwhile, we were edging toward the door and couldn't get out of there fast enough! Working in a library didn't appeal to us at all. Our teachers never suggested that we read current literature. They gave us lecture notes with textbook assignments. In the internship I was too busy to do very much reading. When I got to Rockefeller, a combination of events got me started reading, and I found that I enjoyed it and got great satisfaction from it.

"I don't think I would mention any of my teachers at McGill as having had an influence on my thinking or my career. We didn't see our teachers outside of their professional role. They were good clinical teachers, and they certainly had us on the right track as far as what to read and what the current thinking was, but we didn't see much of them as people. I learned medicine from making rounds with the professors at the Montreal General. Senior medical students were taken on ward rounds at that time, but they were not part of the clinical teams as they are now. This is one change for the better. The professors would stand there and talk about the patients. They would examine the patient, looking for physical signs. Imaging techniques were not what they are today. We had to palpate a spleen or an abdominal tumor or hear something in the chest that somebody else hadn't heard. Looking for physical signs was a big part of the thrust of medical education. We watched them and they helped us to acquire that kind of skill, but none of them stands out in my mind as an influential teacher who had anything to do with my thinking afterward. A big part of learning in medicine is that you learn more from your classmates and from people who are a year or two ahead of you than you do from people who are in exalted positions on the faculty. The things that a resident teaches you are things that stick with you all your life.

"There were two black students in our class. We got along well with both of them and respected them. They went to our parties and we had meals together. There was no distinction on the basis of color. There were three or four women in my medical school class of a hundred. One of them led the class and got the top prize of the Holmes Medal. They were rare birds. I don't recall sharing any projects with them. They tended to sit together, to walk out of the lecture room together, and to go places together. The boys did not go along with them. Women were not looked upon as colleagues, and they were not really accepted. That was in marked contrast to the attitude toward women in medicine now. I still go to the VA hospital [Seattle] every week for their clinical conference in medicine. When a woman resident presents a case she is perfectly at ease, and she is looked on as a colleague and is completely accepted. This was not true even when I was at Yale. There were a few more women there, but they were uncommon.

"There had been enormous prejudice against women in medical school a few years before I entered. The few who tried in the nineteenth century were treated outrageously by today's standards. If they weren't turned down flat when they applied to medical schools, they weren't given hospital privileges when they got out, or they weren't allowed to practice in some states. The fact that a woman made a big financial gift to Johns Hopkins with the proviso that women be admitted there changed all that. Since it was the best medical school in the country, this had a lot to do with things beginning to change. But they hadn't changed all that much even by the 1930s, when I was in medical school.

"I had different jobs during those summers in medical school. One summer I worked as a carpenter's helper on an apartment house that was being built in Ketchikan. And two summers I worked as a U.S. Customs officer simply riding on a Canadian oil tanker that was taking oil to salmon canneries that are all around southwestern Alaska. It was a dandy job. Beautiful scenery. We toured around the Inside Passage. All I had to do was be there to satisfy legal requirements. No other commerce except oil was going on. One summer I worked as a deck hand on a tug boat that was towing salmon traps out to anchor them. The traps were long and made of logs. They had a big tail attached to them and to the land. Towing one of those traps slows a tugboat down to about two miles an hour. Our trips were very long. I did a lot of turns at the wheel, which was not doing much. I realized at the time that this was good experience for me. I was living and talking with uneducated working people who were always going to be working people. I was getting some idea of another group of people that I hadn't had much contact with in my school days.

"In the summer between my fourth and fifth years at McGill, I took a summer internship at Johns Hopkins, in gynecology of all things. My brother had done that and he recommended it. I went down and tried to get one with the medical service. They didn't have an opening. But somebody said, 'I think they need a subintern in gynecology.' So I spent a summer there. That was enough to give me some feel for what the old Johns Hopkins Hospital was like. There is a tremendous spirit that pervades Johns Hopkins: We're the best, we have always been the best, we're still the best. It's a great place.

"After medical school, I also followed in my older brother's footsteps to the University of Pennsylvania for my internship. At that time, the U of Penn had a two-year rotating internship, which was an excellent plan. It was one of the last schools to keep the two-year internship. It kept it up until the war [the Second World War]. I'm sorry that it had to be given up. We had six two-month rotations in specialties such as obstetrics and pediatrics and neurology and outpatient clinic work. In the second year, we had six months of general surgery and six months of general medicine. This was ideal preparation for me, as I thought I was going into general practice. I got a little bit of the hospital wards and the outpatient departments, and I saw something of what medicine and surgery are. At that time, I didn't have any specific goals. I was just following the treadmill that you do to get a medical education. Many of us were uncertain as to what our life work would end up being, and we were glad to have those two years as a logical next step after medical school.

"There were fourteen interns. I think about eight of those were U of Penn graduates, and the rest of us were from schools elsewhere. We had a good time together. We had no salary. We got our room and board and laundry at the hospital. House officers were not married. It was a kind of enjoyable club, because we had common interests and there was not much technological work to be done in the care of patients. Intensive care units did not exist yet. We were in the hospital and had to be on call, but we had lots of time to sit around and talk. We played games and poker. There was no cafeteria; the cafeteria hadn't entered hospital life. We had a nice dining room and we were served at the table. This was in the depths of the Depression. We didn't go out much. No one had any possessions. No one had much money. I was dependent on the little check my father would send to me every month. I did not have a cent for clothes or amusements or anything of that kind. But that was standard with internships then. There wasn't much grumbling. People didn't complain about the conditions of work or anything else. We tried to do our jobs and enjoyed what we had. Later, house officers married. Indeed, a large proportion got married in medical school. They insisted on having nights off. Later came the great surge of technology in medicine and nights on became very hard, long nights. It's a very different experience now."

OLNEY

Pediatrics—Medicine beyond Hospital Walls

"I GREW UP in Richmond, California, a laboring man's town. My father owned and managed a dry goods store. My mother bought and managed a ranch with an almond orchard and fruit trees. My father was on the school board and the grand jury. Both parents were very active in lodge work. All of my summers were busy working in my father's store or helping with the ranch work. I worked along with the farm workers cutting grapes, harvesting apricots, irrigating the land. Gypsies used to come into the store. My father taught me to watch how they would sit down and brush things off the counter, into their laps, into bags that they had brought with them for that purpose. I also learned about short-change artists. I grew up with exposure to a great variety of people and a great variety of occupations.

"I don't think that a doctor visited our house more than twice in all the years I was growing up. Once was when I had herpes stomatitis [an inflammatory condition of the mouth]. The doctor's solution to that was to have me drink out of a moustache cup. I still have the cup. The other time was when my sister had some vomiting at the onset of an illness, and the doctor thought it was appendicitis. Most of the young-sters that we had heard about had died with operations for appendicitis. My mother had the 'courage' to stand up against the convictions of a good physician. She refused to give the doctor permission to operate. My sisters and I were in a panic, because we didn't know which was the right decision. My wanting to go into medicine grew out of a desire to develop a rational basis for difficult and emotional decisions like that in making people well.

"I remember the big influenza epidemic of 1918. Everybody had to wear a mask on the street. We all had 'flu.' My mother bled from her lungs. She was one of the few people who recovered. I had to learn to walk again after that influenza, it was so debilitating. My father's store on Main Street was next door to the funeral parlor. The hearses would arrive six, seven, eight times a day. Hundreds of people in the town died. The undertaker died. Many of the students at school died. I suppose that experience was also some of the background for why I went into medicine.

"In that era, people didn't talk about doctors or being sick. Illness was a skeleton in the closet. To be sick was to admit to inadequacy. I doubt if any child would have known that his grandparents had hypertension or a cardiac problem. I think people accepted the fact that there were a few things a doctor could take care of, but most illnesses were meant to be terminal, nature's clearinghouse. We depended on doctors for doing smallpox immunization, and they were credited with taking care of a cold and pneumonias. Mastoidectomies were new but diabetes, heart disease, nephritis and that sort of thing were conditions that could not be cured, and therefore, they were not to be talked about. The elders felt that illnesses were an adult concern and not to be visited on a younger generation. When my mother had a lung hemorrhage during the influenza outbreak, we were not supposed to know about it. A doctor was not called to the house. Knowledge of scientific things and scientific medicine was sparse. I remember various cultists who canvased the communities. I was curious about the neighbor who had breast cancer. Her husband bought strips of bacon to put on the breast as treatment.

"There were sixty students in my class at the University of California medical school [University of California, San Francisco School of Medicine]. Twelve or thirteen of them were women, the highest number they had had up to that date. The first year was on the Berkeley campus. I did my first year dissection section with three young men who asked me, 'Why do you keep a man out of medicine by taking up a place in the class?' They were angry. I didn't know any appropriate answer, so I didn't make one. I remember in my sophomore year here in San Francisco everyone was pretty congenial. We women were accepted generally pretty well, I think.

"I didn't have a lot of contact with my classmates because I had to work to provide my own room, board, and tuition. I would go from my last class of the day to the San Francisco Public Library to work. I had a job there for the evenings and weekends during my sophomore year and during the summers.

"When I worked at the public library over Christmastime to make my spring tuition, I didn't have quite enough money. That was the only time I had to take a loan from the university. The university would lend it to me if I would repay within a month; I think that was the time specified. I felt pretty low about that, because how was I going to pay my rent and have anything left to live on if I repaid that loan? I talked to one of the fellows about it and he said, 'One of us could talk to the department about it.' That was marvelous empathy I thought, and makes me think that there wasn't a lot of bad feeling towards women. The university extended the loan about a month.

"There was a very strong feeling against working your way through medical school at that time. Two of the internal medicine men said that they would flunk anyone they discovered working. So we kept it all pretty quiet. You were supposed to give your full time to medicine. The professors talked very strongly against anybody who would be presumptuous enough to think they could give medicine everything they had and still work on the outside. Those of us who were working—I guess about twenty of us—sort of faded out of the picture at the end of the day and phased back in again at the beginning of the day.

"The only way I felt handicapped at all was socially. But I don't imagine the other students had much time to have a social life either. One of the most fun things I think in medical school was getting together with classmates and reviewing material before finals. I didn't have the chance to study with other people while I was working during my sophomore year. Then two of my classmates from Los Angeles knew of a woman there named Grace Howland. They got her interested in helping me through my junior and senior years, so I didn't have to work during those years. I have never been able to find out enough about her and her benevolence.

"Several instructors were particularly influential. Dr. Connor, in the Department of Pathology, was one of the finest teachers I had ever run into. He would listen with interest to our student papers and make constructive criticisms. We were assigned a term paper. I did one on skin grafts. He could pick the difficult parts and present them in a way that you knew you were wrong and yet you didn't feel that you had to back off the earth because of unworthiness. It is a beautiful teaching talent.

"K. F. Meyer was spectacular as an instructor. He was the man with the Prussian accent. When he taught about lymph nodes in the tuberculous animal, he would bring a wash tub with lymph nodes the size of the weights that you put on a fish net to demonstrate that this was what tuberculosis did to that animal, and that milk from tuberculous cows was not desirable to ingest.

"I learned what it was not to have empathy. When I worked in emergency, a man on a gurney was lying there complaining of pain. It wasn't his turn yet to be examined. The resident said to him, 'Why don't you get up and go home if you don't like the way we take care of things here?' I was shocked. I wondered how anybody in the world could say that to somebody who was laid out in great pain and in hope of relief. That resident's remark was traumatic for me. I remember saying to myself, 'I hope I never lose my empathy for patients.' I still burn when I think of it.

"I can remember residents who would know they were going to do such-and-such a procedure at a certain time. If I was home studying, I would get back to the ward at that time to see that procedure done. I got to recognize the people who were empathetic and the people who could do things skillfully. Residents are wonderful teachers. They are close enough to having been through training themselves, and they are just recently out on their own doing it, so they are invaluable to students.

"When it came time to choose an internship, I had to make a first and a second choice. I thought if I put down a second choice, that is what I would get, so I put down the same thing for first and second choice. And I did get an internship at San Francisco General Hospital, because I wanted to know a broad spectrum of medicine. I had worked in the fruit sheds on my family's ranch in the summertime. I had worked with the grape pickers and I had worked in my father's store with the gypsies. I knew a pretty big segment of the population, but I wanted to know more. That was a very useful year, because it was a rotating service and you could see so clearly what illness meant to families. No matter what kind of illness it was, it meant a deprivation to a family in some way or another.

"I wanted surgery. I wanted orthopedics. I would have traded anything for more orthopedics. I loved it, the mechanics of it, the challenges of rehabilitation. I wanted to specialize in orthopedics. But I had a very well-rounded experience between medicine, surgery, orthopedics, pediatrics, obstetrics, and gynecology. That was when the prostitutes used to be brought into the hospital for checkups. To see what life had done to some of those girls was very revealing.

"Tuberculosis patients were in a convalescent home in the town of Belmont, a suburb of San Francisco. There was good general medicine between staff and patients who were there, so it was a very challenging experience. I diagnosed an acute appendicitis there. I found out what people complain about and whether or not complaints are real or not real. I considered it a very valuable two months.

"On obstetrical service I did thirty-nine home deliveries in a month. The person who came on after me delivered triplets! That would have been interesting. Sometimes I went into a home where they would say, 'We don't want you. You are from the hospital. We have a midwife here.' I visited the families postdelivery on the third and fifth and seventh day after a birth.

"I remember I had a fifty-six-hour straight session without going to bed. That is when I counted on the nurses to do the driving as we made the calls around town. The car was my only place to sleep. Now, residents and interns both feel that if they have to work for a twenty-four-hour period, they should have some time off. This was still in the time of the twelve-hour shift for nurses. The eight-hour shift didn't come until later, during my instructor years. I think that the twelve-hour schedule may well have been why so many nurses developed tuberculosis on the job. When the eight-hour shift came in, many fewer were afflicted.

"From the beginning, I learned a tremendous amount from the nurses. When I was interning at the county hospital, the nurses taught me all sorts of procedures. They taught me to do circumcisions, how to handle the postpartum patient, how to do dressings. I was always most grateful for that, because I didn't see how I could ever teach a parent to do something if I hadn't learned it from somewhere. How could you ever tell a mother how to do a colonic flush if you hadn't learned how to do it from a nurse? There were ever so many procedures I learned from the nurses.

"There were many deaths from pneumonias before antibiotics. I remember pleural effusions, where they had to open up the chest. I can remember the thoracic surgeons pulling membranes off the lungs to allow them to expand. Children screamed with the pain of having that done. We had ever so many pleural effusions on the ward—as many as six at a time. Tuberculosis wards were full. We knew tuberculosis of the larynx. We had to inject chaulmoogra oil onto the vocal chords. One of the girls in our class got tuberculosis. Enteric ulcers were more common than they are now. In the wintertime, the hospital had beds down the middle of the medical ward, because sick people couldn't sleep in the park anymore or on the library steps.

"Many people were under treatment for syphilis. We treated children for central nervous system syphilis. We used to drive down to Palo Alto to bring back the blood from the malaria patients at the hospital to give the syphilis patients, then allow them to have the appropriate number of fevers and chills to cure them.[1]

"About the only thing I didn't have experience with was tropical diseases. Otherwise, the internship covered the whole span of medicine. It was so valuable for going into straight pediatrics.

"Dr. Leon Goldman, who supervised the interns at San Francisco General, had been asked to find somebody to do examinations and stand by for a Camp Fire Girls camp. He thought that perhaps I could do with a little time in the Santa Cruz Mountains, so he asked me. I found it most interesting. There was a very heavily overgrown area with poison oak. I had upward of twenty dressings to do a day for campers with poison oak.

"One of the CCC boys in the area put an axe through the top of his foot, and I remember being taken to the CCC camp to give directions about what should be done with him. The staff was glad to have a doctor in the area. The camp experience made me feel that I had some extension into the community, and that I wasn't just a hospital doctor."

RHOADS

Quaker Surgeon

"MY FATHER was a general practitioner. It was rather different from general practice today. He did fractures until X–ray was discovered. Then that work became centralized in hospitals, where they had X-ray equipment. He did minor surgery. He did a great deal of obstetrics. Indeed, many of the children I went to school with he had delivered. He was the school physician among other things. As a young boy, I thought I wouldn't want to follow in my father's profession. My sense was that it was an honorable profession and that it was built around taking care of other people. It was not terribly remunerative. I don't think my father ever saved very much money. I think his idea was to keep his charges about as low as he could. For a long time, I think he charged one dollar for an office visit and two dollars for a house call.[1] I think it moved up about a dollar after World War I. I'm not sure how much it moved up after that. I had a sense that my father was greatly respected in the community and greatly beloved by his patients and that it occupied too much of his time. I thought I saw less of him than my schoolmates did of their fathers and that it was a profession I would never enter.

"I think I had a mixed response, over the years, to our insecure finances after my father's health began to fail. On the one hand, I was very anxious to save enough money for old age. On the other hand, I didn't think it was a good idea to try to get as much money as you could from people. I used to take a good deal of pride during the first two-thirds of my practicing years in the fact that, nearly every year, somebody would send me a supplementary check because they thought I hadn't charged them enough.

"My father took the position that you shouldn't go into medicine unless you really wanted to very much. His advice was that one should do something useful. He had very little use for stockbrokers and people like that. He thought you should do something that was, shall we say, palpably useful, like farming or medicine or teaching. I agree with that, I think, because you can always take pride in a job like that, get satisfaction out of it, even if it doesn't pay very well.

"I didn't talk with him much about medical subjects. His office was in the house. He had a laboratory set up and a sink. I suppose the whole laboratory wasn't as large as this table, but he could do urine sugars and urine albumins and so forth. One of my sisters, Esther, was at Drexel studying chemistry, and she used to run these tests for him. Once when I was watching, she found a urine with a lot of sugar in it [indicating diabetes]. My father came in and repeated the test and again it showed a lot of sugar. He looked very grim and I asked him about it. He said that means the patient will almost surely be dead within a year or two. That was before insulin. So I had some exposure to that sort of thing.

"I think my father was very concerned about honesty in medicine. I remember asking him once what he told people who had cancer. He said he tried to be honest. But he also told me that early in life, when he was a house officer in hospital work, he helped operate on a man with cancer. The man asked him about it, and he told the man. Later, the man went out and committed suicide. So I think he modified his willingness to tell people what they had. I think he did it mainly by circumlocutions. He didn't like to lie. He worked very hard. He was very conscientious. I think he accepted the fact that some of the patients were going to die, particularly when they were older. If he felt they could accept it, he probably shared the fact with them.

"My father died when I was a sophomore at Haverford College and that shook me up. I greatly admired him. I still hadn't made a career choice in my senior year. I was thinking about medicine, but I was also thinking a great deal about engineering, particularly aeronautical engineering. I think I finally decided upon medicine rather than engineering for two reasons. I thought I could be more independent as a doctor, and that I could enjoy it at any level of success. Whereas, with engineering, I was afraid that if I wasn't a great engineer I would end up doing various assigned duties in a large, industrial department of engineering somewhere. That didn't appeal to me. I also reasoned that I'd probably do better to go into a profession where I knew the problems. I knew that medicine entailed long hours that are disruptive, and that you don't have much free time in the evenings or on holidays. At least I knew that I could have good relationships with other people and that I could take satisfaction in it.

"At Hopkins, there were seven or eight women in our class of about sixty. All the women were very good students and very capable. Two of them went into psychiatry. My wife and two others went into pediatrics.

"They had recently revised the curriculum in order to give students a great deal more elective time. They had decided to give exams only twice, at the end of the second year and at the end of the fourth year. I found this a psychological hazard. I figured they wouldn't want to flunk very many people at the end of the fourth year, so they would probably be pretty ruthless at the end of the second year. They didn't let you know how you were doing along the way. So, I decided I should devote most of my elective time in the first two years to cramming, and I did.

"Anatomy is always a rather grim subject to start with. You wonder whether you're going to pass out at the sight of all these dead people, stinking, rather reeking with formaldehyde in the embalming fluid. But we all weathered that course all right. Then we had physiology. I received a letter saying my work in physiology was unsatisfactory. I was considerably worried about this and boned up and, in the end, did well with it.

"There were weekly sessions called clinical pathological conferences. They included the first- and second-year students. A patient who had recently died was described by the clinicians. They discussed what they had done, what they had found, and what they thought would be found in an autopsy. Then, the pathologist discussed his findings in the autopsy. They had some very keen clinicians. These were interesting discussions and served as a sort of introduction to clinical problems for the people in the first two years of medical school.

"We had a course in physical diagnosis in which we examined each other. This was a deadly course, because until you see the abnormal, you cannot possibly tell what the normal is. Then we finally got to see some patients. These were Baltimore poor, mostly black, people who came in. We went out to the city hospital, where we saw mainly two things: tuberculosis and aneurysms. In those days, there wasn't much to be done about aneurysms. They were mostly caused by syphilis, and they went on and finally ruptured with a great spurt of blood. That is how some people died of syphilis. The exposure to TB was great. I think 10 percent of our class got active TB, either during or after medical school. One of the people who lived in my rooming house got tuberculosis while in medical school. There was a Haverford graduate a year ahead of me who belonged to the fraternity next door. He got tuberculous peritonitis and died between his second and third years. It was not a very healthy environment, but it was an interesting one.

"I think we all had gone into medicine for better or worse. Medicine was not a money-making game in those days. People who wanted to make money went into another line of work. I think that most of us felt it was a duty to take care of the sick. If we survived, well and good, and if we didn't survive, that was part of our lot. We all knew tuberculosis was a risk. I think we could have been smarter and exposed ourselves less than we did. We could have worn masks and at least reduced the exposure. But actually at that time, a great many people had already been exposed to tuberculosis. They did tuberculin tests on us as freshmen. I was already positive before I had any Hopkins exposure. I don't know where I was exposed to it. It was pretty rife through the community. People all around were recovering from it.

"A generation earlier, the mortality from tuberculosis was nearly 100 percent. Trudeau had it [Edward Livingston Trudeau, 1848–1915, a well-known physician and friend of William Osler]. He thought he would like to spend his last months in the Adirondacks, where he had had some happy summers. So he went up there, but instead of dying, he got better. That encouraged other people with the disease to do the same. And then they started the sanitarium. A great many people started to get better, and the mortality rate went way down.

"The only illness of great note that I had as a medical student was in my third year; I had an acute upper respiratory infection. I had a temperature of 103 degrees, and they put me in the hospital in the isolation area. That's what they did with medical students; I had a separate room at ward rates. That developed into mastoiditis, and I had to have mastoid surgery. I remember being very interested in the mortality rates of mastoid operations at the time. They were about 5 percent. That was not large, but nevertheless people did die from it. We didn't have full confidence that we would finish growing up, but we hoped we would.

"We had our exams at the end of the second year, both oral and written, and got through them all. I don't think they gave us grades. They just told us whether we had passed or failed. I hadn't used much of the free time for research. I was afraid to. I thought I'd just better study my lessons.

"I was moderately interested in getting married, so I sought out some social opportunities. I was interested in a girl I knew here in the Germantown area. She turned out to be engaged to someone else. But she mentioned a classmate of hers at Vassar whose name interested me, a daughter of the biochemistry professor at Harvard, Otto Folin. I had studied his work in biochemistry. The daughter, Teresa, had finished Vassar and had gone to medical school at Boston University. Harvard didn't admit women to the medical school then. I didn't have the highest regard for Boston University medical school at that time. So I took it upon myself to send Teresa a Hopkins medical school catalog. I posted this thing off anonymously in my second year. Lo and behold, she appeared on campus the next year. She had transferred! So she was in my class for the last two years. We married four years after graduating.

"The third and fourth years of medical school were much more interesting, stimulating. We had outpatient work mainly in our third year, and inpatient work in the fourth year. We had a lot of elective time, which I used for selecting various assignments. I transferred to Harvard for two months in my senior year. There was an exchange pattern; a few people did it each year. That was where I met Harry Beecher, who became a very prominent figure in anesthesiology and for a long time later was head of anesthesiology at Massachusetts General Hospital. I lived in Vanderbilt Hall, a student dormitory. I spent one month at the Boston City Hospital, where I was exposed to two very good young clinicians: Soma Weiss, who later became the chief of medicine at the Peter Bent Brigham, and Chester Keefer, who became chairman of medicine at Boston University. The other month I spent at the Boston Children's Hospital. That was probably the best arranged student experience I had.

"I knew I wanted to come back to Philadelphia after medical school, and I got an internship early at this hospital [University of Pennsylvania]. The internship was divided into two-month rotations on the specialty services the first year and six months of medicine and six months of surgery the second year. I had two months of orthopedics, which at that time was largely looking after the disabilities of children who had polio and were left with various paralyses. It was mostly a chronic service. The acute fractures were handled by general surgery at that time. I went on to the laboratory for two months, where we actually did a great deal of the laboratory procedures ourselves, particularly at night. There were no technicians then. We had to be able to do the routine blood chemistry, which, of course, was much simpler than it is now. Then I had sort of a substitute service, partly on medicine and partly on pediatrics. That was followed by the nose and throat service, during which I did, I think, forty-seven pairs of tonsils. That was the heyday of tonsillectomy and adenoidectomy. There was a perception that it was unwise to do these at the time that polio was rife. So most of them were done as school let out, but before the summer season. So I had extended experience there, with no supervision except the visiting man. My two-year internship ended in June of 1934.

"The interns carried a great deal more responsibility then than they do now, because there were very few residencies. We simply had more responsibility for the patients. In medicine, there was only one resident for the whole service. We reported directly to the chief. With the specialties, we saw a lot of the chiefs also. In surgery, there were surgical fellows who were half way between us and the chief, and who were expected to spend half their time in the laboratory and not interfere very much in the responsibilities of the interns.

"This was a comparatively friendly place and much different from Hopkins. The atmosphere in Baltimore was more competitive. There, it was a dog-eat-dog system. They would take a group of people and drop a few out and drop a few more the next year, and end up with one or two. It doesn't improve your relationship with your fellows. We didn't have that kind of competition here. An intern at Hopkins was pretty well at the bottom of the totem pole in the medical hierarchy. They saw the chiefs largely at formal rounds. Here, we worked almost directly with the chiefs, and saw them frequently. I think C. Everett Koop, who came here a little later as a surgical resident, best expressed the internship. He said he wouldn't have missed his internship for anything, and he wouldn't do it again for anything."

HODGKINSON

From Pharmacy to Gynecology and Obstetrics

"I WAS BORN in New Castle, the western part of Pennsylvania. My father was a merchant tailor, and a good one. He did custom tailoring for well-to-do people.

"When I graduated from high school in 1925, I decided to attend pharmacy school at the University of Pittsburgh. I worked in the drugstore at nights while I was attending pharmacy school. My boss, the owner of the drugstore, was a very dominant influence in my younger life. He taught me business practices. He taught me that hard work paid off. He treated me like his son. He was wonderful to me and I worked like hell for him. He had many doctor friends who would come into the drugstore, into the back room. They would talk to me and I always admired them. In 1928, when I graduated from pharmacy school, my boss decided to open a second store and he put me in charge. I was aggressive in merchandizing and the store became quite a success. As time went on, I bought shares in the store. But I wasn't satisfied with the drug business. I decided I wanted to go to medical school when I was twenty-two.

"In the meantime, I had gotten married. I finally decided to give up the drug business and return to the University of Pittsburgh to complete my credits to gain entrance to medical school. After talking it over with my wife, I told my boss. He admired my decision and agreed to repay all the money I had invested in the new store. Giving up the drug business and starting back to school in 1930 for my premedical credits was not an easy road to take. My family was never very affluent and I certainly wasn't very affluent. But by working in the drugstore at off hours, we managed to make it through premed. My wife was a nurse, and she also gained employment at her alma mater, Western Pennsylvania Hospital in Pittsburgh. It took me two years to get my undergraduate qualifications for medical school, and I finally got accepted to the University of Buffalo School of Medicine. Our first child, a boy, was born in September 1932, just a few days before I started medical school.

"I left my wife and son with her folks in New Castle when I entered medical school. I got some grants from various organizations. The Knight Templars loaned me five hundred dollars, a lot of money in 1932. It was very difficult for me for a while. I didn't do anything but study at Buffalo, and I acquired excellent grades.

"When I finished the first year at the University of Buffalo, I wanted to transfer to a medical school in Pennsylvania for financial reasons. I wanted to get a scholarship to a state school. I was working in the summer in a drugstore in a suburb of Pittsburgh, Greenfield. There were two doctors. One of them, Dr. McClenahan, used to come into the drugstore and talk to me. He said, 'I think I can get you into Temple.' I said, 'That would be nice.' I didn't really believe him because he was a very unimposing man. He wasn't very pushy. He said, 'I know Dr. Wayne Babcock down there quite well.' I didn't know who Dr. Babcock was from the man in the moon; he was the professor of surgery and one of the foremost surgeons in the United States at that time. He helped popularize the use of spinal anesthesia in this country.

"So I made out an application to Temple and also to the University of Pennsylvania. I got a letter from Dr. Babcock to come down to Temple for an interview. I went to Philadelphia, and after office hours one evening he interviewed me. He was instrumental in getting me admitted. I transferred my credits to Temple University. I got two loans. Then I got a scholarship, which was a big help. My father-in-law loaned me a thousand dollars. And I worked. That is how I got through.

"I think I was an atypical medical student for a couple reasons. I was a little bit older than most of the students. And most of them were financed by their parents. They were mostly from Pennsylvania; a few came from other states. Out of a class of 186, there were 6 girls.

"At that time, Temple was a young school. It was trying to come up in the world. There was great competition between the schools in Philadelphia. They tried to improve their academic standing by procuring the most prominent professors. Temple had been extremely successful in weaning outstanding professors from other schools. It was a good school and we had good professors. Dr. Babcock was well up in years by the time I was a student. He was a wonderful teacher and I had great admiration for him. He had a tremendous fund of knowledge.

"The Depression was a terrible thing, and I was in medical school during the worst of it. With many homeless and jobless wandering the streets of Philadelphia, and the severe winter of 1933–1934, we saw many afflictions. The Budd Locomotive Works was located in Philadelphia. It had failed because of the Depression. The manufacturing plant was closed down. However, the company maintained a low heat level in the huge building. They turned the building over to wayward men, men without work, without any prospect of work, and God knows, there were plenty of them. They filled the area with cots and blankets. We were taken as a class to minister to these poor men. We observed all sorts of diseases. We observed many cases of pneumonia in all stages. Those were preantibiotic days and many of the men were doomed to die. The hospitals were full. But the Budd plant was a refuge for them.

"We saw patients at the Philadelphia General Hospital [PGH] in inner Philadelphia. It was a fantastic place. It's a big, big hospital, five thousand beds, and it's full of all kinds of medical curiosities. We went to PGH for our clinical conferences. I'll never forget one morning in that terrible winter, the clinic was devoted to gangrene. Dr. Babcock had every different kind of gangrene that was ever thought of to display to this class. Many kinds were caused by frozen legs and feet. I was sitting in the front row of the amphitheater and the stench that came from it—I could hardly stand it.

"The clinical conferences were the most outstanding thing for me in medical school, where we had the problem of making diagnoses and outlining treatments. I think one of the most striking clinics was on the subject of acute appendicitis. Dr. Babcock precisely outlined the details of the diagnosis of acute appendicitis, and I think I can remember every single detail. That proved to be a valuable experience for all my clinical years. I remember one outstanding case that I had years later. A three-year-old boy was brought into Fitzsimmons General Hospital [Denver, Colorado] with nausea, vomiting, and apparently abdominal pain. In a child that age, the diagnosis of acute appendicitis is extremely difficult and often associated with considerable error. I studied the child for over one hour before coming to the conclusion that he was suffering from acute appendicitis. I removed an acutely inflamed appendix, and the boy's recovery was prompt. I feel sure that if I had not had the benefit of Dr. Babcock's lecture, I would not have made the correct diagnosis nor had the courage to operate.

"We saw a lot of infectious diseases which fortunately we didn't get: typhoid fever, a lot of tuberculosis, a lot of pneumonia. On the obstetrics service, we had to deliver six women in order to graduate. We had a little black bag. Sometimes a senior would go with us. We would go to these homes and these women, mostly black, were in labor. We would sit there, forever sometimes. I remember one who I thought was never going to deliver. She had six kids already. I called back to the hospital and said, 'I think this woman is going to need a cesarean section.' They said, 'Go on, just go back there and be patient.' And she delivered.

"I began to see the results of illegal abortions; they were very common. I saw patients who had put all kinds of things up into the uterus to try to abort; coat hangers were very common. It was probably the most dangerous instrument used. The women also used slippery elm bark and they used unsterile catheters. They would start running fevers. They would come into the hospital after they got sick. We had no antibiotics. I saw many, many, many women die from illegal abortions because of septicemia. There was nothing we could do about it, nothing.

"The medical school had a good neurological department, and Temple Fay was the neurosurgeon. He was kind of a wild man but an excellent professor of neurology and a very noted neurosurgeon. He had a theory about convulsions that was dominant at the time. His theory carried over to obstetrics; eclampsia is a very serious convulsive disease. No one really knows what causes it. Temple Fay's theory was that dehydration was the best therapy for eclampsia. They would purge patients with magnesium sulphate, that is, epsom salts. It was a rapid technique to get patients to lose a huge amount of fluid. It did improve the statistics on eclampsia. That theory and treatment were in vogue when I was in medical school. By the time I had decided to go into obstetrics and gynecology, another treatment for eclampsia had come into use and the dehydration treatment had fallen into disrepute.

"I was interested in surgery because of Dr. Babcock. He had a surgical society, which I belonged to. At that time, in order to finish surgery, the students had to scrub with Dr. Babcock on six different occasions. The assistant surgeon told me what to do. I remember once he said, 'Now we are going to do a thyroidectomy and we are going to use silk to tie off all of these vessels. Your job is to take a piece of gauze and everytime he ties a knot and they cut it you swipe his hand with this gauze to get rid of the ends of the silk that might have fallen off. He is not going to wait for you; you have to do it right away.' Dr. Babcock was a very commanding person. He scared people, he was so intense. I remember at one of the surgical society meetings, he called one of the members up to the blackboard and asked him some questions. The guy was so scared, he couldn't spell!

"I was terrifically interested in medicine, and I studied hard and did very, very well. I can't say there was anything I disliked. Some things were more difficult than others. Neurology and neurosurgery didn't command my entire interest like some other subjects. I was always interested in technical things and laboratory experience and in surgery.

"I worked all of the way through medical school. I worked as a druggist during the summers. I used to work in the medical school pharmacy on weekends. They paid me WPA wages; it wasn't much but it was something. I made some money and it was a good place to study. I could take my books over there and, though the pharmacy was open, usually no prescriptions were coming in. I would go in about 10:00 A.M. and leave about 10:00 P.M.

"I graduated from Temple in 1936 with honors. I won the faculty prize for the highest grades in the class. Dr. Babcock offered a gold medal prize and a hundred dollars for the best summary of the Babcock surgical clinics in the senior year. There were two first-place winners, and I was one of them.

"Because I graduated at the top of my class, Temple didn't want to lose me. They wanted me to stay there as an intern. I could have had any internship I wanted. At that time, interns didn't make any money. That was a problem for me. I had to go someplace where they paid some money, because I had to support this family of mine. My wife's parents had been supporting them. At the time, Henry Ford Hospital in Detroit was paying a hundred dollars a month to interns, a fantastic amount of money in 1936. To get accepted at Henry Ford Hospital, I had to take a two-day test. Well, that was unheard of anywhere else. About fifty people took the test when I did, and I guess they all were in the top 10 percent of their classes. There was a lot of competition. That was the toughest test I have ever taken. But I was accepted there as a surgical intern. I have never regretted my decision to come there. From my background in the drug business and knowing the doctors who used to come into the drugstore, I think my objective at the time was to become a good general practitioner.

"I moved my family to Detroit and rented a little apartment and things were all right with us on a hundred dollars a month. In fact, we could start to save a little money and start to pay back some of my debts. We enjoyed it in Detroit.

"Henry Ford Hospital was quite different from other institutions. For one thing, it was an institution made up of specialists. The hospital was set up to have specialties for everything. The lines were drawn strictly, and no one infringed on your specialty. The hospital was built by Henry Ford in 1912 or 1913, who had very definite ideas about what a hospital ought to be. The doctors were on a salary; physicians didn't collect fees from patients. That was unusual. The hospital was always a private institution. Now it is affiliated with the University of Michigan. But during my internship, it was not. It was not a teaching hospital.

"Specialization never dawned on me until I got to Ford Hospital and saw how it worked. In New Castle, most of the doctors were general practitioners. We did have a few specialists. We had an ophthalmologist, and ENT people. We had surgeons, but the surgeons did everything else, too. They did medicine. They took care of everyone who walked into the office. We had one physician who I considered to be a specialist in internal medicine. Everybody had great admiration for him, including me. He didn't do surgery. That constituted all there was in the way of specialization in medicine in New Castle. At Ford Hospital, specialization worked very well. The divisions cooperated with one another. I began to change my objective of becoming a doctor. I wanted to become a specialist.

"As a surgical intern, I spent six months in the surgical specialties: urology, gynecology and obstetrics, nose and throat, and ophthalmology. I think I spent three months in medicine. I got a little bit of everything, but the proportion of services was different in medicine and surgery. There was no limit to the hours we worked. Sometimes the hours were tremendously long. The interns did the preliminary laboratory work for surgery: blood counts, hemoglobins, urinalysis. The nurses weren't allowed to give intravenous injections. The interns had to do it. That was a tremendous chore sometimes, because there were a lot of people, and sometimes it was difficult to get into their veins. Then we had various ward chores—changing dressings and things of that sort. We were allowed to scrub in on operations, but we never did anything much. We worked hard, but it was quite varied and we had many, many different experiences. It was a formative year and helped me mature a bit, medically speaking. I'm sorry they have done away with internships. I think it is a transition period between didactic medical school and practical medicine that is much needed."

ROMANO

Builder of Psychiatry

"I WAS BORN in Milwaukee. My father taught music at home. He taught the violin, mandolin, piano, and accordion. I grew up in an atmosphere of learning. My father was never a successful man in terms of income. We were poor and we lived marginally.

"My mother was an unusual woman. She worked in the family welfare movement, the private philanthropy that started in the 1860s. It started with very wealthy people taking baskets to the poor. Later she worked in organized public welfare. She only had an eighth-grade education, but she knew German, Italian, English, and Polish. She had a certain giving relationship with the entire neighborhood. When the young social workers got panicky because the family was about to cut their own throats or attack them, they would call in my mother as a visiting housekeeper. In about thirty minutes, she had calmed everyone down and created order out of chaos. She would have a pot boiling with soup. She would change the diapers of three children. She was stitching something; she was ironing something. I went with her sometimes to see this. It was magical, fantastic. She had this great gift of giving of herself. Also, people would come to our house and ask for things. I remember one time, I had two sweaters. This boy came over and she gave him one of my sweaters. She told me, 'You know, you had two and he had none.' She was that sort of person.

"As a poor boy, I had all kinds of jobs. I worked in drugstores. Then I piled concrete blocks. When I finished high school at sixteen, I didn't have any money to go to school. I worked for a year in the complaint department of the Milwaukee Gas Light Company. A fellow telephone clerk was about to enter the school of osteopathy in Kirksville, Missouri, and he tried to persuade me to become an osteopath. I remember talking this over with another fellow clerk, a tall, lean, sober character who had attended a Lutheran college in Minnesota, who advised me not to do this. If I wanted to become a doctor, I should follow the traditional path. The manager of the department where I worked offered me a job as assistant manager. They wanted me to stay. I was not quite seventeen. They would have paid me $150 or $200 a month. I was tempted but I didn't stay. I think it took me ten years to get back up to that salary.

"I read Sinclair Lewis' *Arrowsmith,* which was published in 1925, just as I had finished high school. I read it a hundred times. I was so enthralled with Arrowsmith and his wife and her death and all those people. Later on I learned who some of them were. They were modeled after people from the Rockefeller Institute for Medical Research. Reading that book impressed me immensely. I must have had visions of being a research scientist and sacrificing all for the good of mankind.

"I went to Marquette, a private, Catholic college. I only had two years there. In those days, you went into medical school after two years of college. Later on, I took a year out twice. So I actually did have the equivalent of the four-year collegiate experience. I had English, history, math, physics, chemistry, and biology. I had no mentor, no person to guide me. My mother and father couldn't do that. Looking back, I wish I could have enjoyed a more leisurely collegiate experience.

"I was wage earning from the very beginning. I paid my way as best I could, so I didn't burden my parents. The tuition at Marquette was three hundred dollars a year. I worked and I could pay it. In the summertime, I had a job making and piling concrete blocks. I think I made fifty or sixty cents an hour. I worked about ten hours a day. It was about an hour on the streetcar each way. I would pile so many tons of concrete a day at the Marimonte Cement Block Company. I worked with people who were homeless and destitute at times. They would have the job for a few days, get paid, and then go somewhere else. They were vagabonds, on the move. As I look back on it, some were probably simple schizophrenics. Some were psychopaths; some were alcoholics. They would make a few dollars and get drunk again. It opened my eyes to a population I had never known before. Some of them were quite sensitive to human affairs, I thought. Some of the psychopaths had occasional episodes of tenderness that I would see from time to time. It helped me keep away from too rigid a view of psychopathology in my later clinical work as a psychiatrist.

"I also worked on the railroad. I used to go from 6:00 to 10:00 at night and load freight cars with food. I had to leave school and dash down there, put on some overalls and throw huge A & P bread baskets four or five high inside a freight car. I loved the railroads. In my early life I heard the railroad sounds, because in Milwaukee there are lots of railroads. I'll never forget the first time I ever earned money as a doctor. Here I was, a first-year medical student, and everyone called me Doc. A man got off a train with a cinder in his eye and someone said to me, 'Doc, this man needs help.' Well, Helen Keller could have taken it out with boxing gloves, but I scrubbed and took it out with my handkerchief. He gave me five dollars. I thought, 'My God, five dollars!' I think I was being paid sixty cents an hour for the night. Everyone said, 'Well, it's not too bad to be a doctor.'

"Between my first and second year in medical school, I took a whole year out and I was a student assistant of biochemistry for fourteen hundred dollars a year. It was 1929, the year of the crash. I was so poor that the crash didn't affect me. I didn't have anything to lose. My father lost a few dollars in a bank that failed, a few hundred dollars I think. It was a great year for me personally. It was the year I met my wife. She was then at Madison going to school. I would visit her in Madison. I paid back the school debts. I put away some money. I bought a suit. I bought some books. I was just giddy—it was so much money.

"Most of the students weren't working their way through the way I was. There were students from the middle class and lower middle class. They were from Wisconsin, Minnesota, Iowa, North and South Dakota, Michigan, and Indiana. All kinds of ethnic groups—people of Polish, German, Greek, English extraction. There were only three of us with Italian names. There were six Jews. Our class was small, only fifty-two. There were only three girls. There was some kidding with the girls from time to time, but they were all pretty good sports, and the boys were too. Most of our class became general practitioners. After a year of internship, they did minor and major surgery, as well as medicine. They would sometimes take summer postgraduate courses in Chicago, a two-week course on disease of the gall bladder, or surgery of the ear, or something like that, and then they would do that. Most of them went to small towns in Wisconsin, Minnesota, and the Dakotas.

"There was a practicing psychiatrist at the Sacred Heart Sanitarium in Milwaukee. He was a lecturer. He would come and read from a book. Imagine! That was the lecture. The book was a very good book, a textbook of psychiatry by William Alanson White. This fellow would get up there and sonorously read this thing. We would be so bored and disgusted. That was our beginning in psychiatry.

"But there were some very good teachers. Walter Zeit was a young man in anatomy then. Later on he became professor of anatomy. He was my mentor, and later my friend. I spent a great deal of time with him during my year as a student assistant in biochemistry. He and his wife befriended me and later my wife. They would invite us over to supper. He opened my eyes to all sorts of things—German literature, painting, architecture. He was a broadly civilized man and influenced me quite a bit. Yet, I don't remember any discussion with him, or with anyone else, about medical education, medical practice, or medical economics.

"I had a job in my fourth year at the Milwaukee Asylum for the Chronically Insane with my friend Leander J. Van Hecke. This was 1932–1933. It was a very prestigious job because they gave us room and board. No money, but room and board. It was my first experience with chronic schizophrenic patients. During the summer we worked there all day long. We did physical and neurological examinations. There was a medical superintendent, but we never saw him. There was an assistant superintendent, and he tried to teach us something. But there were no nurses at this place for fourteen hundred patients, just orderlies. The pharmacist was an alcoholic. So we had to prescribe and dispense. We pounded pills and made solutions.

"There were men we called Rip Van Winkles. They hadn't talked in twenty years. They were catatonic. Some of them had postural edema of the legs; they used to call them piano legs. They had become rigid because they sat so long. Others had 'buffalo necks' from leaning over in their chairs. The hospital started an occupational therapy program there in 1932. Two young women from Downer College, occupational therapy students, worked with a senior therapist. Together, we took ten of these men. First we began to sing songs with them, like 'Flow Gently Sweet Afton.' Some began to hum a bit and began to make noises. We played baseball with them. At first, they wouldn't even protect their faces or bodies. The ball would hit them and they wouldn't move. After being with them all day long, day in and day out, all summer, three or four of them started to talk with us but not with each other. I realized then that a schizophrenic patient is never dead. They are still alive, but so fragile. Their recovery is fragile. As soon as we had to go back to our school classes in the fall, they regressed and became silent again and just sat.

"But I had a whole year with chronic illness, because when we returned to our classes we were on duty at the hospital from 5:00 at night to 8:00 in the morning. We would have to fix scalp wounds. We boiled our own syringes; there was no nurse around to help with any of that. Many people would fall; epileptics would fall and tear their scalps. We would sew them up. We corrected some fractures. We delivered a few women who went out and got pregnant and had their babies. It was like practicing in northern Alaska, and it was a tremendous experience for the two of us.

"At the end of the fourth year, beer came back to Milwaukee. Pabst, Schlitz, Blatz, and Miller all came back. It was spring 1933. I was on ambulance duty the night beer came back. I'll never forget it. Beer was being given away free. People would spike it with ether, with shaving lotion, with sterno, the solid alcohol. All kinds of fights and troubles broke out all over Milwaukee. I have never been as complete a doctor as I was that night.

"My wife and I got married at the end of my fourth year, 1933. It was the trough of the Depression. We were married on the day I was exempt from final exams, because I had the highest marks in the class in surgery, of all things. Only a few of my fellow students got married. It was unusual to be married in medical school or internship then. Out of a group of forty, only two were married. In those days, medicine was more of a monastic system. William Osler used to say to his students, 'Keep your emotions on ice.' That was his advice.

"The internship was in the Milwaukee County Hospital. It was the Depression, 1933–1934. Everybody was poor. We worked twenty hours a day with maybe one day off a week. The food was terrible and most inadequate. The laundry was destructive. But we arranged to have a series of noon clinical conferences, and we invited part-time and full-time staffs to come in and conduct the conferences. They were very successful.

"Most of America was medically indigent. Middle-class America was coming to the county hospital. The standard of care was quite good. I learned a lot and I saw a great deal of pathology. I saw some good teachers and some poor teachers. There was a lot of indiscriminate surgery done then. I'll never forget one gynecological surgeon who did radical surgery—removed the uterus—on a young woman. She was nineteen or twenty. She came in with a vaginal discharge. After the operation, she had an intestinal obstruction and died. This was a couple of days after she came into the hospital. The doctor had me tell the husband and talk with him about it. I almost cried with him I was so upset about it. In those days, if the uterus was tilted a certain way, they wanted to remove it. There are ridiculous fads that go on in medicine. Even then, I didn't think the surgery done was necessary. I got so mad at the surgeon, I almost got fired. I told him what I thought about his doing this surgery. He was going to throw me out of the internship, but other people came to my rescue.

"We also used to take out tonsils and adenoids. The group of us used to do fifty every Monday, imagine! You go in and scoop out the tonsils of these kids. I used to think, 'What the hell are we doing?'

"We delivered babies. I delivered about fifty babies during the obstetrics rotating internship. Many of them in their homes. There were quite a few Mexican and South American peasants who came up to work in the tannery factories in Milwaukee. In some places there was no electricity, and I had the lights from the car shine on the house so I could see what I was doing. I had a lot of ambulance duty, and a lot of babies were delivered in the ambulance. I had ambulance duty with the women interns. They couldn't lift the stretchers, so I had double duty. The hospital couldn't afford attendants in those days; the interns were the slave labor.

"During the internship I saw a great deal of infectious disease. One must remember this was before sulpha and before antibiotics. If patients came in with miliary TB and with subacute bacterial endocarditis, it was expected that they would die in a short time, which they did. Patients died of lobar and bronchopneumonia, of cerebral hemorrhage, of kidney and heart disease. Sulpha was introduced in the mid- and late 1930s.

"I became more and more interested in psychiatry during the internship. The eighth floor of the county hospital was the psychiatry unit. I called it the sheep dipping place, because the patients only came in for a couple of days. They were then sent to jail, the chronic insane asylum, or back to the courts. A nurse ran it very well. She taught me a great deal. She knew so much more than the interns, and she was patient with us. There wasn't much time for study, but I did begin to develop some psychiatric interests."

DEFINING MEDICINE AND
THE PHYSICIAN'S IDENTITY

HOW DID THE nature, conditions, and goals of medicine in the 1920s and 1930s help shape the moral outlook of these seven individuals? As Shields and Beeson describe, the principal task of medical education in their early experience was physical diagnosis, performed mainly in the context of the charity hospital. Those two factors largely influenced the scope of medicine in the 1920s and 1930s. In a description of medicine between the 1920s and the Second World War, the period these seven individuals were trained, David E. Rogers discussed the eminence of physical diagnosis: "Medicine of the day was a do-it-yourself discipline in which one's own observations rather than those of others or the laboratory reigned supreme. Young physicians soon realized how many times the correct diagnosis could be achieved by trained observation, unaided by much in the way of technology except for a stethoscope, a flashlight, and an otoophthalmoscope, and they strove to emulate."[1]

The importance of physical diagnosis for shaping the nature of medicine cannot be overemphasized. Observation and touch were the primary tools that doctors had. The stethoscope and flashlight were merely extensions of the physician's personal diagnostic capabilities. Physical diagnosis was the sole means by which the puzzle of disease was solved. It took both cognitive and intuitive skills to discover what symptoms related to what diseases, and that challenge is what made medicine so exciting during this era. Physical diagnosis was a test of multiple skills, an integrative exercise.[2]

Today, physical diagnosis has been replaced by the laboratory test, and diagnoses are much more detailed and accurate than ever before. Perhaps most important, laboratory tests are expected as routine. While medicine has gained scientific precision through the reliance on the laboratory, it has lost the necessity of touching and knowing the patient. It has lost the excitement of discovering a disease through a combination of intuition and highly limited instrumental knowledge.

Medical students and interns learned the skill of physical diagnosis on poor patients in charity hospitals, where attending physicians volunteered their time. Trainees gave free care to the indigent in exchange for learning medicine on them. Beeson notes the attitude of doctors of the day was that patients were lucky to be receiving care at all. Doctors and students thought themselves to be kind, charitable people. Those who volunteered their time to teach were especially so, and they were a medical student's first influence.

Along with physical diagnosis and charity work, medicine's identity was shaped by the doctor-patient relationship. Communication in the form of explanation to patients was largely nil, but this was not perceived as negative or thought to reflect negligence on the part of the doctor. Explanation as we now define it—in the context of a patient's right to know and right to information—was not considered an integral part of medicine. Beeson wrote about the nature of the doctor-patient relationship during his training years at McGill. He was embarrassed to recall the moral superiority that doctors in training assumed and the ways in which that attitude infused doctor-patient relationships:

> . . . the teaching hospitals were true charity hospitals. My recollection is there was a real social gap between the providers and the clients. We thought of ourselves as kindly people and also as charitable people. Indeed most of our teachers were doing their teaching on a volunteer basis and making their livings in private practice. Medical students never saw the doctor-patient relationship in the private practice situation. During internship there was some exposure to this, but the thing I am emphasizing is that we considered ourselves in a different kind of society from our patients and I suppose there was some unvoiced assumption on our part that they were lucky to have us giving them care. I recall one Sunday morning when I had to go down to the medical ward at the Montreal General Hospital for something and took along a couple of preclinical fraternity brothers who just wanted to see what the Montreal General wards were like. I took them on a ward round myself and stood at the end of each bed, probably without nodding to the patient in that bed, and told them quietly what was going on with each patient. We moved along from bed to bed all around the ward and I remember feeling quite smug when one of the freshman medical students said to me, "It's interesting how impersonal you were and how you could stand there talking about each patient without any feeling of embarrassment." Well, I am embarrassed about it now.

Similarly, our teachers, when they made ward rounds with a larger group, did not usually say much of anything to the patient as they moved from bed to bed. We all prided ourselves on those code words which we could say within the patient's hearing, assuming that the patient would not understand—works like lues, mitotic figures, and so on. I'm quite sure that when the attending man left the bedside he did not put a hand on the patient's arm or look the patient in the eye or stop to say anything about what was going on. The main function of the attending physician in medicine then was to demonstrate physical diagnosis since we had such inadequate diagnostic technology.

Another thing that I regret is that we never told patients when the prognosis was unfavorable. We did indeed tell the families, but in nearly all instances this was a conspiracy to be kept from the patient. In rare instances when the patient would ask right out what the outlook was we lied about it and our teachers lied about it. I remember once . . . when a patient had read her chart saying that she had an inoperable cancer. When the attending surgeon came along with his troop of followers she stopped him and asked about that and without an instant's hesitation he said, "that's fine Mrs. (   ), that means you don't have to have surgery." We sailed on thinking what a great bit of quick wittedness that had been.[3]

The use of medical terminology so that patients would not understand, avoiding disclosure, and an attitude of moral superiority were givens, accepted features of the doctor role that were not criticized within the profession or condemned publicly. Fifty years later the contrasting values of physician honesty and directness, patient involvement in therapeutic decision-making, and the moral equality of doctor and patient are standards against which the quality of health care is measured.

Contemporary notions of the need for patients to make informed and educated therapeutic choices were not part of the cultural repertoire in the era in which these doctors were trained. With little technology and few curative drugs, there were not many treatment choices for patients to make. Nor did patients hold expectations that doctors would discuss the ramifications of a diagnosis or explain the course of a disease to them. Explanation as part of the doctor's task and understanding as a patient's right (or even as a prerequisite to patient compliance) were not attributes of the doctor-patient interaction and therefore were not goals to which medical students aspired. The lack of importance paid to direct communication, honesty, and openness in the doctor-patient relationship in no way contradicted the notion of medicine as service and the physician as empathetic toward the community at large. For one could work toward the common good by treating the indigent without having to assure their individual understanding of disease, its treatment, or its outcome.

Underlying the absence of explanation was, as several of the doctors state, the knowledge that doctors and patients were from different social worlds. Doctors were predominantly male, white, middle or upper class, and Protestant. Jarcho, Romano, and Olney were exceptions to the norm. The hospital patients that medical students observed were largely poor and from the variety of ethnic groups that resided in the area. Medical knowledge, authority, and a sense of duty to serve the indigent separated both doctors and medical students, by a vast cultural gulf, from the general patient population. With what were considered to be profound socioeconomic, educational, and attitudinal differences between practitioners and patients, it was assumed that patients would not understand the nature of disease processes or prognosis, and therefore that explanation was unnecessary and usually not appropriate.

Romano recalls that a lack of explanation accompanied by a lack of empathy frustrated him when he witnessed an unnecessary surgical procedure performed on a young woman who subsequently died from its complications. In that case, the tragedy of the death, caused by the surgery, was compounded in Romano's eyes by the fact that the attending physician refused to discuss the case with the woman's husband, sending Romano to explain for him. Romano publicly protested against both the unnecessary surgery and the doctor's avoidance of informing and empathizing with the husband, an act that endangered Romano's own career. Olney, too, vividly recalls lack of empathy on the part of a resident toward a patient in pain. Fifty-five years afterwards, the resident's verbal cruelty still upsets her viscerally. At the time the words were spoken, they taught her a great deal about the range of physicians' attitudes toward their involvement with patients and the importance of empathetic doctor-patient communication.

The diseases students and interns observed were a fourth dimension of medicine. They defined the range of problems with which doctors dealt. The prominent diseases remembered by all doctors include tuberculosis, the pneumonias, and aneurysms resulting from syphilis. Not much could be done for tuberculosis or the complications caused by advanced syphilis. Pneumonias, too, were treated primarily by bedrest and nursing care, though Shields speaks of the use of antitoxin, and Olney recalls the use of drastic surgical measures. Those diseases constituted a large part of the subject of medicine. Before antibiotics existed, doctors did not have the power to cure patients routinely. The natural progression of the disease, not acts performed by doctors, was the omnipotent factor in medical outcomes during these doctors' early training years. Doctors could offer only limited treatment with the hope of avoiding complications and potentially aiding the body to rid itself of disease, and they could make the patient as comfortable as possible in the hospital setting. It was hoped that their treatments would strengthen the body and comfort the spirit. But none of their activities routinely resulted in cure, and there was no expectation, by doctors or patients, that they could or would.

Observing the range of diseases in others is quite different from personal exposure to and experience with a potentially fatal illness. Rhoads best describes the relationship of the physician's own illness to commitment in medicine. Doctors of his generation do not often discuss the significant health hazard tuberculosis posed at the time of their training, or their own confrontation with a potentially fatal disease. Tuberculosis posed a health risk to medical students generally, as both Rhoads and Olney attest.[4] Rhoads has eloquently summed up the moral outlook of the era: ". . . it was a duty to take care of the sick. If we survived, well and good, and if we didn't survive, that was part of our lot."[5] Duty in the face of exposure to disease was expressed as the commitment to giving medical care to sick members of the community regardless of the health risk to oneself. Exposure to infectious diseases, especially tuberculosis, could endanger one's life, but that was the risk one took to serve the sick. The physician, as well as the patient, was vulnerable to disease and death. Social class and education separated the patient from the doctor, but life-threatening illnesses did not.

A fatalistic attitude pervaded medicine: death was part of life and could and did strike people at any part of the life span, not only in advanced age. Death was not a disease to be cured or a mistake to be avoided. It simply happened. Part of the doctor's role was *to stand by and lend support as it happened*. When people were sick enough, they died. It was inevitable. Yet fatalism in medicine was accompanied by a tempered optimism. After all, these individuals had witnessed the recent, great decrease in mortality from tuberculosis in the twenty or thirty years preceding their own medical training. Diagnostic and surgical techniques were improving steadily as well. Rhoads articulated the general existential attitude toward illness of the 1920s and 1930s when he reflected upon his own mastoid surgery: "We didn't have full confidence that we would finish growing up, but we hoped we would."

Diagnosis and treatment involved the performance of tasks no longer included in the student and intern repertoire. These physicians all spent many hours doing the routine blood work of the times. Shields spent the first six months of his internship as a laboratory technician. For Romano, medical work also included the chore of sterilizing instruments and the pharmacist's job of preparing and dispensing medications. He also played baseball with and sang to chronic schizophrenic patients. Olney recalls learning a great many procedures from nurses and driving from hospital to hospital to bring blood from malaria patients to those who had syphilis. Hours spent in performing those mechanical tasks were a fifth dimension of medicine that contributed to the responsibilities of being a doctor.

During the late 1920s and 1930s, the identity of the physician and the nature of medicine itself were shaped largely by the following taken-for-granted features: the primacy and satisfaction of physical diagnosis, charity patients who were lucky to have care, a sense of public duty and personal empathy coupled with a feeling of social distance, lack of explanation to patients and families, potentially lethal infectious diseases for which there was no cure, hope invested in medical research, and finally, certainty that the natural progression of the disease determined medical outcome.

DIMENSIONS OF DISCONTINUITY

Medical school was a process of digesting material that was seemingly timeless in its content. Little new knowledge that would alter day-to-day practice was being produced, and the body of relevant knowledge to be learned was contained in textbooks. The culture of medicine was characterized by its continuity and its assumption, held from the late 1880s, that the doctor's role was to diagnose disease, offer treatment and comfort, and stand by the patient. Medical students were to learn the specific ways in which to carry out those activities. These doctors' collective goal when they began medical school was to become general practitioners as had most doctors before them. The point is that doctors of the preceding generation could and did serve as role models, because there was no gap between their fundamental experience of medical practice and the experience of those doctors trained in the early 1930s. To be sure, some changes had appeared within medicine; new diagnostic tools and therapeutic regimens had appeared in the years since their fathers and others of the preceding generation were trained.[6] But medicine's essential responsibilities, problems, and goals—its very nature and definition— were understood and remained stable. These people had no expectation during their early training years that characteristics basic to its practice would be later transformed. Medicine maintained a strong sense of identity between its recent past and its expected future.[7]

Medicine's unchanging scope and highly limited powers affected these doctors' expectations in profound ways. I asked Dr. Beeson to talk about the "permanence" of the material he was learning and his ability to master the material in light of today's knowledge explosion. He replied: "In medical school I had the feeling that there was much skill and experience to be acquired, but did not have the feeling that new 'bits' of knowledge, often without relevance, were going to swamp me. I have just been looking at the 1931 textbook of medicine that I studied and practically memorized, and it is quite clear from my underlinings and margin notes that I thought this was about 'it,' and that I would be using that dogma the rest of my life. Later, at the Rockefeller Institute, 1937– 1939, I was thrown among people who were producing new knowledge, and began to realize that I would have a hard time keeping abreast of new developments."

The early understanding of continuity and permanence in the body of knowledge and skills these doctors were acquiring is in marked contrast with assumptions about the stability of medical knowledge, and thus the goals of medical practice, today. Questioning the relevance of the ever-burgeoning and detail-overloaded curriculum today's medical students face and making attempts to revamp medical education in light of constant new biomedical knowledge are two results of the lack of stability and constant growth in the information that constitutes medicine. Melvin Konner pondered the impact the biomedical knowledge explosion is having on understanding what the practice of medicine is actually about when he reflected upon his own experience as a medical student between 1981 and 1984:

> Consider a few of the changes that have occurred just within four years of my first day at medical school. Liver transplants, previously a rarity, have become relatively practical and commonplace. The immunosuppres-

sant cyclosporine has dramatically altered the success rates of all kinds of transplants. Traditional antacid therapy for ulcers has been laid aside in favor of systemic drugs like cimetidine, which within two years of its approval became the most frequently prescribed drug of any kind in the United States. Calcium-channel blockers, a completely new class of drugs, were approved and became a mainstay of cardiology. Noninvasive widening of clogged arteries in the heart began to rival bypass surgery as a treatment method for one of our most common serious illnesses. AIDS, a new and fatal disease, was identified, shown to be taking on dangerous epidemic proportions, and linked to a virus not just of a species but of a whole biological category previously not considered to be among the causes of human illness. Lithium, an extraordinarily simple elemental substance, overtook antischizophrenic drugs as the treatment of choice for intermittent forms of psychosis. Alzheimer's disease was recognized as the leading cause of senile and presenile dementia and a major health problem of our time. The basic science of recombinant DNA became an essential part of every physician's knowledge, promising as it does a vast variety of new and powerful drugs, as well as the imminent prospect of that science-fiction therapy "gene surgery." Magnetic resonance imaging—known also as nuclear magnetic resonance, or N.M.R.—became the gold standard of radiology, promising to replace CAT scanning (itself a quite new modality) in several important areas of diagnosis. And in vitro fertilization made the transition from a science-fiction laboratory technique to a proven and accepted method of treatment for infertility, making hundreds of "test-tube babies" a reality. These are only a few highlights of the new knowledge discovered or made practical while my graduating class was attending medical school. In most cases they were not, and could not be, taught to the students who graduated the year before we entered. Those students thus had substantially less to learn than we did, although they must have been equally bewildered trying to keep up with discoveries made in their four years and equally suspicious of the validity of textbooks just published. Neither they nor we had an education that taught us in any significant way the skills needed to evaluate and master this always-emerging new knowledge.[8]

But it is not only an exponential growth in information to be absorbed that is troublesome. It is also, as Lewis Thomas informs us, the fact that today, contrary to the stability of medicine during the era in which he and the doctors here were trained, "nearly all the usable knowledge came in a few months ago. Medical information does not, it seems, build on itself, it simply replaces structures already set in place . . ."⁹ So medical knowledge is transient. New scientific information and practices are always emerging to replace the old, so that current medical truths will become antiquated when they are supplanted with new frameworks of understanding. This fact is fundamentally unsettling and impacts the work of physicians in ways that are almost entirely unexplored today. The discontinuity between the known past and unknown future makes certainty about medicine's goals and responsibilities, and thus certainty and stability about the individual physician's responsibilities, impossible.

PART II

Specialization: 1930s

In the early 1930s it was not clear what a
specialist was, or should be, let alone how he
should be trained.

> —*Rosemary Stevens,*
> *American Medicine and the Public Interest*

We have instruments of precision in increasing
numbers with which we and our hospital
assistants at untold expense make tests and take
observations, the vast majority of which are but
supplementary to, and as nothing compared
with, the careful study of the patient by a keen
observer using his eyes and ears and fingers and
a few simple aids. The practice of medicine is an
art and can never approach being a science even
though it may adopt and use for its purposes
certain instruments originally designed in the
process of scientific research.

> —*Harvey Cushing, M.D.,*
> *"Medicine at the Crossroads," presidential address,*
> *Congress of Physicians and Surgeons, 1933*

COMBINING CARE AND SCIENCE

The Residency

ONE OF THE early and notable features of medicine's transformation was its embrace of the scientific enterprise. That process began to occur dramatically during these physicians' advanced training years. Medicine was depending more and more on science—on laboratory experimentation and the application of laboratory findings to the treatment and cure of patients. What sets these physicians apart from others of their era is that their advanced training included participation in some of the major laboratory discoveries and clinical insights of the time. Moreover, they had the chance to observe the direct application of those discoveries and insights at the bedside.

CHOICES

Before the Second World War the decision to specialize was uncommon.[1] All seven of these doctors became specialists. Shields and Jarcho specialized in internal medicine but did not have added years of formal training beyond the two-and-a-half-year internship. They both describe the last six months of their internships as equivalent to a residency today. They had great responsibility in making treatment decisions, and they served as teachers and models for the newer interns. The other five doctors had formal residency training.

There was no way to predict the specialties these physicians chose. Beeson realized while working as a general practitioner that he had no talent for surgery and thus chose to specialize in internal medicine. Romano did well in surgery during medical school but became far more interested in psychiatry. Rhoads, interested in both psychiatry and internal medicine, finally chose surgery. Hodgkinson, starting out as a general surgeon, switched to gynecological surgery and obstetrics.

Olney is the only one of these physicians who describes her choice of specialty as determined by constraint rather than by interest. She could

111

find no program in the United States that would fully accept a woman in orthopedics (that is, she would be allowed to walk in the door, but would not be permitted to touch patients), so she decided on pediatrics, the most common specialty "chosen" by female physicians of her generation. Though the number of women in medical schools throughout the United States remained around 5 percent during the 1920s and 1930s, a smaller percentage were admitted to internships and residencies during this era. The prevailing assumption of the period was that women were less committed to medicine than men and that they would eventually drop out to marry and raise children. Their education thus was considered by some institutions to be a waste. Internships and residencies at elite hospitals were simply not open to them, and high-quality residency training was extremely difficult for them to obtain. Seventeen states had no hospitals at all that would accept women into their internship and residency programs. California and Illinois, where Olney received all her training, were among the few states that offered advanced training opportunities to women.[2]

Although she considered marriage during this period, Olney decided against it, because she felt it would be impossible to devote a full-time career to medicine and be a wife and potentially a mother as well. Women physicians of her era faced an either/or choice: give up medicine to marry or practice medicine and do not marry. The very few female physicians of the 1920s and 1930s who were wives or who were both wives and mothers generally worked part-time in the public health field or in community or school jobs.[3] Rhoads's wife, a pediatrician, continued to work part-time in clinical research while rearing four children—a highly unusual path—though she ultimately terminated her career. The cultural assumption that a career in medicine and family life were mutually exclusive was not shattered until the rise of the feminist movement in the 1970s.

Men, on the other hand, could marry and have children whenever they chose without jeopardizing or limiting their opportunities in medical education, choice of specialty, or training experience. Although it was unusual for men of this era to be married in medical school or during the internship, Hodgkinson's early marriage and family did not constrain his career, nor did Romano's marriage before his internship.

Beeson, Olney, Rhoads, and Hodgkinson had mentors during the residency years, individuals who acted as teacher, advisor, inspirational guide, and role model all in one. The mentor played a very powerful part in these doctors' professional development. All four describe their mentors as vibrant, extraordinary people who expanded their horizons about medicine's purpose and possibilities. Romano, alone, regrets the lack of a mentor. He recalls his need for one when he was struggling to define subjects of psychiatric research and the nature of psychiatric practice for himself.

As the first major choice in medicine, the residency was a rite of passage from generalist to specialist, apprentice to authority, novice to expert. The mentor served as a much-needed practical guide through the many unknowns of medical work. But more than that, the mentor was an exemplar whose moral and intellectual attributes the residents sought to emulate. Though the scientific fields were producing new techniques and procedures that changed many aspects of medical knowledge and practice, the very nature of medicine—to cure sometimes, to help often, to comfort and console always—*was still assumed to be changeless*. And the experience of elders was critical to the skill acquisition and attitude formation of the next generation of doctors. The period of these physicians' residencies can thus be characterized by the historical convergence of two features: medicine's turn to scientific experimentation and method in order to solve day-to-day problems in patient care, and the assumption that medicine's overall goals and purposes were timeless. The relationship of those two features would begin to change during the Second World War.

Turning now to the narratives, we can begin to see how the relationships between science and caregiving were carried out in daily work during the 1930s, and how the mentor was an inspirational guide to physicians who were becoming both future-looking scientists and traditional humane clinicians.

BEESON

From General Practice to Camelot

FROM HIS comfortable childhood in Anchorage, Alaska, Paul Beeson followed in his older brother's footsteps to the University of Washington, McGill University medical school, and the University of Pennsylvania for his internship. Through his internship training, he had no specific career goals. He assumed he would be going into general practice as had his father. Beeson told me about his false start in private practice with his father and brother in Wooster, Ohio. Tears appeared in his eyes and he became visibly emotional when he vividly recalled an example of his father's miraculous heroism at the bedside while he was incapable of acting at all: with no anesthesia or antiseptic, his father quickly and efficiently sutured a woman's ruptured cesarean wound. Beeson was in awe of his skill and knowledge of what to do. His father was an extraordinary role model. But Beeson knew he did not have the talent or inclination to be that kind of physician.

By a lucky break, Beeson went from a short stint at the New York Hospital on the not very desirable private service to two years of residency at the Rockefeller Institute (1937–1939). There he was exposed to the worlds of clinical and laboratory research and realized he wanted a career as a researcher as well as a practitioner. He spent an additional year as chief resident under Soma Weiss at the Peter Bent Brigham Hospital in Boston. He idolized Weiss and emulated Weiss's clinical skills. Beeson would pass those skills on to his own students in the future. He characterizes both the Rockefeller and Brigham experiences as Camelot-like— precious opportunities to learn from great individuals.

"I was at Rockefeller from 1937 to 1939. It was a glorious time to be there. I was put on the pneumonia service, to take care of pneumonia patients. This was prepenicillin. Just the year before, researchers there had developed a way of making type-specific antipneumococcal serum for many different types of pneumococcus. Serum therapy in that disease is very difficult, because there are sixty or so types of pneumococcus.

Maybe ten of them are clinically significant, and we had little supplies of specific antiserum for all of those. We were getting patients with clear-cut pneumonia who were referred to us from all over New York. We would type the organism that was causing the pneumonia, then treat them with the rabbit serum. We were getting spectacularly good results, as good as you can get with penicillin. But it was time consuming and expensive and not as simple as penicillin, and so it lasted a very short time. The clinical work was wonderful there.[1]

"The head of our department was Oswald Avery. He was the man who discovered the role of DNA in genetics. Avery, MacLeod, and McCarty published the paper in 1944 that started the revolution in molecular biology that is still going on.[2] He was in a cubbyhole office right across the corridor from me. Right next to him was Rene Dubos. They both worked by themselves. Neither one had a technician. I saw a great deal of them. One morning Avery was good enough to spend a couple of hours telling me what he was looking for and why this was significant. I can remember the experience very well. The thing I remember best of all is that it didn't mean a thing to me! I couldn't see why he found it so exciting. Of course, a couple of years later, they found that the transforming principle of pneumococcus was DNA, and they reported it in 1944. It took the scientific world another six years or so to really recognize the importance of this and to begin to transfer it into other genetic research. Avery died before he could get a Nobel Prize for that work.

"I did get in and do some laboratory work there with a man named W. F. Goebel. We were working on the pneumococcal polysaccharide, which is the capsular material around the pneumococcus. That is the substance responsible for the differences in types. We were studying one from Type 14 pneumococcus, because it cross-reacts with one of the blood group substances, Blood Group A. They are very similar in their construction. This was an exciting problem to get into, and it did give me a taste of laboratory work. The typing of the pneumococcus, all of the bacteriology, we had to do ourselves.

"Those two years at the Rockefeller were a marvelous, lucky experience for me. For the first time in my life, I saw that you could get great satisfaction from studying and learning. I was appointed to go on for another year, but the offer came to be chief resident under Soma Weiss, the new chief of medicine at the Peter Bent Brigham Hospital in Boston. The Rockefeller Hospital was very specialized. It was a clinical research center with five different kinds of disease and that was all.[3] I still saw myself as a clinician, and I knew I needed a lot more training in clinical medicine. I wanted to be a good internist. I wasn't sure that I wanted to stay in academic medicine. So when the opportunity came to be Weiss's chief resident in 1939, I jumped at it.

"Soma Weiss was a great man. He was a Hungarian Jew who had come to America after receiving his university training in Hungary. He obtained his M.D. at NYU and got a job at Bellevue Hospital in medicine and clinical pharmacology and later moved to the Thorndike Memorial Laboratory at the Boston City Hospital. There, he became a very popular clinical teacher. He used to give special rounds at Boston City Hospital on Tuesday nights. Doctors from all over Boston would come and go around to see patients with Soma Weiss. When he moved to the Brigham, he immediately picked up a contingent of doctors in the Brookline area of Boston. His grand rounds on Saturday morning were great spectaculars. At least a hundred people went around those wards to see patients and hear Weiss talk.

"Everyone who met him can remember the exact circumstances and what he said. He had great charisma. He was intensely interested. He worked very hard at being a doctor and being a teacher. His passion for medicine came through very clearly. At morning report, Soma sat there intensely. He never took his eyes off the person who was reporting a case. He often made interesting and instructive comments about the condition. He also often said, 'Just give me that patient's name and hospital number on a slip of paper. I want to file it away because I'm interested in that.' He had broad interests and wrote on a broad range of subjects. He had a very heavy Hungarian accent that people laughingly said he never made any attempt to change. It was his trademark. For me to be his chief resident that first year was a great good fortune. I adored him. He made medicine so exciting and so important to learn. He was certainly one of the most influential people in my life.

"He drove the staff hard. He didn't approve of ski weekends and he let that be known. He didn't want somebody coming back with a broken leg and needing a substitute for a few weeks. There was a tennis court on the grounds of Brigham Hospital, and when he walked down the long corridor, he never failed to say, 'I see you have some time for tennis.' But he could do it in such a nice way that nobody resented it. He worked so hard that he could command work from the rest of us.

"He was interested, too, in human beings generally. He met my family briefly, and when he did, he had something nice to say about me. He remembered them, what they did, where they lived. He knew a little about the personal family problems of many of the house staff.

"He was willing to give important assignments to young people. I learned that from him. For instance, he put Eugene Stead in medicine and John Romano in psychiatry into very high visibility spots. I think Weiss was the first person who brought a psychiatrist into a department of medicine. They talked at grand rounds on occasion. He gave young people great opportunities. I think this is one of the things that made it sort of a Camelot-like experience for all of us. We all realized it at the time. We realized that this was a precious experience and to work under Soma Weiss was a great privilege.[4]

"Soma Weiss died, unfortunately, at the age of forty-two. Otherwise, he would have been an enormous towering figure in American medicine. There is no telling what his influence would have been had he lived longer. He was becoming in great demand to give talks at other schools. I remember, as chief resident, I resented this a little bit. His presence was so important; I always wanted him to be there. That was something I kept in mind when I became head of a department. I turned down lots of committees and visiting lectureships, because I think the house staff do know it when the head of the department is not there.

"I was starting a second year as chief resident when World War II broke out. Conant, the president of Harvard, wanted to make some gesture of support for Britain. With the American Red Cross, he sent a unit over to Britain to work in the field of infectious diseases [American Red Cross Harvard Field Hospital Unit]. It was thought that with air warfare, which everyone could see would be important, there would be a lot of bombing of sanitary facilities and water supplies. Epidemics might be a great problem. In the fall of my second year, I was asked to go over to Britain and I did. I was concerned about the war. I was glad to get in and play some little part. This was before Pearl Harbor. I went over in December 1940 and stayed until July of 1942 as head physician of our little unit. Soma Weiss died while I was in Britain."

OLNEY

Vision of the Whole Child

DURING MEDICAL school and internship training at the University of California in San Francisco, Mary Olney sought out experiences that would not only contribute to her medical education, but would also broaden her knowledge of people and of family life beyond her childhood experiences with socially marginal people in rural California. "To comfort and console always" emerges as a guiding principle when she remembers the lack of empathy she saw on the part of some physicians and how important empathy was in patient care. This became even more important to her as a pediatrician when she had to comfort parents about the terminal illnesses of their children.

When Olney realized that no hospital residency program would take a woman in orthopedics, she chose pediatrics and calls that decision the biggest turning point in her career. She spent two years in training at UCSF, followed by another year at the Bobs Roberts Memorial Hospital, University of Chicago. Her experiences in the outpatient clinic, home, and community settings influenced her decision to practice medicine outside as well as within hospitals. She did not have much laboratory experience during this period of her career. But during her advanced training years, she was influenced greatly by a visionary mentor.

"I was busy enough in pediatrics and didn't spend any time regretting that I wasn't in orthopedics. But I was still attracted to orthopedic problems in pediatrics and that compensated in some way for not specializing. Pediatrics was pretty much an all-absorbing specialty. I spent my time at night trying to read Holt's text on pediatrics so I would be one step ahead of the admissions that were being made. With the advent of the sulfonamides, antibiotics, and new diagnostic methods, everything was advancing very rapidly and there was little time to spend regretting choices.

"Things were really not very good before the antibiotics. Looking back, it seems it was a matter of desperation for something to do. Young

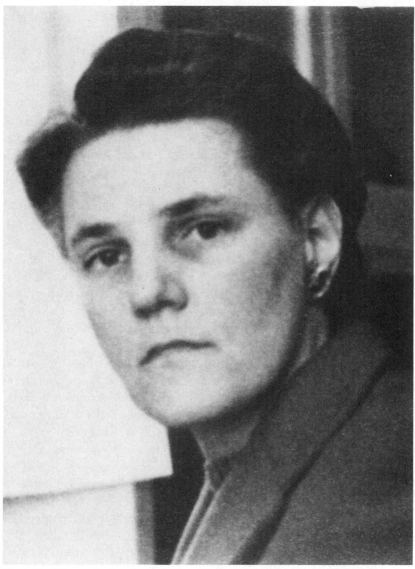

Mary B. Olney, during her advanced training or early instructor years, 1930s. Courtesy Alumni Faculty Association, University of California, San Francisco.

people today have no concept of what it meant to have to plant maggots in bone lesions in order to remove decayed tissue. Or the scraping out of bones as the treatment for osteomyelitis. The treatment of impetigo used to require the removal of infected skin crusts with the youngsters crying with every motion. For subacute bacterial endocarditis we used gentian violet intravenously, which was terrible. There was tremendous excitement when the sulfonamides arrived; we began to see cures. I can remember the first case I saw of subacute bacterial endocarditis that was treated with sulfonamides, and the patient was cured. Later, when antibiotics became available, it was such a marvelous advance. Being able to treat with oral medication and local application was truly marvelous.

"Francis Scott Smyth, the department chairman, was my greatest inspiration during my residency and later when I became an instructor. He believed in treating the whole child, everything concerning the child. Dr. Smyth had children referred in from all over the state and from other states. If things were not taken care of while the child was hospitalized here, there was no recall to get the child back to do things that were very necessary. He felt this was the one and only contact that he had, and he felt responsible for returning the child to the community without deficits.

"Dr. Smyth could not see fit to discharge a child with serious dental caries who might develop gingival abcesses and not be able to chew food and be properly nourished. He wanted it taken care of on that hospital visit. The same was true for problems in orthopedics. If a child was very flatfooted and was going to have trouble with walking later in life or have arthritis in the ankles, he wanted the feet seen and prescriptions made by an orthopedist. The same was true for a child who came in for some other reason but needed to have his tonsils taken care of. If a child had a speech defect, he wanted treatment instituted for that child so he wouldn't be made fun of in school and so he wouldn't develop psychological problems about having to recite in front of other children.

"Dr. Smyth was one of the early users of child psychiatry. He had a very close association with Olga Bridgeman, who did a lot of the early work in child psychiatry. He had very strong feelings about correcting and getting plans laid out for the bedwetter and the child who was a chronic vomiter. Our department was one of the very early ones to recognize and treat dyslexia. Dr. Smyth made us do a lot of thinking about it. We came to realize that a lot of adults took jobs that they could work at without being able to read. And they stayed with a job they didn't like because they hadn't been able to read. I was very interested in following the course of dyslexic children after I read a report about the high incidence in prisons of dyslexic individuals who had tangled with society, being unable to cope because they could not read.

"We were very close to the patients. For example, if Dr. Smyth thought that you should go out and see an asthma patient and see how the home fell short of carrying out the regimens you were giving in the clinic, you went out to the home. If you had a new diabetic and the family didn't know how to set up a home-care center for taking care of the diabetic routines, you went. In the cases that involved psychiatric care, it was important to see how the family functioned, and you went.

"Dr. Smyth also believed in sending children to summer camp when they had few other opportunities for contact with children outside of their own social class. So, we had a very rich inheritance from Dr. Smyth. There wasn't any part of the child he overlooked. Dr. Smyth was also very wise in seeing that we had experience outside the department. He liked to place his residents in a clinic like Telegraph Hill, which was 'Little Italy' then. There were language barriers, but that was another type of experience. Then, of course, I had the privilege of doing home visits on children with diabetes and with rheumatic fever. Each one furthered my experience."

RHOADS

Research Surgeon—From Patient to Lab and Back Again

JONATHAN RHOADS'S Quaker background and admiration of his physician father were the deciding factors in his delayed choice of medicine as a career. After the Friends School in Germantown and Haverford College, two Quaker institutions, he attended Johns Hopkins University School of Medicine. His experience with his own serious mastoid infection and related surgery and a classmate's death from tuberculosis contributed to a sense of duty to care for the sick, regardless of the risk to oneself, and to the knowledge that there were no guarantees that one would live to see old age.

Rhoads did not choose surgery as a specialty until his exposure to I. S. Ravdin, a charismatic professor of research surgery who became his mentor at the Hospital of the University of Pennsylvania. Under Ravdin's guidance, Rhoads plunged into a career in academic research as well as surgery. While Rhoads was in the middle of his residency, the time required for surgical training changed from three to five years. He decided to take advantage of the added time and complete a doctorate in medical science—conducting research on plasma and plasma proteins—while continuing with the residency. He was always glad he had completed the extra work and earned a doctorate "that was something more than a professional degree." He, like Beeson, embarked on a full-scale career in research as well as clinical medicine.

Here he talks about Ravdin's influence on him. He describes the integration of laboratory research, surgery, and patient observation in order to provide breakthroughs in postsurgical patient care. He also describes the major diseases general surgeons saw and treated during that era and the surgical techniques that were available at the time.

"I met Dr. Ravdin when he was thirty-five. He was an exceedingly vigorous man, short, stocky, full of energy, full of ideas. He had almost a genius for drawing younger people to him, for inspiring younger people. He was good about letting people do the things they wanted to do if they were reasonable. He was very generous about putting the names of younger men first on scientific papers. I think this was part of his technique of encouraging young people. I don't think he was the first author of the best papers he wrote. They were his ideas, his plans, his laboratory, and his organization. But he would get somebody engaged in it who would spend hours working at it, and then Dr. Ravdin would give him the primary credit. He was quite a taskmaster in his way, but on the other hand, he would come up with an idea that would fire you up and you would want to take off and explore it.

"Some people used to describe Dr. Ravdin as a one-man employment agency. All kinds of people would come to him for suggestions about where they could get a job, and he would recommend them for jobs. They hardly ever let him down. That was one of the amazing things about it. People thought he was overvaluing some people that he recommended, but they almost always measured up to what he predicted.

"The residency was originally a three-year program, but in 1937 the American Board of Surgery was established and it required five years beyond the internship. It became clear to us that if we did not go ahead and pass our boards, we wouldn't really be credentialed as surgeons. I either had to give up what I had already invested or else agree to take two more years. So I agreed to take two more years.

"As residents, we lived out of the hospital, so we were in and out. We made rounds in the morning and we operated. We went to the laboratory. We came back and made rounds again, usually in the late afternoon. Then one of us would come in and make rounds in the evening with the interns, and then we would be on call at least every other night. So, life wasn't too hard but it was busy. Those were still the Depression years. We were sort of glad to be indoors and to have something to eat. I had a little money, a few hundred dollars a year perhaps, which was more than most people had. I think I got paid $105 a month and had to provide my own board and keep.

"Appendicitis was frequent in those days. If an appendix was allowed to rupture, the individual had a very significant chance of dying. So our attitude then was similar to our attitude toward a breast lump now: you didn't wait and watch it. You took it out, and if it was benign you didn't apologize. So we took out a great many normal appendices from people who had sort of miscellaneous pains in their abdomens as well as those that were acute. We tried to hold back a little. I remember I had one that ruptured because I thought the symptoms were so slight that we ought

to wait. Fortunately, he recovered. We did a vast number of appendectomies at all hours of the day and night. For some reason, there seems to be
less appendicitis now.

"We had quite an elaborate routine to treat people if we weren't
going to operate on them. We sat them up partway in bed so that the pus
would tend to gravitate into the pelvis, where it seemed to be better
tolerated and more easily drained. We'd give them morphine, which
seemed to keep them from getting too distended. Then we would give
them nothing by mouth and put them on suction drainage.

"Then we did a good many acute gallbladders and many more
chronic gallbladders for gallstones. Our diagnostic precision was less
than it is now, but it wasn't too bad. Then there were people who got
jaundiced, and some of these had stones in the common bile duct; others
had stones in the lower part of the hepatic duct or tumors in the pancreas
surrounding the duct. We still combat those. Then there were ulcers. We
did not have Tagamet or any of the newer drugs. Many ulcers came to
develop complications that required surgery, and many different operations were developed and compared.

"We had cancers. We had some terrible skin cancers in those days—
great, raw, bleeding cancers. We excised them and grafted some of them.
There were some over the scalp that invaded the skull. Then we had
cancers in the mouth and the tongue, and we did some of those. For the
sinuses we usually called in the nose and throat people. We were not at
home in the sinuses, but we didn't mind taking out half a tongue. If there
were nodes in the neck we would often take those out. Sometimes those
were due to tuberculosis; some were due to cancer. Then the cancers
occurred right on down the gastrointestinal tract, small bowel rarely,
large bowel commonly, including the rectum. We would take out spleens
sometimes, because they were ruptured from accidents. Sometimes we
would take them out for various hematologic disorders.

"We didn't do very much in the chest. We would drain pus collected
between the lung and the wall of the chest. We had a good deal of that
until we got the drugs that attacked pneumonia organisms. Then we
would have lung abcesses. We would drain some of those. We removed a
great many thyroids. Surgery was then the treatment for hyperthy-
roidism. There were tumors of the parotid gland. There were nasty
infections of the floor of the mouth. If you didn't drain them they would
lead to swelling of the larynx and suffocation of the patient. We would
sometimes open the trachea and put a tube in. Then there were a galaxy

of local tumors occurring in other parts of the body, the arms and legs and back and so forth.

"We did the acute fractures for a good while. It was a much wider field than general surgery is now. Later on we began to do operations in the chest. The orthopedists took over more and more of the fractures. Now they do most of them. We did not do backs. I never opened a skull. Some of the surgeons would drain a subdural hematoma after an accident if they diagnosed it, but I never got into that. There were a lot of other things to do.

"The first important technical innovation that affected surgery was air conditioning. In the days before air conditioning, we used to cancel operations on hot, muggy days, because we felt the patients didn't tolerate heat well. With air conditioning, we were able to operate all year round without feeling that summer weather induced any increased risk to the patient.

"We used to be more afraid of electrical apparatus explosions in the operating room, because the anesthetics were explosive. We used to put metal grids on the floors of operating rooms so we could ground everything. There have been advances in lighting. Many surgeons now use head lamps that project light from between the eyes. Wherever they look, there is a bright light shining.

"The instruments are much the same that I used when I started out, except that more use is now made of the automatic suturing instruments. We got our first automatic suturing instrument in the mid-1930s. There have been advances in retraction or mechanical devices that hold the wound open so you don't need as many assistants. Then came the flexible endoscopes for the stomach, the trachea, the large bowel. These are tremendous diagnostic aids which have supplanted a good deal of open abdominal surgery for removal of polyps in the large bowel. The development of intratracheal tubes taught us a lot about the control of intrathoracic pressures. With those tubes, the pressure of air into the lung could be controlled and the lung kept from collapsing when the chest was opened. Because of negative pressure in the chest, when you open the chest, the lung collapses, so that thoracic surgery was then very hazardous. I suppose that for every innovation that has endured, there are a hundred that were invented and discarded.

"Operating room technique for sterility has fluctuated a little. It was originally a ten-minute scrub and then a rinse in alcohol. After we had antibiotics, it became a five-minute scrub. There was a rash of antibiotic-resistant staphlococci that resulted in a number of deaths in the 1950s, so we went back to the ten-minute scrub and used various solutions for our arms and hands. Whenever there are postoperative infections, one tends to go back to the longer scrub. It currently is a five-minute scrub.

"AIDS worries people. I recently wrote an editorial suggesting that it was time to give up the use of wire sutures, because they tend to prick through a glove after they are cut off. If you pick up discarded gloves at the end of an operation and blow them up with water, it is suprising how many of them will have a leak. So that is a new problem in operating room technique. Some surgeons are reluctant to operate on people who haven't been tested for AIDS. Actually, there are on record only about three cases of health professionals who have caught AIDS from their work [as of 1987], but presumably there will be more.[1]

"In the experimental work that I did as a resident, the general pattern was to recognize the problem in the hospital while taking care of patients. Then, if there seemed to be a possible surgical solution, we would try it out in the laboratory, usually on dogs. If it seemed to work in the dogs and it appeared safe enough, we would try it out on patients. To give you an example, one of the first problems Dr. Ravdin recognized was the tendency of patients to vomit after they had had a new opening made from the stomach to the upper, small intestine. Those operations were done for ulcers, particularly those ulcers that resulted in scarring of the lower end of the stomach, the pylorus. The patient would come in vomiting, having lost a lot of weight. Surgical openings were made, and instead of the food going out through the opening, the patient would continue to vomit. There were various theories about this. Dr. Ravdin got the idea—partly from his reading, partly from observation—that this was due to the fact that patients developed a nutritional deficiency during the weeks they were vomiting. They didn't have enough protein to keep the water in the body properly adjusted between what was in the circulation and what was in the tissues. Therefore, the tissues swelled up, particularly around the recent operative site so that they shut it off. That's why the patients continued to vomit.

"Dr. Ravdin decided that nutrition would be a good field to devote the efforts of the surgical research laboratory to. He took the problem to the laboratory and adopted a technique that had been developed by Dr. George Whipple at Rochester, New York, for producing hypoproteinemia—low-serum proteins—in dogs. Whipple shared the Nobel Prize with Minot and Murphy for the work on pernicious anemia, but he also did an enormous amount of work on nutrition, specifically on plasma proteins. Ravdin used Whipple's technique to lower the plasma proteins and then operated on the dogs, doing the gastroenter-ostomies. Their stomachs emptied very slowly. Then he did it on some dogs that the surgical class had operated on the previous year, and their stomachs emptied slowly. Then they did it on dogs that hadn't been operated on at all, and it still held true. His team, which included Dr. Paul Mecray and Dr. Robert Barden, showed that the small intestine was slow in transporting the food from the stomach to the large intes-tine if the proteins were low. By putting the dogs back on a good protein diet—by giving them plasma protein—he was able to reverse the condition.

"We utilized this in taking care of patients. If the patients got into this difficulty, we gave them some transfusions and raised their serum pro-teins, and a number of them straightened out. One dramatic one, I remember, was a patient in Florida. A doctor there had a postoperative patient who was vomiting away. He knew Dr. Ravdin and called him. Ravdin told him to transfuse the patient several times with plasma pro-tein. The doctor called back three days later and said the vomiting had stopped. That was a good example of seeing a problem, taking it to the lab, and bringing it back to patients. Later on, we did that with intrave-nous feeding techniques."[2]

HODGKINSON

Surgical Expertise and All the Emotions

SPECIALIZATION HAD NOT occurred to C. Paul Hodgkinson until he saw how it worked at Ford Hospital. After his internship and two years as a general surgery resident, he decided to specialize in gynecological surgery in order to work with Jean Paul Pratt, a brilliant surgeon, clinician, and researcher. Like Rhoads, he pursued an academic degree while completing his residency, writing a thesis on cancer of the cervix.

Here he describes Pratt's innovations and the impact they had on his career. He talks about attitudes toward anesthesia in labor, cesarean sections, treatment of breast disease, the impact of the Pap smear, and the use of diethylstilbestrol (DES) during those years. Although he claims that obstetrics was never as interesting or scientifically challenging to him as were problems and surgical techniques in gynecology, he was the most animated during our interviews when he recalled obstetrical cases and the range of emotions he had seen and experienced while delivering babies. For he expresses a deep involvement with the women who were his obstetrical patients.

"My residency years were very busy years and we worked very hard. We were always under supervision. We assisted the various surgeons in their operations. My experience with Dr. Pratt was the most valuable part of my residency. He was my mentor. He was a stimulating man who taught mainly by example. He had little patience with formal teaching. He always insisted that each resident have a research project. I spent six months in the laboratory trying to perfect a test for the blood determination of adrenaline, and did other general pathology work as well.

"Dr. Pratt was an expert gynecologic surgeon. He had trained under Dr. William Halstead at Johns Hopkins. He was a keen clinician and had excellent technique. He was a good diagnostician. He was an excellent gynecologist and never minded spending long periods of time counseling his many grateful patients.

"Early in his career, Dr. Pratt developed an interest in basic reproductive gynecology, particularly in the field of ovigenesis and reproductive endocrinology. With a couple of other investigators, he devised a program to recover unfertilized human ova. He operated on patients who had to have hysterectomies. He carefully timed the date of the hysterectomy to coincide with the early postovulation period. By then the ova should have escaped from the follicle and gotten into the fallopian tube. When the uterus was removed, a technician flushed the uterus and tubes with saline solution. The flushed fluid was collected in Petri dishes and carefully searched with a microscope for ova. In all, he recovered seven unfertilized human ova in various stages of maturation. He recovered the ova at Ford Hospital. The microscopic work was done by his co-investigators working in Barnes Hospital and Washington University School of Medicine in St. Louis. These techniques laid the groundwork for the subsequent recovery of fertilized ova and, eventually, for in vitro fertilization.

"When I began my residency, we usually used sedation for labor. We used a lot of scopolomine and some barbital; the idea was to obliterate the woman's senses. Those drugs were given by hypodermic needle. Scopolomine made women crazy and wild; they would scream and yell during labor. Scopolomine and atropine given together were known as twilight sleep. It became routine to use them. I knew a doctor who used to meet his patients at the front door when they were coming in to deliver and give them a shot of scopolomine on the way up to registration. That was how hepped people got about that drug. Scopolomine is not a dangerous drug if it is used properly; it is a very good drug. Many patients would go through labor with very little discomfort and have a perfectly normal course, and the baby was fine. A lot of different sedatives were experimented with then. The idea was to make the labor as comfortable as possible and have the patient not recollect any of it. But gradually, people began to see that too much sedation was a bad thing and sometimes babies were born partially anesthetized.

"I remember one incident that really impressed me about drugs and labor. I had a patient who became addicted to Miles Nervine, a patent medicine. It's largely made up of a sedative, potassium bromide. The patient was pregnant, and she had been taking this by the bottle, just tipping it up and drinking it. Her membranes ruptured one day, when she was about seven months pregnant. I delivered this little premature baby. It screamed as soon as it was born, and I was very happy. I thought that the baby was going to be all right. But right after that the baby went to sleep and never woke up. We took a blood bromide level on that patient and on the baby. The baby's bromide level was higher than the mother's. The baby was anesthetized and died.

"Anesthesia has progressed a great deal. There are safer anesthetics now, and the techniques of giving anesthesia to a pregnant woman are better understood. I think that most patients now will accept minimal anesthesia, and I think that is a good thing. The doctor sometimes needs anesthesia to do a good job, and when he needs it, he needs it—for instance, in repairing an episiotomy. Many forceps deliveries can be conducted without anesthesia, but sometimes you have to have anesthesia for that too. I think the biggest danger of anesthesia nowadays is in the cesarean sections. Sometimes women in labor don't progress very fast and gastric juices collect in the stomach instead of passing on into the intestine. After a woman has been in labor eight or ten hours, her stomach may be pretty full of very acidic juices. You have to be very careful that the patient doesn't aspirate those gastric juices; that can be fatal. It takes a very good anesthesiologist sometimes to prevent that. There have been some suits over that. As someone said, 'There is such a thing as a minor operation, but there is no such thing as a minor anesthetic.'

"During my residency, the cesarean rate was way down. It usually was down around 5 percent. The Joint Commission on Accreditation of Hospitals, a governing body sponsored by the American College of Surgeons and several other national organizations, would come around and inspect hospitals. One of the things they would look for was the percentage of cesarean sections. If it got over 5 percent, you had to explain it or risk being discredited. So everybody tried to keep cesarean section rates below 5 percent. Our rate at Ford Hospital was about 3 percent most of the time. Prior to the advent of antibiotics, cesarean section was a relatively serious operation. It carried a death rate, a very substantial one. Doctors balanced one thing against another at that time. They did not want to do a cesarean for fear that the mother would die from the operation.

"Now, of course, it's quite a safe operation. And the cesarean rate is out of hand, 15 to 20 percent sometimes. It is atrociously high. It's up because of malpractice. That is the worst kind of suit, because it is very emotional. If the baby died, or suffered, or was damaged mentally or physically, the lawyer can really make a big show and say, 'If you had done a cesarean section, this would not have happened.' So doctors get scared. If anything goes wrong during labor, they jump to cesarean sections. I think any obstetrician will admit that the cesarean section rate is way too high.

"We didn't do very many prophylactic examinations. Women didn't come in for that. They came because they were sick, something was wrong. We saw patients for various gynecological conditions. We saw cancer of the ovary and various infections. Gonorrhea was common, and we would see an occasional case of syphilis. A lot of people developed intra-abdominal conditions like ovarian cysts or uterine fibroids. Cancer of the cervix was a major problem then. We saw much more of it than we see now. It's not so much of a problem now because of Pap smears. But Pap smears weren't invented during my training. Dr. Papanicolaou came out with his test around 1940.[1] It began to be used at Ford Hospital toward the end of my residency, just before I went into the service in 1942. Most cancers get detected very early now. But then they didn't get detected until it was too late. Women would come in having had a bloody vaginal discharge for a couple of years. It was terrible.

"Radium had been discovered in the 1920s. Ford Hospital started to use radium for the treatment of cancer of the cervix in the early 1920s. They had no guidelines, and they did a lot of damage. People were burned because of too much radium. During my residency, the standard treatment for cancer of the cervix was insertion of radium capsules. They came in various shapes and sizes. After we removed them, we would give a short course of X-ray treatment. Later, we would usually operate on the patient to remove the uterus. The results were fairly good compared to earlier treatments, but they weren't good compared with improvements later on.

"The idea of routine physical examinations for women didn't develop until after the Pap smear was invented. It took about ten years before people began to see that prophylactic examinations and the Pap smear were a good thing. It was a long time before Pap smears were finally accepted by women and by doctors.[2] There was a lot of trouble because some people didn't know how to read them. You got false-positive and some false-negative tests. I can remember many times taking Pap smears right off a very obvious cancer, and the laboratory reported back negative. When the war came along, there was a lot of neglect of Pap smears, simply because there wasn't enough manpower. I think Pap smears generally got tossed along the wayside until after the war. Then people began to get interested.

"One of my special interests was breast surgery and examination of the breast. No doctor has the opportunity to do prophylactic breast management like a gynecologist. When I first started, many gynecologists didn't want to bother with the breasts, and the reason was purely mercenary: the hospital rules didn't permit them to operate. Their thinking was along the lines of, 'Why should I examine someone's breasts if I can't do anything about it? If a woman has a problem with the breasts, she should see a general surgeon to start with.' Of course, in the early years, no doctors were examining the breasts.

"Dr. Pratt was a general surgeon before he took over the Department of Obstetrics and Gynecology. He had to go take a special course in obstetrics in order to be head of the department. In giving up his general surgery, he extracted the promise from the head of the surgical department that his service would include breast diseases. So my experience with breast cancers is probably unique. I was trained in breast cancer work, and I always had an interest in trying to detect breast cancer early. In those years women didn't like to have their breasts examined, and doctors didn't want to bother with it. It has taken a lot of medical publicity to get gynecologists particularly to examine breasts. Now they all are doing it. Yet very few gynecologists do breast surgery, even today. I was doing it early because of Dr. Pratt. I liked to do breast surgery and I did a lot of it. I'd try to get other people to do it, but they didn't want to bother with it.

"In my early years with breast cancer the standard treatment, regardless of the stage of the disease, was the Halstead radical mastectomy. That involved the removal of the breast, removal of the large pectoral muscle, the pectoralis minor, which is the smaller muscle underneath, and then cleaning out all of the lymph nodes along this chain. It was a formidable procedure. I was in practice forty-seven years, and the Halstead radical mastectomy was the standard treatment for about the first thirty of those years. Not enough time has gone by to evaluate other treatments. Breast cancer is a very, very peculiar disease. It does funny things. Most cancer statistics are based on a five-year cure; that is not enough for breast cancer. Twenty-one years after I did a radical mastectomy on a patient, she developed a recurrence. She got along fine until then. Five years is not enough.

"I don't think the incidence of breast cancer has changed very much over the years. It is a very common disease. In the old days, I would see patients whose breast cancers were inoperable. Those patients would come in with great big ulcers on their chest wall from cancer that had been there for ten years maybe. There is nothing you can do for a patient like that; it has already spread too far.

"During my residency years, drug salesmen would come around and talk about this and that new drug. They wanted to have clinical studies done: they would provide the drug, and the doctor would give it to the patient. The patient would report back, and the doctor would determine whether the drug was any good. Of course, this isn't done now. But sometime around 1940, a salesman came around and got Dr. Pratt to do a clinical study on diethylstilbestrol [DES], one of the first synthetic estrogens ever discovered.[3] Dr. Pratt was well-noted nationally as one of the first gynecologic endocrinologists. He also had a keen interest in psychosomatic gynecology. He decided to run a study to see whether or not DES prevented hot flashes in menopausal women. He devised a double blind study. The 'blind' drugs for the study were 0.5 grain pheno-barbital [the placebo], 0.1 milligram DES, and 1 milligram DES. The greatest relief in hot flashes was in those patients given 1 milligram DES. But patients who received the phenobarbital and 0.1 milligram DES had some relief also, and Dr. Pratt concluded that much of the benefit from the drugs was psychosomatic.[4] In those days of relatively low-potency drugs, Dr. Pratt found it difficult to believe that 0.1 milligram of any drug could produce positive pharmacologic effects. We only used it for menopausal patients.

"About that same time, a doctor in Boston came out with a very detailed paper showing that, if you gave DES in large doses in pregnancy, it caused an increase in secretion of the corpus luteum, or progesterone, and that prevented spontaneous abortion. That paper was quite uniformly accepted, and patients who had diabetes mellitus or any patient who had a threat of miscarriage began to be given huge doses of DES, sometimes as high as 40 milligrams a day. I never accepted this DES theory, and I never gave DES to my pregnant patients. I just never thought it prevented miscarriages.[5] DES was given for years. Then papers began to be published showing that DES was of no value in the prevention of miscarriages. In the meantime, thousands of mothers had received this drug. In Boston they began to see some carcinoma of the vagina in young girls. It was found that most of their mothers had been given DES. DES was causing cancer of the vagina in those young girls. There was no way of predicting this. By that time, the drug was stopped. I'm glad I never used it, because I received a lot of letters when this became publicized. I got letters from mothers asking me if they had ever received this drug.

"After my residency, I drove to Atlantic City to take my American Board Examinations in Obstetrics and Gynecology. When I got back to Ford Hospital, there were two letters of importance. One was from the American Board that I had passed my exams. The other was from the draft; I had to go into the service."

ROMANO

"Brain Spot or Mind Twist"— Attempts to Understand Psychosis

JOHN ROMANO observed and worked alongside the chronically mentally ill and the destitute from the time he was earning his own way through Marquette University and School of Medicine in Milwaukee. When he tells the story of his early training years, he recalls the jobs he held along the way in much greater detail than his formal educational experiences. For those jobs provided him great exposure to the range of human problems.

Hodgkinson's total of six years in residency training and Rhoads's five years of training at the University of Pennsylvania are the longest among these doctors. All seven doctors' residencies are in contrast with Romano's in psychiatry, his being the least well-delineated during that period. He was at three institutions. He had a year at Yale followed by three years as a Commonwealth fellow in psychiatry at the University of Colorado School of Medicine (1935–1938). Wanting further training, he spent an additional year on a Rockefeller Fellowship in neurology at Boston City Hospital affiliated with Harvard. With relatively few methods of actually measuring accomplishments in neurology and psychiatry training during the 1930s, Romano was, relative to the others, left to his own devices.

When he describes his psychiatric training, what stands out are specific patients, the cases he observed, attempted to treat, and struggled to understand. Through his care of individual patients, Romano constructed research problems and carried out some research projects. He had a strong desire to explore biological dimensions of psychosis, but there was no precedent for that kind of work in psychiatry. No one around him at Yale or Colorado was conducting psychiatric research. Neurological research, however, was making great strides, and at Harvard Romano was able to work with two of the greatest neurologists of the time.[1]

"At Yale, I became interested in a young patient who was going to a school in Farmington, the most prestigious private school for girls in

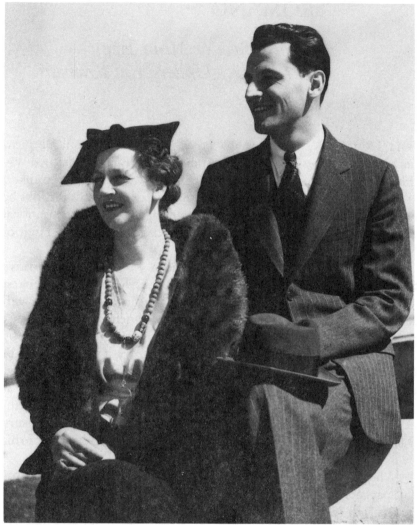

Dr. and Mrs. John Romano during his Commonwealth Fund Fellowship at Colorado Psychopathic Hospital, 1935.

America. Shortly before her menstrual period, this girl became psychotic, excited, assaultive, obscene, restless. Then, as soon as her menstrual flow started, she became calm. So we hospitalized her, and as soon as her menstrual flow came she went back to school. Then four or five days before her next period we hospitalized her again. I realized that there was something very interesting here. I thought it had to do with estrogenic hormones or gonadotropic hormones. I persuaded the professor of anatomy at Yale to undertake some studies of this patient, which were never completed.

"Another patient was a young woman who had grown up in Tibet; her parents were missionaries. The psychiatric staff thought she was a deteriorating schizophrenic. I didn't think so; I was so naive. At the case conference I was the only one who thought she had any hope of recovery. I worked with her and she got better. Thirty-five or forty years later she came to see me in Rochester. She had gone into psychology because of her interest in me, she said. She was married and had children. There was something peculiar about her, maybe schizoidlike about her. Still, she had lived a good life. No social deterioration. I was pleased to learn of her life course.

"There was another patient, an elderly woman who had taught school in the New Haven area for years and years. Late in life she married, and on her honeymoon she became psychotic, with a cyclic type of mania. In the evenings she was well enough to go out. At midnight, like Cinderella, she had to be back in the hospital, where she took all her clothes off, became manic, excited, jumping and yelling until maybe 11:00 the next morning. Then she would quiet down and have breakfast. At 4:00 P.M., she became calmer. And this cycle would happen every day. I thought this was amazing. I tried to study her and I tried to get help, and I did some studies on cyclic mania later in Colorado. I never published them. I also studied twenty-four-hour urine samples from manic women. Of all the difficult things I've done in my life, to get a twenty-four-hour urine sample from a manic woman is really something! I studied the women and kept a protocol of their behavior over a certain period of time.

"I could have stayed at Yale, but then the Commonwealth Fund asked if I could come to Colorado the next year. I was in Colorado for three years. In Colorado I continued that research. I met Reuben Gustavson, who was then professor of chemistry at Denver University. I went to him and said, 'I can get the urines of a number of women in mania. Would you be interested in working with me doing rat studies on the extracts in their urine, assaying estrogenic and other sex hormones?' He said yes. So we worked together for a long, long time, but we never published the data. I didn't publish a number of things I probably should have way, way back.

"We showed that in the premenstrual period there were certain hormonal changes in the manic woman that were different from such changes in normal women. I was interested in finding out if the change in motor acceleration, the restless mind, restless body, had something to do with some of those hormonal changes. That was my question. I never really answered it to my satisfaction. The data were never completely analyzed. We had some trouble because somebody made an error in labeling the urine samples. We were so disappointed with the labeling thing, we almost killed the person who made the mistake. I guess it was an honest mistake on his part. So we never really came through with the data.

"Unlike the others with whom I worked in the psychiatric group at Yale and at Colorado, I believe I was the only one doing what passed off as research. It wasn't very good research. I was really interested in asking questions, really interested in trying to systematize what I saw and to reach some general conclusions about it. There weren't many mentors. There weren't many researchers in the field of psychiatry. I wish I had had a mentor. I was naive and unlearned. I didn't have any preparation in statistics. I didn't know epidemiology. I didn't know sampling. I didn't have anybody to guide me as to method and discipline. I learned it from the seat of my pants. I began to write some papers. I did some studies on alcoholic neuritis. I studied a man with hemophilia, with a delirium. I wrote some case histories.[2] During that period I became interested in the Rorschach and also interested in psychoanalysis.

"Today a young man or woman has a much better time. There are more role models. In America from the 1920s to the 1950s, psychiatry didn't have any Rockefeller Institute to groom young professors as there was in medicine, physiology, pediatrics. We had to wait years to have the National Institute of Mental Health. University departments [of psychiatry] were very small and not very prominent. In Europe they were quite prominent because of national subsidies. The psychopathic hospitals of Europe were university hospitals, a hundred beds or less, with a professor as director. While they gave service, their primary thing was research. We didn't have that for a long time here. We still don't in many places.

"In Colorado, I used to run the neurosyphilis clinic. Patients would receive arsenicals, Tryparsamide and other arsenicals. There was also fever treatment. It all changed later with penicillin. A major psychosis was eliminated by biochemical means.

"I took it upon myself to do various things that patients experienced.

I sat in the continuous tub for two hours. You lay in a hammock in a tub and there was a flow of water at body temperature, 98 degrees Fahrenheit. It was sedative. You could use this tub for a couple of hours to get old people to sleep and rest and stop their excitement. That way, you wouldn't have to give them more drugs and cause more delirium. I went into a cold wet pack. Then I had the Scotch douche, a spray of water about ten feet away. It's very sharp on you. It's supposed to be stimulating. In those days, hydrotherapy was still used. I did all those things to learn something of what patients experienced.

"To try to quiet disturbed patients who often were suicidal or homicidal, all we had were bromides, barbiturates, chloral hydrate, and paraldehyde. I had a patient named Roberta. She was a very attractive schizophrenic girl who used to write long essays to me. Fantastic imagination. When I was younger and thinner I looked more like the devil. One day she said, 'There he is, the devil.' I used to make 9:00 P.M. rounds. She threw a cannister of hot cocoa at me, and it burned me a little bit. Then she came over to see how I was. There were people in acute terror, acute furors, acute rages. Sometimes with syphilis a paretic would have a sudden unpredictable rage reaction, tear a chair apart, take the legs off the chair and strike people with them. So there were hazards at that time. It still can happen, but I think it happens less now because of modern psychotropic medication.

"We had techniques to protect ourselves, for example, a single bed or cot mattress. We had some straps put in the middle so we could use it as a shield in approaching a disturbed patient. I helped design one. You put your hand through the middle of it, because otherwise, with the handle on the ends, you can't use your hands. We could use one hand to placate somebody on the other side.

"One time in Colorado a man came in with a gun and brandished it at me, a paranoid patient. I was very scared, and I sat there and kept on talking with him. He wasn't my patient, but I knew him. I kept talking to him and finally he put the gun down on the desk. I said, 'Would you give me the gun?' And he gave it to me. I was really scared to death; I thought I was going to be killed. Those are things that happen.

"During that same period, there were many conjectures about schizophrenia. Henri Claude, a Frenchman, thought schizophrenia was a variant form of tuberculosis, because schizophrenics were highly tubercular, probably because of their long institutional care. Many schizophrenic patients didn't live long because of the tuberculosis. In 1913, Hideyo

Noguchi and J. W. Moore had found a spirochete in the brain of syphilit-
ics. So they thought, 'Aha! All madness is due to organic disease. We'll
look for the bacteria.'

"With the advent of psychoanalysis in the 1920s came a wave of
'psychologicalness': To what degree is aberrant behavior due to hidden
infections, genetic factors, constitutional factors, environmental factors,
life experience? Ernest Southard, one of Karl Menninger's teachers at
Harvard, used a very good metaphor to describe this thinking of the
time: 'brain spot or mind twist.' Either something [bacteria] is up there
doing all these bad things, or it is due to life experience from childhood
on. Throughout my professional life the debate has continued: Is it
nature or nurture?

"They asked me to stay at Colorado on the faculty following my
fellowship. But I applied and was selected for a Rockefeller Fellowship
in neurology, as I wanted further training. I went to Harvard in 1938. I
was at the Boston City Hospital. I could do as I saw fit. I spent a lot of
time there and learned a lot about neurology. I saw many patients and
read a lot. Boston City Hospital was like the Arabian Nights. Fantastic
place. Everything unexpected in the world happened there daily. It was a
treasure house of medicine. I remember a man who had some injury to
his cervical spine. After discharge as a patient, he lived in the hospital, in
some nook or cranny in the basement. And he went on rounds with the
medical students. Boston City Hospital was full of people like that; they
just lived in catacombs through the whole place and stole food, or were
given food and money by the house staff.

"William F. Orr was the chief resident in neurology. He was from
Nashville, Tennessee, from Vanderbilt. I worked with him. I used to see
ten or twelve patients a day. Most of them were psychiatric but not
diagnosed as such, because in those days the prefix 'psyche' was more
forbidden at the City Hospital than I found it to be in Moscow some
years later. It was called the nerve service. Later they called it psychiatric.
Ward One was the alcoholic drying-out place. Half of the patient problems I saw were psychiatric problems: acute psychosis, delirium, and
panic and hysterical behavior.

"Tracy Jackson Putnam and Houston Merritt were at the Boston
City Hospital. Putnam was a Boston Brahmin. He was related to everyone. He was soft-spoken and very aristocratic. He was a professor of
neurology at Harvard, head of the Department of Neurology. Putnam
did all kinds of venturesome, radical, imaginative neurosurgery. Cut-

ting the cervical cord at a certain area to relieve unilateral dystonia, unilateral disturbance of movements. He did many of those things at that time. He was a very fine man, a great scholar, and an outstanding clinical investigator.

"The person who most influenced me there was Houston Merritt, Putnam's associate. Houston Merritt was more of a Sancho Panza to Tracy Putnam's Don Quixote. Merritt was from North Carolina. He was probably the greatest neurologist of this century. A very good diagnostician. I used to make rounds with him. When I went to the Peter Bent Brigham Hospital to be a neurologist and psychiatrist after my year at Boston City Hospital, Merritt used to come over every Tuesday at 5:00 P.M. and see eight or nine patients with us as a senior teacher. We would make rounds with the Harvard students.

"In 1938 Putnam and Merritt reported their studies of anticonvulsant drugs, which led to Dilantin, and I worked in that first clinic.[3] They used a system of creating electric convulsions in cats and then used drugs to find out which drug would diminish the convulsion. That was the method used. Merritt was pilloried in Boston by the antivivisectionists, who had pictures of him and the cats in their storefront lobby on Park Square.

"I also spent four weeks one summer modeling the human brain, in a course of anatomy and physiology at Harvard. I spent every day working on this project, four times actual size with spaghetti wires and plasticine. I learned the nervous system by this reconstruction. I brought the model home on the streetcar; I didn't have a car. We used to call it the Huntington Avenue Chorea streetcar, because by the time you got off, you were shaking like a chorea patient. The brain model, about ten inches high, sat on a wooden platform. The several colors of plasticine and the wires emerging from the base were quite striking. There was a drunk sitting opposite me on the streetcar. He kept looking at it, and he just couldn't make it out. Finally he said, 'I can't stand this anymore, what is that?' I said, 'This is a human brain.' He got off at the next stop. That year in neurology was a very good year.

"I was certified in both psychiatry and neurology in 1940."

BECOMING AGENTS
OF CHANGE

MENTORS AND THE VISION OF
CLINICAL MEDICINE

"Genius," "charisma," "inspiration," "intellect," "dedication." These are the words used to describe the characteristics of these doctors' mentors: Soma Weiss for Beeson, Francis Scott Smyth for Olney, I. S. Ravdin for Rhoads, and Jean Paul Pratt for Hodgkinson. All professors and department chairmen at the time of these doctors' residencies, the mentors exhibited an extraordinary ability, energy, expertise, and dedication in their work. They were on the leading edge of their fields, engaging in pathbreaking research and clinical activities that were revered and emulated by many others. *Their vision of medicine's possibilities as a clinical science* and their enactment of that vision through their day-to-day work left a lasting impression on these doctors. Beeson and Rhoads, especially, speak of their mentors with great admiration. They portray Weiss and Ravdin, respectively, as having been generous with young people by giving them responsibilities and by putting them in important, high-visibility positions to advance their careers. The mentors had high expectations for their trainees, and they apparently were never disappointed in them. Romano, alone in this group, talks about the need for and lack of a mentor during the Yale and Colorado period. He feels that he floundered while he sought information and guidance. He recalls that he wanted an inspirational figure during that period in his life, a personal guide to the conduct of research and a key to unlocking the direction of his career.

The mentors significantly influenced the goals of the others. Through Weiss's encouragement and model, Beeson decided to build a career in academic medicine. Weiss's way of being a doctor and teacher—listening carefully to patients, families, and staff, paying close attention to variations in pathology and to the diagnostic process, giving young people a chance to perform and succeed—were emulated later on

142

by Beeson. Rhoads's relationship with a mentor was the most prolonged and intimate among this group. Ravdin involved him in research that he was to build on for the rest of his career. Hodgkinson, too, was deeply influenced by the surgical skill and innovative research projects of his mentor. Though he did not pursue the same areas of research, the desire to do work that had direct clinical applications was nurtured by Pratt. Both Ravdin and Pratt insisted that their residents conduct research, thus setting the stage for Rhoads's and Hodgkinson's careers of laboratory and clinical research combined with surgery.

Olney's career was shaped by her mentor Francis Scott Smyth's holistic approach to the child: any problem that affected the child's optimal development was the physician's responsibility. Allergies, dyslexia, behavioral disorders with a psychological cause, the need for summer camp—all were problems that would benefit by a pediatrician's intervention. Smyth viewed the child as a developing organism, not as a miniature adult, whose fulfilled potential depended on the growth and health of all its parts, psychological, somatic, emotional, social. Smyth was no doubt influenced by the groundbreaking work in normal child development carried out in his era by Arnold Gesell.[1] Olney put Smyth's legacy into immediate and lifelong practice in treatments fostering the broadest possible physical, psychological, and social well-being of children in spite of their diseases and problems. Beeson, Olney, Rhoads, and Hodgkinson each absorbed and internalized the personal virtues, dedication, and achievements of their mentors to become, in some sense, like them. Then they placed their own imprint on the mentor's legacy to give direction to their specialty in the years ahead.

SCIENTIST CAREGIVERS

These narratives are examples of development within the specialties during the 1930s. The Rockefeller Institute was the leading medical research institution in the country when Beeson worked there, and it was the model for the conduct of medical research well into the twentieth century. Activity at the Rockefeller Institute was based on the premise that the diagnosis and treatment of disease in patients would be combined with the study of diseases in the laboratory, an innovative idea at the time it was implemented. The hospital of the Rockefeller Institute had opened in 1910, and from that time on, its integrated laboratory research and patient treatment services provided the example for clinical investigation in academic medical school departments. Residents were hired to conduct independent research in addition to their responsibilities in the treatment of patients.

The first immune serum against one type of pneumococcus was developed by Rufus I. Cole, the first director of the hospital of the Rockefeller Institute, and his associates, in 1912. Oswald T. Avery joined the Rockefeller staff to conduct research on pneumonia in 1913. Over the next decade or so, Avery and his colleagues isolated and extracted the chemical substances in the pneumococcal polysaccharide and determined their immunological specificity for four types of pneumococci. Their contributions are considered the basis of contemporary immunochemistry, and their work was one of the early demonstrations of the importance of clinical investigation for basic biological science.[2] In 1932, a method was perfected for rapid typing of the pneumococcus.[3] The understanding of lobar pneumonia and the development and use of type-specific antiserum begun by Cole and carried forward by Avery and his group have been called by one medical historian "one of the most elegant performances, from the standpoint of both theory and technique, in the history of medical science."[4]

Beeson's work at the Rockefeller Institute carried that research forward. He played a part in a very important moment in the history of clinical investigation.[5] That bacteriological research was made obsolete a few years later with the advent of the sulfonamides and penicillin, both of which proved to be effective against all types of pneumococcus, thus doing away with the need for specific antiserums.

The links between research and care had begun to be appreciated throughout the medical world only in the 1920s. Aside from a few isolated pathbreakers in the generation before them, Beeson and Rhoads were among the first cohort of physicians who were able to see the direct results of their laboratory experiments and procedures in patient recovery rates. Experimental laboratory research and treatment approaches at the bedside had become integrated activities; the first fueled the second.

Yet there was no biological psychiatry. Compared with Rhoads's training—learning to recognize a problem in patient care, conducting experiments on animals to create and then rectify the problem and finally, taking the solution back to patients—Romano's independent forays into research during his fellowship years seem naive and highly unsystematic. His experience reflected the fact that psychiatry simply was not a scientifically based field of medicine at the time. And there was no precedent in 1934–1938 for conducting psychiatric research, especially biologically grounded psychiatric research, in the United States. At the bedside, Romano saw the psychiatric outcomes of infectious disease, especially neurosyphilis and deliriums. He also saw cases of bizarre psychoses and manias. Diagnosis and treatment were his challenges. For infectious diseases, he used the standard treatments then available. But disease processes of psychiatric disorders per se were not understood. Treatment was implemented on a case-by-case basis and often consisted only of hospitalization and bedrest. Psychiatry was not yet exploding with new drugs that could revolutionize the treatment of mental illness. Those treatments, in the form of the major tranquilizers, would not arrive until the 1950s. Psychoanalysis had arrived from Europe, but it could not cure psychosis, and, from the beginning, it had a highly specialized clientele of both practitioners and patients. Psychiatry as a whole was not driven by experimental laboratory research that had a clinical impact.

Pediatrics, on the other hand, benefited from the discoveries made in medical research. The use of the sulphonamides fundamentally changed the treatment of many diseases affecting children during Olney's residency years. She was standing at a crossroads, watching treatments she had learned to give in medical school become obsolete when the antibiotics arrived. The old problems and old treatments that Olney describes declined or vanished completely during the 1930s, causing the pediatrician's activities to change dramatically.

Disease prevention had been instituted as a goal of pediatrics by the 1930s, the only specialty that identified prevention as part of its training agenda.[6] Though they had been taking their children to the pediatrician for routine checkups, adults did not view prevention for themselves as part of medical care. Hodgkinson mentions that women did not come to gynecologists (or to any doctors for that matter) for routine examinations prior to the Second World War. His own early interest in prophylactic medicine both extended the doctor's role and predated the postwar cultural trend.

The career tracks that they all chose, but that Beeson, Rhoads, Hodgkinson, and Romano emphasize—combining clinical and/or laboratory research with patient care, publication, and teaching in the academic setting—were extremely uncommon through the 1920s in

American medicine. The subordination of private practice to teaching and investigative work within an academic institution was still very much a minority career path during the 1930s, and it was to become the elite of medicine. Individuals who were able to create the links between investigation, teaching, and treatment by combining all three activities in one career were acting as agents of change within their specialties and were contributing to medicine's transformation.

PART III

Generalists, Scientists, and Curers: 1930s and 1940s

By the 1940s virtually everyone had heard of miracle drugs and many people knew they owed their lives to them.

—*John C. Burnham,*
"American Medicine's Golden Age: What
Happened to It?"

CURING AND OTHER TRENDS

MEDICINE'S IDENTITY further evolved during the 1940s, when physicians began to be able to cure diseases *routinely*. This feature of medicine's transformation occurred while these seven doctors were completing their formal training and embarking on their careers as practitioners and researchers, and as teachers and mentors of younger physicians and students.

This section begins with the first jobs these doctors held following their internships or residencies and includes their experiences through the Second World War. It describes clinical practice, research, teaching, and career decisions made during the late 1930s through the 1940s, the influence of war work on professional development, and discussions about the doctor-patient relationship, including the ethics of experimenting on patients. The moral confusion created by contemporary medical knowledge and practices begins to have visible roots in the forms and values of medicine described in the following sections of the narratives.

Though their broad specialties had been chosen, the physicians developed particular clinical and/or research interests during these years. They made decisions about which jobs afforded them the greatest opportunities for continued growth, challenge, and economic stability. They also faced decisions about emphasis: how much time to devote to private, university-, or hospital-based practice, clinical and laboratory research, teaching, and community service. Shields and Jarcho, who did not have formal residency training, both chose to remain in the community as practicing internists; Jarcho continued to teach as well. Beeson wanted a wide range of clinical and research experience. Hodgkinson and Rhoads both continued with research in order to solve problems in surgery and patient care. Olney chose to combine a half-time private practice with a university career of teaching and working in the clinics. Research she conducted was secondary to both those tasks. Romano's interest in teaching medical students began during this period. He started to integrate psychiatric and psychological concepts with the rest of the medical curriculum, pushing teaching to the forefront of his work. Both Olney and Romano took their specialties out of the clinic and into the community during this period. In order to promote the self-esteem and overall adjustment of diabetic youths, Olney started a summer camp. To ease psychological burdens created by the Second World War, Romano applied principles of psychiatry and psychology to problems encountered by local welfare organizations and community agencies.

At least four trends in medicine's development during the 1940s are important to these doctors' careers and narratives. First, specialization increased dramatically. The number of full-time specialists increased from thirty-seven thousand in 1940 to over sixty-two thousand in 1949.[1] Medicine was on its way to becoming a profession of specialists. Indeed, Olney remembers older general practitioners who returned from the Second World War and committed suicide, so distraught were they by the pressure to specialize and seek advanced training and by the necessity of mastering more and more scientific information.

Second, for the first time in history, medicine totally embraced science when thousands of scientists, doctors, and technicians confronted the medical problems created by the war. The Second World War gave scientific research in general and medical research in particular a high national priority and wide public recognition.[2] The federal government began its multimillion dollar support of scientific medicine, pouring money into laboratory and clinical research in the effort to solve a multitude of combat, injury, technical, and survival problems faced by the armed forces. Physicians such as Beeson, Rhoads, and Romano, who worked in university settings, became involved in various war-related research enterprises. For some doctors, this led to a career-long interest in a specific topic (Rhoads). For others, this research contributed to growing professional and scholarly reputations and set the stage for additional research in a variety of fields (Jarcho, Hodgkinson, Beeson, Romano).

Third, during the 1940s the hospital was fully established as the center of the medical world.[3] Fourth, with some regularity, doctors began to cure diseases. Sulfanilamide was found to kill bacteria in humans in 1935. Along with the related sulfa drugs, it began to be used from 1936 to treat a variety of streptococcal infections, peritonitis, mastoid infections, and some forms of pneumonia and meningitis.[4] In 1942 penicillin became available for military use. In 1945 it began to be produced in large quantities for civilian use. More widely effective than the sulfa drugs and less toxic, penicillin began the "new era" of medicine: large numbers of infectious diseases were now routinely curable.[5]

SHIELDS

"Any Kind of Work"

SHIELDS FONDLY recalls his training at Tulane University School of Medicine in New Orleans and his internship at St. Luke's Hospital in New York. What stands out for him was the impotence of medicine during that period. It was "an era of very little light." Yet he struggled to save lives and had enormous faith in the possibilities of medical research.

Here, in describing his early years of private practice in Concord, New Hampshire, Shields continues the theme of medicine's powerlessness in the prewar period. Concord was a small town when he arrived there in 1933. He did not have formal residency training, but he was determined to become a specialist in internal medicine. The most valuable thing he learned, he recalls, was to sit down and listen to the patient, for that simple act embodies the time-honored values of medicine—"to comfort and console always." Its importance runs through his narrative. He shudders with embarrassment, but laughs as well, at the memory of his jack-of-all-trades practice. From dental anesthesias to psychoanalysis, he did everything, except deliver babies.

Shields is the only physician in this group to have seen combat during the Second World War. The war interrupted his career but added to his medical experience. He served as a physician in the navy and treated the wounded in two of the bloodiest battles of the Pacific—Iwo Jima and Okinawa.

"After a couple more months at St. Luke's, I had to go to work. I put out some feelers and found out about a doctor in Concord, New Hampshire, who wanted to have somebody join his practice. I was interested. Don McIvor was a Scotchman, born and raised on the Canadian border at Swanton, Vermont. He came down to Concord to be connected to the state mental institution. He came down as a general practitioner, not as a psychiatrist. He was doing general practice completely. He had no special training in anything. He was very successful in spite of the fact that most of the doctors here said he would starve to death. He gradually

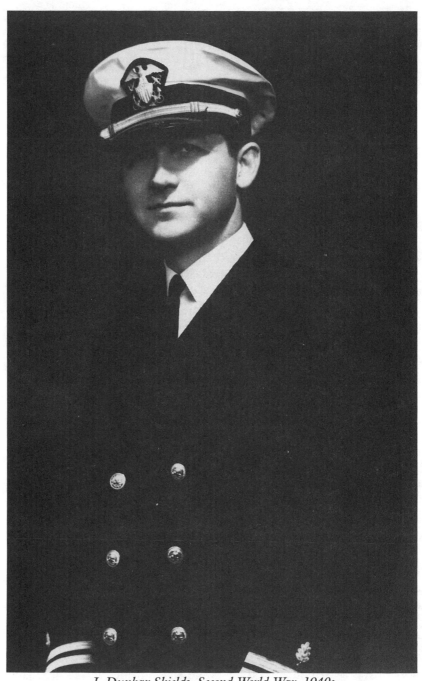

J. Dunbar Shields, Second World War, 1940s.

worked into surgery. In those days, people could teach themselves surgery to some degree. He did it by assisting others. He began to do minimal things—appendectomies and hernia repairs. Then he began to go to meetings and find out how to do surgery. He got to be good. He wanted to drop medicine and just do surgery. And he wanted somebody to come in and take over the medical part of his practice.

"Don McIvor and his wife came down to New York to meet me. I liked them both tremendously, particularly his wife. He would pay me a terrific salary of $250 a month. That sounded good to me. I decided to come to Concord, I thought for perhaps six months to a year. I wanted to make enough money to go back to the South and practice.

"I came to Concord in September 1933. Dr. McIvor was about forty at the time I joined him. We hit it off beautifully. He was a remarkable guy. What he did in surgery was remarkable. He loved people, although if he disliked you, he'd probably throw you out. He had very little patience with people he didn't like. He could be a gruff and abrupt individual, but not with his patients. Underneath he had a tremendous amount of compassion. His patients were extremely loyal to him. I learned how to listen from him. I went on house calls with him when I wanted to know what was going on. He would come into the room. Instead of being restless, or standing up, or breaking into a conversation by asking questions right away, or being tense and nervous, he would always sit down. He would sit down and look as if he had all the time in the world. The patients immediately felt comfortable, and they immediately talked to him.

"I was so pleased after the first year because things were going so well. I went back to Mississippi and got married the following June, 1934, and brought my wife back up here. I did not remain in the South, because I wanted to do internal medicine exclusively. In the South they didn't know what an internist was. I wanted to be the best internist in the state.

"Instead of exploiting me as people were doing so much in those days, Dr. McIvor paid me for a year and a half, and then called me in and said, 'I just went over the books and last month you made money for me. I can't have that. You start on your own now, and you make your own money.' That's the way I started out. I remained with Dr. McIvor until he retired, a total of more than twenty years. He retired at about sixty-five, when he began to have coronary disease. He was marvelous during the time I was gone during the war. He even did some of my work for me.

"During those early years, I was doing everything except obstetrics. I did pediatrics. I was seeing the ordinary garden variety of things—sore throats, bellyaches, and so forth. With children, I saw the usual child-hood infectious diseases. The most dramatic thing I saw perhaps was pneumonia. I was also assisting Dr. McIvor in surgery. And that stood me in very good stead later during the war. I helped him a lot with orthopedics cases. I'd take the X–rays and help him put on the casts, but I did not set the fractures. So I was doing every kind of medicine. I was doing general practice out of financial necessity.

"To really see the full picture, we have to take economics into account again. I think there were about twenty doctors in Concord when I first arrived; we had fifty-five new ones come in last year [1989]. Although we didn't have many doctors, there seemed to be very little work, and we competed for it. When I got a house call, I wondered whether I could get there before another doctor did. Sometimes I would find two or three doctors already there when I arrived. That wasn't a bit unusual.

"We did any kind of work we could possibly do. I assisted in surgery because that was good money. I did insurance exams. I examined for so many companies—about eighteen of them. I used to do dental anesthe-sias; the thought of that makes me shiver today. I would use up a certain amount of gas and oxygen, and I would get five dollars. I had a gadget with two tanks, two great big tanks, one oxygen and one nitrous oxide. Then I had an anesthesia machine, a gadget that I put over the patient's nose with two pipes that came behind. There was also an ether attach-ment, because we couldn't get them to sleep enough on nitrous oxide, so we added ether. I used to carry all this up a flight of stairs to the dentist's office, or it was also done in people's homes. I would put them to sleep. I had a gadget that would make their mouths stay open. Then I'd take a big wad of cotton and stick it in the back of their throats so they would breathe through their noses. Often, the dentist would have his fist in the person's mouth, so I couldn't keep a decent airway. And now, airway is everything. How I didn't kill a whole bunch of people, I don't know. I came awfully close a couple times. One time I had to give a patient artificial respiration and jump in the ambulance with him and get him to the hospital. It is just horrible to think about.

"Some of those dentists were very unskillful, and most of the work was extractions. They didn't try to save teeth much then; they just yanked them out. I remember once going to a home, and this very nice old lady was having her teeth out. In that particular case, the dentist was having a hard time. He had both hands on the forceps—going back and forth, trying to get the tooth out, and shaking and shaking the forceps. Finally, it came out. He held up his forceps and he had the tooth, but a big piece of mandible as well.

"In the early days in Concord we had undulant fever. It was caused by a bacteria that was carried in milk. This was a dairy area, and cattle had the disease; it produced abortion in cattle. People got the disease from drinking raw milk. It was difficult to diagnose unless you thought of it. There was a test we could use to diagnose it. But it was very difficult to treat; there was no drug that helped. It lasted for months and months. People would have the symptoms of a low-grade fever and just feel lousy and mean and have generalized aches and pains. It was difficult to distinguish it from psychosomatic problems. When we were able to diagnose it and told the person, it made their distress a lot easier to handle. It was a disease which was peculiar to that era. With pasteurization, it was eliminated.

"I made one great mistake early on in medicine because I was interested in psychosomatic medicine. I had had some psychiatric training, but psychiatry then was mainly labeling. I dabbled in psychiatry, really. It was an era of psychoanalysis. Many people were being analyzed. The analyst of course had to be analyzed. It was a fascinating facet of medicine at the time. I read enough about it to feel that I wanted to help people, because their pains were real. There were no medications that helped them. I thought I could listen to people and explain to them how their psyche was disturbing them and why they were ill. And I would spend time with them. That was at the time when I didn't have a lot of patients. I fell into the trap of getting too deep into analyzing them and not being skillful enough to handle it. I got in trouble, because there was some transference. That was very bad, very embarrassing, and very difficult. I took care of a few women who tried to pull me in bed with them.

"I can remember one of the first cases that shocked me. She was an extremely beautiful woman. She had psychosomatic illnesses. She came to see me in the office several times, and things got a little sticky. One day I made a house call because she was supposedly quite ill. I was leaning over to examine her, and she just grabbed me by the neck and pulled me down in the bed. That was not common, but it did occur and I had to stop that foolishness. I had to keep from getting too deep in the situation. The doctor becomes not only the father but also the lover if he doesn't watch out.

"That was before the era of the tranquilizers and, more particularly, the mood elevators. We couldn't treat depression. The patient might be suicidal, and we could get into real danger there. We did have psychiatrists, of course. And when we got in too deep we tried to get the patient to go to the psychiatrist. But often, they didn't want to go to a psychiatrist. They were frightened by the term 'psychiatrist.' That was a tough part of medicine, it really was—treating both the psychosomatic problems and the real psychotics that we didn't recognize as psychotic.

"Eighty percent of the medicine I did was treating people who were not actually organically ill. Those are by far the hardest people to take care of. Later on, the fact that we got drugs that we could use was very helpful and made us see things a little differently. And I think we learned more about psychosomatic illness. But over the years, I don't think the basic psychosomatic problems have changed, or their causes.

"Dr. McIvor wanted our office to be able to do most of the work so we wouldn't have to send patients to the hospital or out of the office for lab work. He had an X-ray machine. I did a lot of lab work and I did radiology as well. I was glad I had taken a little extra radiology. I was taking X–rays of extremities and the chest. Later on, we had an eye man in the building. I became interested in a very complicated X-ray procedure to localize foreign bodies in the eye. I learned to do that for him.

"We had the first electrocardiogram machine in the city, a string galvanometer. It was a beauty, manufactured in France. It had a regular electric light that shined through a string that was in a magnetic field. There was a moving photographic film that focused the action on this string. It was portable, which was quite unusual. The machine that I worked with when I was at St. Luke's was an immense thing. We had to put the patient's hands and feet in water that had a lot of salt in it. The electrodes came off from that. That string galvanometer was on a big concrete base, and there had to be a whole room for it. The French portable instrument was a very new thing. We had trouble with it all the time. Dr. McIvor used to laugh because I had a screwdriver and a wrench that I was using all the time in order to make it work. We'd take the ECG and then have to take the film into the darkroom and develop it.

"I used to do a lot of consultation work. I went to about twelve small towns in an area of about fifty miles. I did all the consultations in that area for all the doctors except one. I borrowed money from my aunt to buy a car. I used to go quite frequently to Antrim, about thirty miles from Concord. I was called over there to see a man who had chest pain. I went over to see him in consultation with the local physician. I took my machine in and examined the patient and took the cardiogram. I said to the doctor, 'I bet I'm going to find that he's had an infarct. I'll call you after I get back and develop the film.' I went back to Concord to develop that film, and there was not one thing on it. The ECG had gone bad, as it so often did. Well, I had to fix it and go back and do the whole thing over. That was 120 miles I had to go for that one house call. It took most of the day. That was an example of the vicissitudes of practice.

"I was doing a great consultation practice. The transportation to the hospital wasn't the same as it is today. And the doctors in the small towns weren't trained that well. They were taking care of their patients in their environment and doing a great job. But when a patient had a coronary or got pneumonia, I was called in. Also, when they had a surgical procedure, I did the consultation.

"But I did absolutely anything. In those days we worked seven days a week, and we were on call twenty-four hours a day. I had night office hours five days a week. I was there. I was available. It was an interesting time. But there was so little that we knew and so little that we could actually do."

JARCHO

Independence in Internal Medicine

SAUL JARCHO'S physician father was the dominant force in his youth. He dictated his son's career and in retrospect was the primary influence on the younger Jarcho's medical education. Jarcho learned ethics and therapeutic methods from him and recalls his physical strength, conscientiousness, integrity, and humane attitude as essential to being a physician.

Trained in classics, literature, and languages at Harvard and Columbia, Jarcho brought his own unique capabilities to the study and practice of medicine. He cites two of his Harvard professors as more influential in his development as a physician than any teachers he had in medical school. The Harvard professors taught him the importance of observation. He had an interest in the relationships among ecology, the social conditions of patients, and disease. His study of Spanish and tropical diseases in Puerto Rico served him well; throughout his career in New York, he treated Hispanic patients with tropical diseases.

Jarcho studied and taught pathology at Johns Hopkins for two years following his internship, commenting that pathology was considered the basis for internal medicine during that era. Though offered opportunities to go into academic medicine, he declined, adopting his father's view that a Jew must forge an independent career. He was aware that Jews were regularly blocked from advancement or promotion in academic life—in classics and in medicine. Antisemitism could destroy a career in the years between the two world wars.

Jarcho returned to New York in 1936 and began the private practice of internal medicine. Until 1942, he also directed an outpatient clinic at Mount Sinai Hospital and taught pathology at Columbia's College of Physicians and Surgeons. Because of his skill with languages, he was employed in medical intelligence during the Second World War and served the war in Washington, D.C. There he conducted medical surveys of the Balkan countries, supervised the examination of medical equipment captured from enemy countries, and studied the geographical distribution of diseases. Toward the close of the war, he became chief intelligence officer.

"Many of the men felt that, after their internships at Mount Sinai, they should seek additional training in Germany or Austria, which were then regarded as leading countries in medicine. In this way, they learned the very latest and best medical methods. They also established personal connections with leading men in all fields of medicine, and they learned German. I had already decided to be an internist, and felt that pathology was the basis of internal medicine. During 1933–1934 I worked in pathology at Mount Sinai under Dr. Paul Klemperer, a Viennese, one of the best. He became noted for his study of connective tissue diseases. He was a jovial man and a very good teacher.

"I went on from there to the pathology department at Johns Hopkins [1934–1936], where I worked under Dr. William G. MacCallum, a Canadian like so many of the Johns Hopkins people. He was an excellent teacher. He said very little to me during most of the two years during which I served first as assistant and then as instructor. I was deeply interested in teaching and became known as a good teacher of pathology. I also did research. There was no salary the first year, and no room and board. In the second year, a professor found five hundred dollars in a special fund that had been lying around, and gave me that—in other words, ten dollars a week.

"I was strongly impressed by Johns Hopkins and am certain that it merits its very large reputation. William Welch died in 1934, a few months before I arrived. The reputations of Osler and Welch were a living fact, not just a traditional myth. They were talked about very often. Their characteristics were remembered by older doctors on the staff and were an actual living influence.[1]

"The medical school classes each numbered seventy-five students. I knew every student by name. By the end of two years, I knew almost everybody in all four classes. The importance of a small class was brought home to me after 1936, when I transferred to the College of Physicians and Surgeons at Columbia, where the classes were over 100, perhaps 110 or 120. That difference was notable. It was impossible or very difficult to know 110 students by name and certainly not possible to know the names of those in other classes. The teaching was necessarily less personal, therefore much less valuable. I'm convinced of the personal presence in medical teaching. It influences the student forever, for good or ill. It is grossly underemphasized nowadays.

"I did autopsies with the second-year class, which was divided into groups of about a dozen students each. As an instructor, I was with those students for the entire year. When I did an autopsy, they would be present. In addition, the instructors divided the burden, or the pleasure, of lecturing. I found it to be one of life's greater pleasures. I loved to prepare and present lectures. Once a more highly placed member of the pathology staff said to me, 'Don't you think you're wasting too much time on the students?' I realized that the medals went to those who did research. Teaching was lower in the rank of esteem. That situation is worse now than it was in 1934. Professors may not belittle teaching overtly, but it is lower in their unspoken system of values.

"I received offers and hints, first at Johns Hopkins, later at Columbia and elsewhere, to get on the academic ladder. But I knew then that I would have a boss, especially in the earlier stages of academic life, and one could be destroyed because of antisemitism or caprice. At Johns Hopkins for example, Dr. Max Wintrobe, one of the nation's leading hematologists, a Canadian Jew, found himself blocked and went off to Utah, where my brother, also a physician, soon joined him in the Department of Medicine.[2] The same reasoning about being my own boss, which was so important to my father, determined my purposeful avoidance of an academic career in medicine, as it had in literature or classics. It was not accidental; it was purposeful.

"After two years at Johns Hopkins I went back to New York and entered the practice of internal medicine. I became at first instructor, then associate, in pathology at the College of Physicians and Surgeons, my alma mater. It was now on 168th Street and Broadway. The pathology course would take up about half a day, three or four days a week. I worked there part-time for six years [1936–1942], not a bit of it with salary.

"I also headed an outpatient clinic at Mount Sinai Hospital before the war. When I became a visiting physician at Mount Sinai [1940], that is, adjunct, the lowest rank of the attending staff, I was required by my chief to be present during visiting hours in order to see the visitors of each patient. I would confer with the social worker. That was an unusual practice—requiring the staff to get to know the families of patients and to discuss cases with the social workers—and was greatly to the credit of the hospital. It was of the greatest value to me as a physician. The chief of my medical service was a remarkable man named George Baehr. He maintained very close ties with the social service department, which was large. It must have cost the hospital a lot of money. We also had a good psychiatry department, which had close contact with the Department of Medicine—an extremely important connection, used actively.

"I practiced medicine in New York from 1936 to 1942. I did not join my father's practice, but I had space in his office. I worked alone, as most practitioners did in those days. It was before the era of groups. But I did have the great advantage of my father's very large experience. He pressured me if he thought a certain treatment I had advocated was ill conceived or if he was not pleased with a dosage. Some patients came from my father. However, even with that it was a solo practice. I did things my way. One difference between us was that he kept his records on five-by-eight cards. This would not do for the kind of history I had been taught to take. I kept detailed files. I was probably excessively conscientious. Another feature was that I recognized that some of his prescriptions were obsolete, as mine would later become.

"I was thirty years old when I started to earn anything. I had to assume that I was charging about as much or as little as my contemporaries were charging, and I was paid either in cash or by check. I'd send out bills at the end of the month. A good many people I treated for nothing, because they were poor. A good many cheated me or would say after they had received their treatment, 'I'll only pay you half.' I got along reasonably well. Money was far from being an important object.

"The diseases I saw included malignancies, heart disease, the occasional case of exophthalmic goiter, and a great many diseases ascribable to emotional disturbance. For cases of infection, there were no antibiotics when I first started in practice. I would try to support the patient's nutrition and morale and physical cleanliness. We considered hygiene very important. With malignancy, one had to decide whether an operation was called for, and we had marvelous surgeons. Almost all organic diseases of the nervous system were untreatable. There was a great deal of psychic trouble, emotional trouble, economic trouble. The psychic troubles I helped as well as I could by conversation or by referral to a psychiatrist. I tried to determine which patients needed psychiatrists. Some patients who I referred didn't come back. I found that one psychiatrist had said, 'Your attachment to Dr. Jarcho is an obstacle to your progress in psychoanalysis.' I would lose them. I lost ever so many before

I woke up. If they needed a psychiatrist, that's only fair, then they need the psychiatrist and they don't need me. But some of the patients also had physical needs; they needed an internist at least occasionally.

"Then there was preventive medicine. We gave vaccinations and immunizations where such were available. We advised people about diet, about bad habits. We made efforts to get them to stop smoking. Some of us stopped ourselves, as I did.

"I had seen at Mount Sinai the abdominal organs of a person who had approximately seventy small spleens. This was a man who, as a child, had gone sledding and hit a post, rupturing his spleen. He had had a splenectomy. Pieces of splenic tissue implanted in the abdominal cavity, and many of them developed into small spleens. Some years later the man died of appendicitis. The autopsy showed this magnificent display of small spleens. I saw another similar case in the Dominican Republic. I used to go to various Latin American countries for vacation, and I would frequent the autopsy room because I had nothing better to do. Then there was a third case at Columbia, which, with the collaboration of a noted pediatric pathologist, I published.[3] All this came from a simple observation in a museum. The disappearance of such collections is another example of unwise changes in medical education.

"At Columbia I also did experimental work on the spleen. I procured a small grant from a patient to support the experiment. I would take the spleens out of rats and divide the tissue into small pieces, which I reinserted, trying to get the pieces to grow. Then I gave the rats injections of a radioactive substance to see if it would locate in the little new spleens. I used to go back to the laboratory at night and work on the animals. I didn't think I had brought the work to a sufficient degree of perfection, and so I never published it.

"At that time I began to work actively in the history of medicine. I began to look up the history of the spleen. I found that the first splenectomy had been done on experimental animals by an Italian named Zambeccari; this was published in 1680. I felt that I had to learn Italian, and I began to work in the history of Italian medicine. Since I had a fairly good background in the classics and in literature, those inclinations were easy to follow. This background, plus an interest in medicine and pathology, explains some of the early writings.[4] That was the beginning of my work in the history of medicine, which has continued up to the present.

"Shortly after the war, I was asked to come down to Washington, because our forces had captured all the records of the German surgeon general, and our people wanted an opinion on them. I came down and went over them. There were other special problems I was asked to consult on over the years. For example, when the Korean War broke out, they called me. They were suddenly short of staff. I went back there as an intelligence officer, as did my wife. We were in Washington for a month, doing duties which resembled what we had done during World War II.

"About the time I was leaving the armed forces, I was offered several jobs. I was offered the job of continuing as director of medical intelligence, either as a regular army officer or as a civilian employee of the War Department. I was offered the job of heading a project in the American Geographical Society in New York on the cartography of disease. I was offered also a very curious job described as having to do with a museum that was about to be formed. That one was disturbingly vague. I later found out that I would have been working for the CIA, which was just about being formed then, or it could have been the Office of Strategic Services [OSS].

"Instead of all those attractions, I came back to New York in 1946. I sat myself down in an empty room at a desk with a pad and a pencil and asked myself, 'What do you want in life?' I didn't leave the room until I had settled that. I drew a vertical line on the paper and made columns to show what I did and didn't want. It was much easier to list what I didn't want. I didn't want an automobile or a country home, the trash and toys of life. What I did want was knowledge. I decided that I would continue being a physician and do the best that I could do in medicine. If I made an adequate livelihood in medicine, as was probable, I would be able to develop and assist my desire for knowledge. That was it. I'm rather astonished at the extent to which I have been able to carry out this simple plan, which many people would laugh at. It has the backing of Plato, however."

BEESON

Infectious Disease Expert

DURING HIS RESIDENCY training, Beeson acquired experience as a laboratory researcher at the Rockefeller Institute and worked closely with Soma Weiss, a legendary teacher, bedside doctor, and chairman of the Department of Medicine at the Peter Bent Brigham Hospital affiliated with Harvard. Beeson was unusually fortunate to be exposed to some of the most important biological research of the day, as well as to an outstanding clinical role model. He made the most of both those advantages. He was to become a highly regarded researcher and clinician in the years to come.

In this section, he describes his first job as assistant professor of medicine at Emory University School of Medicine in Atlanta. He taught medical students, treated patients, and conducted pathbreaking research in the field of infectious disease. He provides a picture of academic medicine during the war years, the social climate of practicing medicine in the segregated South, and the monumental changes in medicine that occurred with the introduction of penicillin.

"While I was in Britain I had wanted to return to the Brigham. After Soma Weiss died, Eugene Stead, who had also been at the Brigham as an attending physician, was offered the chairmanship of the Department of Medicine at Emory in Atlanta. He wrote to me in Britain and said, 'I could give you an offer of an assistant professorship, and you would be the infectious disease man.' Stead was to be the first full-time chairman of the clinical department at Emory. At the same time, I had been corresponding through a Rockefeller friend with David Barr about going to the New York Hospital in infectious disease. At the time I wanted to go to the New York Hospital. It had a greater name. I had known it from my previous experience. And the Rockefeller group was next to it. Stead had to have my answer by a certain date. I sent him a cable accepting his offer. The next day I received the formal offer from Barr, but of course it was too late.

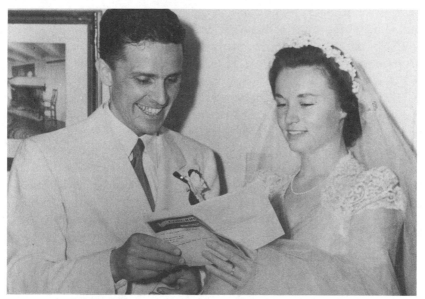

Dr. and Mrs. Paul Beeson, Buffalo, New York, 1942.

"So, I went off to Emory. It turned out to be the luckiest thing in the world for me. I was better able to function—and had much more visibility as practically the only infectious disease person in the Southeast of the United States—than I would have been in New York with that whole crew from Rockefeller and the New York Hospital. Fortune was again working on my side when I took that opportunity. I was there ten years, from 1942 to 1952.

"I met my wife, Barbara, in Britain. She was a nurse in the same unit in 1941–1942. We did all of our courting in Salisbury, where our hospital was located. We came back to the U.S. together in a convoy during the height of the submarine activity, although we didn't see any submarine action. She went to her home in Buffalo, and I went to visit my family in Ohio. A couple of weeks later we were married in Buffalo. We drove from there down to Atlanta to start the job at Emory.

"When Barbara and I got down there we went and had dinner with the Steads. Gene remarked in the evening after dinner, 'Paul, I've got a lab for you and a technician.' I was so naive. I hope I didn't show it too much, but I was flabbergasted with the thought that I would be expected to do research. I could see myself teaching and taking care of patients, but it never occurred to me that I would be expected to do research also. Still, I had done some at Rockefeller and had done some more in the course of my residency at Brigham. I knew some of the techniques of bacteriology.

"A few weeks later, there was no one to run the bacteriology lab of Grady Hospital, our teaching hospital, because someone there had quit. It was a big city hospital, completely divided into two parts—the black wards and the white wards. Our offices and labs were in the basement of what was then called the old colored nurses home. In fact, some earth had to be dug out in order to make ceiling room, but we had offices and labs down there and you could walk into it. It was a wonderful experience for me day after day to see the bacteriology. I was going to be an infectious disease expert. To see all the cultures that came into the lab and become a lot more familiar with general bacteriology, which I had to read about and teach myself, was a precious experience. And I found where the interesting infections were: around the orthopedic service, or the urology service, or obstetrics. It was perfectly all right for me to go see those patients, and I did. By giving me a research lab, and letting it be understood that I was expected to do research, Stead put me in a very favorable position. Infectious disease was not much of a recognized specialty, and I was virtually the only one in the southeastern United States who professed to have a special expertise in infectious diseases.

"Stead had a tiny department with two or three other full-time people. I was an assistant professor. It was war time. Many of the best teachers and practicing physicians in the town had gone away to war. We were exempt because we were in medical education. We had a busy time of teaching and investigating. I owe an enormous debt to Stead for taking me and giving me my first academic job and for setting the conditions under which I could work and work productively. Eugene Stead was, in his own way, just as much of a leader and exciting teacher as Soma Weiss had been. Being in his department for four years taught me a great deal. I saw the way his students reacted to him, how he could make the dullest case seem interesting. He could always find something to talk about at the bedside.

"I wanted a lot more clinical experience in a variety of kinds of infection. Instead of concentrating on one or two diseases, I deliberately tried to study fairly intensively a wide variety of conditions and to write articles about them. My first publications show a great range of interests. I have always been glad I did that. I didn't set myself up as a pneumonia expert and nothing else at that time. The research I did involved a variety of infectious diseases, doing special cultures, serologic tests, and so on. The important questions for me at the time came out of bedside discussions, arguments that arose there, wondering how something happens. Then I would go and try some experimental infections to see what I could learn about them. By that time, I did want to stay in academic medicine, and I did want to become chairman of a department. That's what everyone wanted then.

"My first real hit was in terms of serum jaundice, or hepatitis. While we were in England we had gotten the idea of trying to protect some young British soldiers from an epidemic of mumps that was springing up in a training camp near us in Salisbury. So we got the idea that, since we had some mumps patients in our hospital, we would bleed them, collect their serum, and give it to a bunch of new trainees, and they would therefore have antibodies against mumps. This had been done in the case of measles already. Nothing was known about the danger of transmitting hepatitis. We managed to transmit hepatitis through the mumps serum, and this produced an epidemic of jaundice in those trainees.

"Soon after I got to Emory, I was having lunch in a little cafe across from the hospital with a junior medical student who said he had an interesting patient with what was called toxic hepatitis. The patient had been in the hospital three months before with burns, and they had treated him with tannic acid, the standard treatment for burns. They thought a late tannic acid poisoning had given him the jaundice. With my guilty feeling of having produced hepatitis in those soldiers in England, I asked him, 'Did he get transfusions?' The medical student said, 'Oh yes, he did get transfusions.' Well, transfusions were new at the time. Blood banks were developed during the war, and they were only one or two years old. I looked up the patient's record and, yes, he did get transfusions. Then I rushed to the record room and looked up all the recent cases of jaundice and toxic hepatitis and found six more. They all had this peculiar, long incubation period—two to four months between the time of the transfusion and the time of the clinical hepatitis. I wrote a paper on the transmission of hepatitis by blood transfusions. Stead helped me again. The president of the AMA was an Atlanta physician, Dr. James E. Paullin, who had been Franklin Roosevelt's physician. Stead spoke to Paullin and Paullin spoke to Morris Fishbein, who was editor of the *JAMA,* and they got the paper I wrote on the subject published in no time. That caused quite an uproar: the transmission of hepatitis by blood transfusion. That paper gave me a lot of notoriety.[1]

"I got into other things as well. In the prepenicillin days, the best treatment for syphilitic paresis, or general paralysis of the insane, was fever therapy. General paresis and tabes were the late forms of central nervous system syphilis, and they were very common. You could walk down the streets of Atlanta and see somebody shuffling along with the typical gait of tabes. We always had on our wards two or three patients, white or black, with general paresis who were getting fever therapy.

"To give fever therapy we used typhoid vaccine intravenously. The interesting thing is that you start with a given number of organisms, and you get a chill and fever. It will go up and stay up at 103–104 degrees [Fahrenheit] for some hours and then come back down. In order to get that much fever with the next treatment, you have to give at least double the dose. You keep giving double and double the dose in order to get a total of forty hours of fever over 104 degrees. This worked. This was effective. It began with the use of malaria. A physician in Europe, Julius Wagner-Jauregg, got the Nobel Prize for thinking of deliberately innoculating syphilitic patients with malaria and curing or greatly improving some of them. It worked with the typhoid vaccine therapy as well. I got fascinated when I saw the amount of typhoid vaccine we were giving. I remember so well one patient whose last course involved 200 cc's of undiluted typhoid vaccine intravenously. For an immunizing dose, you usually give ⅛ of a cc. We injected bottle after bottle of this awful-looking material right into this man, and he got the usual fever but no worse. So I took that into the lab and started giving rabbits the same dose of typhoid vaccine in daily injections and following their temperatures.

"Then I read something about reticuloendothelial blockade. The reticuloendothelial system of the body is the one that removes foreign particles from the circulating blood, dead blood cells, bacteria, or whatever. You can block it by giving certain agents such as Thorotrast. When I gave my rabbits Thorotrast and then typhoid vaccine, they got big fevers. What this seemed to demonstrate was that the tolerance to the endotoxin in the bacteria was not an immune phenomenon due to antibodies. It was a phenomenon of the reticuloendothelial system enhancing its ability to remove these foreign particles. I published several articles on various aspects of that phenomenon.[2]

"Another thing that worked out well for me was studying the

bacteremia of patients with bacterial endocarditis. Bacterial endocarditis is an infection on a heart valve which is usually caused by a simple streptococcus, the kind that you carry in your mouth. These are harmless elsewhere, but if they can lodge in a little collection of platelets on a heart valve they can survive there, because white blood cells can't get at them, as there is no circulation in there. They grow and eventually the valve gets destroyed; emboli break off and damage the brain and the kidneys and so on. Over a period of months the patient dies. As I saw it in my internship, this was a uniformly fatal disease before penicillin.

"I had an argument with one of my friends there about whether we would do any better to take arterial cultures rather than venous cultures in order to demonstrate the bacteria in the blood. I happened to be on the right side in that argument, but it didn't make any difference. By that time Stead, who was a cardiologist, and his colleague Jim Warren were using cardiac catheterization in their studies of the circulation. They used the procedure in the study of congenital heart disease, and showed its value in diagnosis of patent atrial septum. I went to them and said, 'Could we take a patient with bacterial endocarditis and put in a catheter and get samples of arterial blood—which we could do with a needle in the femoral artery—and at the same time take the samples from different parts of the venous circulation and see whether there is any difference in the number of bacteria?' In particular, I wanted to go down into the inferior vena cava, go right on through the heart and get some blood samples from there. I also wanted to get some samples from the superior vena cava, which was draining the head mostly. Stead and Warren said, 'Sure, go ahead.'

"The patient would be taken to this special study room which had a fluoroscope and put on an X-ray table. It was well-padded with pillows and so on. Putting a needle in the femoral artery is not very painful; they put novocaine in first. You get a needle in there with a canula inside it, pull the canula out, take your sample, and put it back in. Threading the catheter in through an arm vein sounds bad, but many people have had it done. Everybody who has coronary bypass surgery goes through that, and you don't hear much complaining about the arteriograms. So it wasn't really so bad, except that the patient had to lie on the table for one to two hours. However, they didn't seem to complain. They were all awfully sick. They had been ill for months, and what we hoped was that they felt that someone was trying to do something for them.

"Stead and Warren and a fellow there named Emmett Brannon did the catheterizations. I was in the room the whole time, taking all the samples and timing them. I would put each one in a separate test tube and in an ice bath to keep any bacteria from growing until we could take them back to the lab. There we would pour agar plates, exactly 1 cc of blood from each specimen, and incubate them overnight to see how many colonies we could count on the plate the next day.

"The results were simply spectacular. The blood coming through the liver had virtually no bacteria as compared with the arterial blood that was leaving the heart. The thing we lucked into by trying to go down into the vena cava was that we found we could get into the liver. That discovery opened up a whole field of liver metabolism, because we could get samples from there. By angling the tip of the catheter a few weeks later, Stead and Warren found they could get into the renal vein. Kidney physiology could be studied that way. It turned out to be a very useful technique.

"It was just a little window of opportunity. The technique was there, but penicillin wasn't there. We would never have done those experiments then if we had had penicillin for these patients. I didn't know that penicillin was coming.[3]

"Some of the ethical problems about that sort of investigation that trouble us now never dawned on us then. There wasn't much clinical investigation as such in the early 1940s. There were very few people engaged in full-time clinical research anywhere. We never asked the permission of those patients to go through this procedure. We certainly never explained it. We never told them, 'This isn't going to help you a bit, but it may give us a better understanding.' No patient ever refused to participate. It wouldn't have occurred to them. We would go by the night before and say, 'We are going to do a special study on you in the X-ray department tomorrow,' and they would say, 'All right.' In that way they were like the British. British patients are completely complacent. They never challenge what a doctor is going to do. We had grown up in a tradition of charity hospitals and felt we were giving these patients our time and our skills. They were not paying anything for it. And, there was a social gulf between us. This was part of the reason that we felt we could study them.

"As I look back on it, I think we did more of our studies on the black wards. There were more patients and they were closer to us. Atlanta was a segregated city. Our hospital was segregated. One of the things that annoyed all of us who had come there from Boston was that the black patients always had to be called by their first names. It didn't matter how old they were. 'This is Sarah and she is complaining of shortness of breath.' On the other side of the hospital, 'This is Mrs. Jones and she is complaining of shortness of breath.' They had to be kept separate. They had separate nursing staffs and really separate nursing schools. The facilities in the black wards were not as good as those in the white wards.[4] In our relationships with other doctors and with social acquaintances in Atlanta, we had to learn not to let the race problem get into the conversation or it would get us nowhere. We were completely outnumbered, and there was nothing we could do about it. There were no black medical students. Grady Hospital is no longer a segregated hospital. They have black and white patients on the same wards.

"When penicillin was becoming available and small amounts were being allocated for civilian use, Stead did another thing for me. Most penicillin was allocated to the military, but Stead, through a contact in Washington, D.C., made an arrangment for me to be the 'czar' of penicillin in the southeastern states. I was the first person to use penicillin at Grady Hospital. I also was allocating its use elsewhere in the area and talking to doctors on the phone, saying, 'We haven't got any, and we aren't allowed to use it for this disease or for that.' It was used for pneumonia, hemolytic streptococcal infections, and for staphlococcal infections. An episode I remember with clarity is that of a practitioner in another town calling me and saying he had a patient with syphilis and wanted to use penicillin for that, and I said, 'No way. This drug is not to be used for syphilis because it has not been proved that it would be any good.' My goodness, it just revolutionized syphilis. Syphilis clinics had been places where patients would come back week after week for intravenous arsenic over periods of a year or a year and a half. It was a tedious and not very successful therapy. To be able to clear it within five days or so with penicillin was just stupefying. Being the penicillin czar certainly gave me a lot of exposure to the medical public and was a wonderful opportunity to know what this amazing drug was going to do. It was a very heady thing for a few months.

"Then, in 1943, supplies became bigger. By late 1943, penicillin was in general civilian use. There wasn't any Food and Drug trial of penicillin. It was so harmless and so good that you didn't need to do controlled, clinical trials. It was such a thrill to be able to save the life of someone with meningitis or bacterial endocarditis and to bring syphilis to a halt in a few days. I think we realized that this was a tremendously exciting new development. When it was followed by streptomycin, and then the tetracyclines came along in another year, we realized that we were going into a whole new era. The treatment of infections up to that time had been almost nil: bedrest, nutritious diet, and quiet. Sometimes attempts were made with antiserum, but they were only effective in a few things such as pneumococcal pneumonia. The use of antiserum against most things turned out to be a great disappointment. So there wasn't a lot of drug therapy until all of a sudden we realized that we were going to be able to treat so many things.

"We were beginning to take things away from the surgeons. We treated empyemas ourselves, putting penicillin by needle into the pleural cavity. Before that, treating empyema, carbuncle, or abdominal abcesses had required surgical drainage. The only thing they could do was drain the pus and hope that the natural defense mechanisms would take over. There were these debates going on between the medical people and the surgeons about who ought to treat this or that.

"During the Second World War, there wasn't a push to make medical schools enlarge their classes. The period of medical training was shortened by what they called the nine-nine-nine program, nine months internship, nine months assistant residency, and nine months of senior residency. At the end of twenty-seven months you were eligible for military service. The point was to get them out of the residency training program a little quicker, so there would be a larger pool eligible for military service. Everyone, except those with physical handicaps or those with full-time teaching jobs, did have to go into the military. Things did change during the war in that some of the full-time and many of the voluntary faculty went into the service. A lot of research programs had to be put aside and halted. But at the same time there was money available, and the government was asking for the investigation of certain things, for example, treatment of infection and treatment of shock. That's why Stead and Warren got their catheter research going, to study patients in shock. They were chosen to do that research because Grady Hospital saw a lot of trauma; there were a lot of stabbings on Saturday night. The emergency room at Grady was like a wartime casualty department. So the shock team was always there. They spent Saturday nights there and studied patients in shock with cardiac catheterization to see what was going on with the circulation. Later they used the technique for other kinds of investigation.

"It was abundantly demonstrated during the war that if you put enough money into a big problem, you could solve it: radar, jet propulsion, penicillin. Government researchers developed a good treatment for malaria, because our troops were going into malaria areas. In war ads in the magazines, General Motors would say they were making tanks now, but just wait 'til after the war and see what our new automobiles are going to be like. The whole country was anxious to channel money out of wartime expenditures and into good living. There were a lot of influential people in Congress who saw that things could be done to improve the nation's health if enough federal funds were put into it. The NIH [National Institutes of Health], a branch of the public health service, began to give out large grants to the universities of the country. All of a sudden we had this big explosion of academic medicine—in surgery, medicine, whatever—with full-time departments growing.[5]

"There was federal financial support for people who were working on infectious problems and testing penicillin and the new antibiotics that began to arrive. The government was a source of research support for my work. We had a very small number of clinical teachers. We all carried a heavy teaching load, just because there were so few full-time people in the department. While Stead was there, until 1946, our full-time department was six people. Stead surprised us all by accepting an offer to go to Duke in 1946. He had put so much into Emory and had just revolutionized the place that we couldn't imagine him leaving. When he left for Duke, he took three people with him. That left me and one other full-time person. I was made chairman of the department at that time [1946], and remained chairman for the six years until I went to Yale in 1952. In the Soma Weiss tradition, we used our senior residents as assistant professors, and they taught and helped conduct research as well as care for patients. I was forced to rely heavily on young people, on the resident staff, and some research fellows that I was able to recruit to do a lot of the academic work. I was lucky in getting a couple of very good ones to work with me.

"Since the war was over, the practitioners—internists—in Atlanta came back and reopened their offices. They wanted to teach and they were an exceptionally good, well-trained bunch of people. With the aid of these volunteer clinical instructors, it went very satisfactorily. I went on with the same kinds of research that I had been engaged in before. The department was small enough so that I wasn't seeing people and sitting on committees all the time. My life didn't change greatly after Stead left. I got elected to the two societies in academic medicine that everyone wants to be elected to, the American Society for Clinical Investigation and the Association of American Physicians. I gave a couple of papers before the association, which went well. I am sure that as a result of that I was approached by Yale."

OLNEY

Diabetes Camp—"Not Just a Hospital Doctor"

TREATMENTS BEFORE the sulfonamides and penicillin seem primitive and even barbaric in retrospect. Olney describes the transition from primitive treatment to actual cure that occurred after she entered the field of pediatrics in 1932. Through her work in the outpatient clinics at the University of California, San Francisco, she was introduced to pediatric diabetology and cardiology. She describes how social workers enabled pediatricians to know the patient and family well and to carry out treatment plans in the home successfully. During the time Olney was in her residency, the social worker was an indispensable resource for the physician, an extension of the physician.

Here Olney talks about teaching nurses and medical students, the only one of these physicians to talk in some detail about both teaching methods and subject matter. She also speaks of her indebtedness to nurses over the years. In conjunction with her specialization in diabetes, she headed the diabetic outpatient clinic at UCSF for many years and was among the first to carry out research with protamine insulin.

In 1938, at the suggestion of a nurse, Olney began the first summer camp for diabetic children. Under her leadership the camp grew, enriched the lives of hundreds of children and their families, and contributed to physicians' understanding of diabetic reactions and their control. The campers and counselors are Olney's surrogate children.

In the years before good control of diabetes, taking care of a diabetic child was a strain that many families could not handle. Olney learned that, as a result of that strain, some parents abandoned children or were completely unable to cope with their physical, psychological, and social problems. She recalls the profound and positive impact the camp experience had on the children. Many of them were in a supportive environment for the first time, where they had the opportunity to run and play like normal children. When we talked, Olney's eyes filled with tears when she recalled how camp was a more nurturing place than home for

175

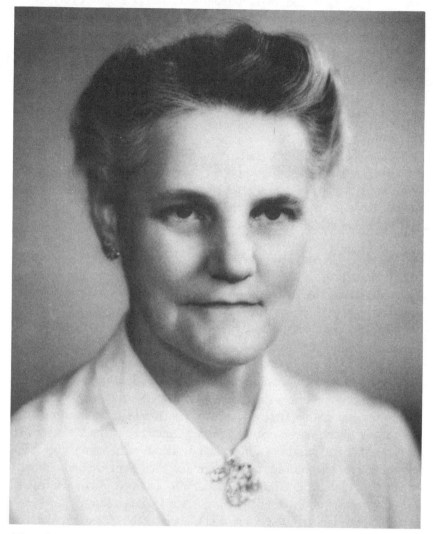

Mary B. Olney, 1940s. Courtesy Library, Special Collections, Archives, University of California, San Francisco.

some of the children. Through the creation of the diabetic camp, Olney truly healed the whole child.

"I came back to UCSF from Chicago as an instructor [1935–1942], and then became an assistant professor [1942–1947]. I taught nurses and medical students and worked in the clinics. Nobody teaches doctors how to teach. You are expected to teach interns and house staff and medical students. For years I tried different teaching methods at different times. There simply isn't a way of evaluating what you teach to know whether it sticks. I would sometimes get depressed because the method I used that particular day was not good. I had not put over my points. I tried not to teach a lot of minutiae. I tried to teach people how to think about problems they were going to encounter. I tried to teach medical students to think about what is the next step and how they can proceed from there. The nurse is going to go to work long before the doctors are there, and she needs information she can use immediately, information she can teach. So the approach is quite different in the two kinds of teaching. If you once hear yourself misquoted by a nurse to a patient, you realize that you are a total failure.

"I taught general pediatrics and contagious diseases to the nurses when I came back from Chicago. I had taught nurses in the Chicago Lying-In Hospital and had lecture notes that I had reviewed many times, and that made it easy to get started. I gradually worked into teaching third-year medical students and giving occasional lectures on specialties like diabetes and cardiology. Instruction in the well-baby clinic at San Francisco General Hospital was lots of fun, because there were students who were not going to go into pediatrics. I wanted to instill in them an interest in the process. It was a real challenge to teach them something they could apply in specialty areas. Students are so satisfied when they find they can manage things. When they aren't learning from patients, they should read medical articles in popular magazines to develop the vocabulary that people are using, not medical vocabulary, which only shows you are trying to be superior. How does a layman describe epilepsy?

"I taught medical students procedures for many years: how to do deep jugular punctures, spinal punctures, and bone marrow taps. Often we would get reports from referring physicians that they couldn't do a diagnostic test because it was a baby and they couldn't get a specimen. To be able to send students out to practice with the confidence that they could succeed with transfusions on infants, for example, was really exciting. Besides teaching them what procedures they could do in a treatment room, I taught what they should do at the bedside. Students don't know what is going to shock all the rest of the youngsters on the ward or how important it is to have a little serenity on the ward—for kids to be able to sleep during rest hour.

"Clinical teaching is great fun, because the child is there. I taught medical students how to be in control of the situation, which for pediatrics is so essential. I tried to show how much you can learn from the laying on of hands, how much a child can tell you. I taught by asking questions. What is the child telling you? What could you do to have him tell you more? How could things be presented differently so the students could learn faster?

"During the war years, I felt very guilty about being here when my associates were overseas. I asked one of the doctors in charge of enlistment whether I should be with the service or stay here, and he assured me that it was better to stay here and take care of the children of the men who were overseas. It's interesting what I remember about the shortages. We did not have any adhesive tape. We had to learn to use and tie bandages. That had been done before, of course. We would take the tongue blades home at night and boil them so we could use them again the next day. There are certain foods that people want for their children. Bananas couldn't take up ship space, and sometimes people thought there wasn't anything they wanted as much as a banana. It's just the sum total of little annoyances like that that set people off. Wives had to go home to their parents so they wouldn't have to maintain a household. We told them what to do to help children make the adjustment to the move. We told them how to put babies to sleep in dresser drawers in hotels during travel.

"One of my first opportunities was to take over the practice [in 1943] of Dr. Meryl Morris, who had been a pediatrician in San Francisco for many years. She expressed the opinion that she was tired of practice, which she was entitled to be after so many valuable years. My first reaction was that I didn't want to be tired of practice. I wanted to accept all the new challenges that came along. I expected the challenges to be greater in the university setting than in private practice. So I have never done more than half-time private practice. That allowed me much more contact with students and with what has to be known.

"I didn't feel there were constraints on going into private practice as a woman. I think constraints were much more manifest in the East. The pioneer spirit seemed more prevalent in the West, and women were allowed to do what they could. Perhaps I felt that way because Francis Scott Smyth was always very fair-minded toward women. I recall his holding up Dr. Olga Bridgeman, the child psychiatrist, as an authority. Whenever it was appropriate to recommend a woman for some position, he did it. When I was at the University of Chicago, it was always a man who was selected to do new and different things. Dr. William Deamer, who followed Dr. Smyth as the head of the Department of Allergy and Pediatrics at UCSF, was the same sort of person, always fair-minded.

"During the war, we had offices at the university. When the men came back, they were moved into the university offices, and those of us who had been there were asked to move out. So I moved into a little cottage across from the university. A contractor turned the basement into an office. To get it all equipped with a table and drapes and all of the things I had never done before was quite an adventure. Then I had to hire somebody to work in the office. I had never done any hiring before in my life. I found a very interesting woman who had worked in a doctor's office. Her first question to me was, 'Do you ask the patient to put the money on the desk before you examine them?' I said I didn't think we would do it that way. I had to get used to a person serving me in the medical office.

"My back window in the examining room looked out on a hill. I didn't realize how the office would look to a child until one of the mothers told me that her child wanted to go back to the place where the cars went up to the sky, which was of course, the cars going up the hill that you could see out the window. It was a nice little office, and we enjoyed twenty-one years of practice there.

"Early on, most of my practice was the children of nurses I had worked with. They wanted their children seen early in the day before they went on duty, and I could accommodate that type of visit. My association with Crippled Children's Services helped support my half-time practice. They frequently would refer a child with a genetic anomaly from a rural area where there might not even be a general practitioner. I would recognize that this anomaly was like that one from somewhere else. It was totally fascinating to identify, to remember what could be done for the previous patient and applied to this patient. It was like having a gold mine at my disposal.

"I worked at the county hospital teaching medical students five afternoons a week, so I could see patients in the morning. There were six or seven house calls to do in the evening. After the war, as the university personnel grew, the pediatric department grew. Some of the new people took over some of the teaching I had been doing.

"The research that was being done at the animal house was interrupted during the war, especially procedures on dogs. It was sad to see essential efforts interrupted. I did research with protamine insulin on dogs. I had two animals that had pancreatectomies. We had to give them insulin to manage the diabetes. At that time, the protamine was in a vial separate from the insulin. We had to mix our own. We had to calculate how much the diabetic dogs would need. We learned a lot about the effects of hypoglycemia and developed a profound respect for insulin by seeing how helpless the animals were and how upsetting reactions could be. The data we needed required taking blood sugars at two-hour intervals around the clock. I could get the blood sugars every two hours during the day. That was easy. But the all-night specimens were a little difficult. It gave me the opportunity to learn about people in the research unit, which was headed by Karl Meyer and his assistant, Bernice Eddy.

"That was the beginning of showing that you could combine regular and protamine insulin to prolong the actions so that children didn't have to take injections so often. A physician decided to premix it—two parts regular with one part protamine, producing NPH insulin. It was fun to have been in on the groundwork for proving that you could combine insulins in different ratios for different kinds of action. I was pleased to have had that experience. We used that insulin in our clinic and had a lot of appreciation from parents who would say, 'This is the first time since my child has been diabetic that I haven't had to get up at midnight to give the dose of insulin.' They used to have to give it before each meal and at midnight. So that was an exciting revolution. Of course, after that, they developed all sorts of insulin. They wanted to see if they could delay or prolong the action for ninety-six hours, but people could not always remember when the end of ninety-six hours was; they would take it a day too early or too late. So that wasn't very practical.

"It is so difficult now to watch the efforts to stop all animal research because, when it comes to a choice between an animal and a child, I really do favor sparing the child the experimental work. Cardiac surgery would be nowhere without animal research, and that is true for so many other types of research. You cannot set up an artificial dog on which to do cardiac research. I can't see any common ground for discussing essential things with people who are altogether opposed to it.

"I continued to learn a lot from the nurses. The county hospital nurses were wonderful to work with. They had to be dedicated to work there. I was very dependent on nurses' observations when I wasn't on the ward, for seeing how a patient fared with medications and treatments of various sorts. I've always felt a tremendous debt to the nursing profession for its contributions and to nurses for putting me closer to the patient. I always enjoyed their questions and concepts while I was teaching them. When the nurse practitioner program came in, I was impressed with how much responsibility, from the standpoint of liability, they could be entrusted with. They are fully aware of the pitfalls and know how to protect themselves and the patient and the physician. I've always been very impressed with the little personal things that nurses were able to do when a very low-income baby would be going home. Someone would always be donating some fancy little dress, or contributing some toys to the ward. They had ingenious ways of teaching parents to do things and getting them to cooperate. When I started working in schools, the school nurses made a big contribution to my education, and they let me know what problems were foremost in their school experiences.

"I was in charge of the diabetic [outpatient] clinic at UC for many years. Children came from all up and down the coast, because the average family practitioner would practice for twenty years and rarely see a diabetic child. So they didn't know the routine for taking care of them. I had only one child in my own practice that developed diabetes, and I've seen many, many children. The diabetic clinic served a very good purpose for many years.

"Dr. Smyth's head nurse, Alice Henry, was completely dedicated to this approach to the child, to the plans for handling children and accepting families. She said to me, 'Since you have had four years experience with summer camps, why don't you start a camp for the diabetic children?' It was her idea. We tried to find out where there were camps. New York had camps for inner-city children. A nurse took about seven diabetics to little cabins in upper New York State and it rained every day, so they had to have lots of indoor activities. I didn't get much information about how to conduct a western camp from them. We were offered a camp site in Napa County that we could use after the 4-H camp finished its season there. We decided to take it. That first year [1938], every child had to take his knife, fork, and spoon from home, because we didn't have any equipment. We learned more about diabetes in the two weeks we held camp than we learned on the hospital wards.

"We learned a lot about the timing of reactions, when insulin acts most and when it acts least. When the children went home, they had to teach their parents and their doctors. We learned how restricted children were at home. Some were allowed to go to school, but when they came home they had to sit in a chair until suppertime, because if they were active they might have a reaction. Children were on very, very limited diets. Some were fed on the wash tubs on the back porch, because the family did not want them to see the foods they were indulging in. A meal as a social experience came slowly for them. The thought of going out and carrying a bag lunch and going on a hike was brand new and wonderful.

"Before the discovery of insulin [in 1921] children with diabetes were frequently thought at acute onset to have pneumonia because of hyperventilation. The parents assumed the child died with pneumonia and didn't know that he had died with diabetes. If diabetes was diagnosed, the child lived only weeks or months on a starvation diet. When insulin was discovered, children were on three or four injections a day. Families had to learn that when you had too much insulin you had low blood sugar and had hypoglycemic reactions. When there wasn't money in the household to buy insulin, or when insulin was not given for a period of time, children went into a state of ketoacidosis and dehydration. Even though they went to the hospital to have the ketoacidosis corrected, some did not make it.

"The early treatment of diabetes was largely a matter of trial and error. Children who were trying to go to school were told by other children that they couldn't play with them because they might catch diabetes. That idea persisted up to the time we established our first camp. Advances in the care of diabetes were very slowly accepted between 1921 with the discovery of insulin and 1937 with the development of protamine insulin, a long-acting insulin. Efforts have been made ever since to develop an insulin that could be given by mouth. They have tried giving it under the tongue in capsules so it might be absorbed. There are trials underway administering insulin intranasally. Who knows how those things are going to work out. Recent evidence points to an autoimmune disturbance in the causation of insulin-dependent diabetes.

"Most young people who grew up with diabetes in the early days had to accept the fact that childbearing in a woman with diabetes involved significant risk to the mother and child. Self glucose monitoring and the use of the insulin pump gave a woman a chance of being accepted by her physician as a candidate for having a pregnancy. With the pump, there is a constant, twenty-four-hour distribution of insulin, with provision for appropriate additional insulin before each meal, so that it makes a person essentially nondiabetic. Women managed their own diabetic control, their own regulation, day by day. They did not have just one child but usually two, as they wanted them to have the company of another child growing up.

"For a long time, the attitude was that the diabetic child was just too much trouble to take care of. I have had many referrals because the doctor would say, 'I don't have time enough to take care of a diabetic child. I don't want to be called any time of the day or night about the problems of a diabetic.' Now, with good control, life expectancy is well into the sixties. I'm sure it can get into the seventies with better controls that are made possible by new techniques—being able to control diabetes by blood sugar monitoring instead of urine sugar testing—and better knowledge of nutritional requirements and the role of exercise. We don't have all the answers yet, but it is going to get better. But we do lose some patients. We lost a little girl from last summer, from our camp population. She got an acute acidosis for whatever reason. We had to let all of her counselors know, because they will feel the loss very keenly. We will lose some patients because we can't disseminate the knowledge of how to control diabetes as fast as we want to or as well as we want to. The advent of nurse diabetes educators has been a valuable contribution to diabetic management.

"In youngsters, diabetes occurs at times of rapid growth when other hormones are beginning to enter the picture. The ages of four to five years and ten to fourteen years have the highest rate of onset. The self-image of the developing adolescent is damaged the most and in part is why we started the camp. At that time, the youngsters with diabetes had a very dim view of themselves. But they began to look at other children who were learning to cope and said, 'If they can do it, I can too. I'm not doing it for my godparents, my grandparents, or my parents. I'm doing it because I want to be like that fellow.' So peer pressure was something we needed to develop carefully to its fullest possible extent.

"The first year of camp, in 1938, we had nineteen children from our own clinic at the university. The parents knew us personally. For the second year, we had to go to a different campsite. It was harder then with new families, because there were parents who didn't believe that anybody would take the trouble to take care of a diabetic child properly, and they just couldn't see facing the consequences of having care violated. Some diabetic children didn't have normal outlets for energy, as they weren't allowed to play with nondiabetic children. So they found other things to do which frequently got them into trouble. We had fifty-two children from around the state the second year of camp.

"Then we got letters from all sorts of groups. Could we take hemophiliacs? Could we take orthopedic cases? asthma groups? epilepsy groups? We had to make our biggest decision in our first years at Whitaker Forest [beginning in 1939]. Would we just take diabetics or would we diversify and take all these other things? We felt that our deficits were so great in handling the diabetic that we had better do a good job with diabetics and let somebody else handle the other things. It was a terrible decision to have to make because of the need, and we could see what camp did for the youngsters. Now of course, there are all kinds of camps, but at that time there were not. Over the years, we went from one two-week session with 19 children to four two-week sessions with as many as 152 children in a single session. There is a disadvantage in having 152 youngsters in two weeks. You can't consistently learn 152 names and personal things about the child in two weeks time. You can't give enough individual attention to the child. You can't make sure his bed is tucked in at night. If you are giving insulin in the insulin line, a child may answer to a name, but you have to look very carefully to make sure that it is the right child.

"We were at Whitaker Forest for twenty-one years. Whitaker Forest is in Tulare County. It's a 360-acre tract that belongs to the University of California and was willed to them by Horace Whitaker. We were there during the war when there was rationing. We even had difficulty with transportation when tires and gasoline were rationed. The diabetic had extra ration points for meat and for all the other things that he needed for his diet. The rest of us were quite a bit short on those things. It was a wonderful lesson. We spent our evenings counting ration points so we could send people into town for supplies. We had medical students and house-staff-level individuals from different colleges or different medical schools. They came from all over the United States.

"The children are ages six to eighteen years. We feel that they learn from each other. The older ones will never complain about getting insulin injections when they see how the little ones take them. And the little ones want to show off in front of the big ones how well they take their injections. The older ones are models for the little ones. We feel that when they get to be fifteen they should be junior counselors in training and return to the camp some of the things that have been done for them. They accept that as a great challenge. Then when they get to be seventeen and eighteen they may be senior counselors in training and be assigned a young camper to be their buddy. The buddy system works very well. A lot of single children in families who have missed all of the companionship of a sibling love having a teenager as a buddy. It's a wonderful experience. The counselors in training come down to see us at headquarters at night and say, 'I got Johnny up to go to the bathroom, but he didn't go very much and I wonder if I should get him up again.' Or the comment would be, 'I'm not sure that I'm going to get married and have a child; they are a lot of responsibility.' For them to learn in their teens that children are a responsibility is probably the best kind of teaching they could ever have. It brings out the best in the older group, to have to watch out for the younger ones. We never put them in complete charge.

"Many camps are not coeducational, but we feel that if boys and girls live together at home they should be able to live together in a camp. They need that exposure desperately. They need to develop respect for one another, and I think they do it there. It builds self-esteem.

"Since 1969 we have had a camp yearbook. The book can be shown to people at school without saying that this is a diabetic camp. Although it tells a diabetic story, it doesn't exhibit the diabetic story. Diabetic aspects are mentioned but not emphasized. It shows what they have learned from crafts they've participated in, trips they have taken. They can say, 'We went to Morro Rock. We hiked to various lakes. We made our own encampment here and there.' Overnight hikes were an innovation at camp, and they are such a rewarding thing.

"We have many children from broken homes, many more than the average in the community. So we have a lot of mending to do. It is terribly important that our older diabetics and our counselors be role models. We have had either mothers or fathers who say, 'This is not on my side of the family. It's not my responsibility,' and they abandon the family. When the child is in the hospital, the mother is usually free to be instructed. The father is not. Fathers can react in a number of ways. Frequently they take the child out on Sunday for a binge, because they don't understand the reasons for limitation of food, and they return the child to the mother in a state almost requiring hospitalization.

"In order to get the mother and father together, Dr. Ellen Simpson, who is my direct assistant, decided we should have a family camp [begun in 1976]. We have four-day periods in which families can interact as they learn and share knowledge and experiences on all aspects of living with diabetes. We don't keep a diabetic in the hospital for three weeks as it used to be. A one-week stay in some institutions will cost eight thousand

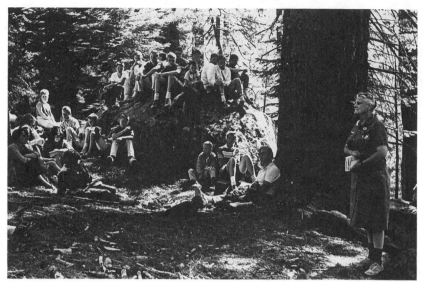

Dr. Olney speaking to campers about diet and diabetes. Bearskin Meadow Camp, 1964. Photo: Bob Clark.

to ten thousand dollars, but you can take a family to diabetic camp and do four days of educating for the cost of food only.

"In 1959, we had to leave Whitaker Forest. We traveled over six thousand miles trying to find a new campsite. Dr. Clarence Nelson, who was conducting research in the UCSF animal lab at the time, took time from his work to help us. Although he was a surgeon, he had more empathy for what we were trying to do than any other physician I worked with. We spent a dozen weekends looking for sites. We finally wrote to the state senators to ask the forest service to help us. They had been using the campsite at Bearskin Meadow for a work camp. When they told us we could have the campsite we could have kissed the ground, because we had a new camp coming up in 1960. We had to be ready.

"It's been our blessing that we have had such understanding and empathetic counselors. We are dependent each year on the talents of those counselors who apply to us. Sometimes there is someone who does woodworking and can teach it. Sometimes it is someone who can do copper enameling or puppetry. My sister, Grace Muma, has done general crafts. We send all the homesick youngsters to her for treatment of their homesickness. After they make something for Mom or Dad or brother or sister the homesickness is all gone, because they want to see how much more they can do while they are there. One of the reasons we had puppetry is because it is a good way of exteriorizing yourself. The children did very well with it. We had one little boy who missed his family very much, and he would go up to the craft hall and sit in front of the case with the puppets in it. He had made puppets—his father, his mother, and his sister—and he would talk to them every morning through the glass case. It takes somebody in crafts who understands what the needs are in order to meet them.

"We hear from the campers over the years. We hear about their graduations, their engagements, their babies. It is such a rewarding thing when the counselors come back and say, 'I want to volunteer my time, because I looked at my old yearbook and I realized that there were counselors who volunteered their time.' We have one girl who has come back and done clerical work for us three years now, because she got a scholarship to camp when she was a youngster. She married a fine man and works in his organization. She has her own child and did not have to have an insulin pump to have him. When she gets her vacation time, she comes to camp and does clerical work and counseling. One of the boys was just a total loss in his camping years. His father maintained a couple of households, and the kid didn't know a home life or who he belonged to or what his future was. His father turned him out in the street a few times. When he got a job after his camping experience he would come by motorcycle to the camp every year to touch base, that was his home. He came back last year with his son to learn to be a counselor. To see him with his youngster, giving him all the tenderness that he was deprived of, was just so beautiful. And a girl who works downtown worked these last three years to save a thousand dollars to give us this year for camp. She came to camp when she was a very shy, timid youngster. She told me, 'I realize that I wouldn't be working and I wouldn't be enjoying life as I do now if it hadn't been for my experience at camp.'

"I was foolish enough in my younger days to think that the time would come when we could turn camp over to the diabetics, because they would understand how to run it. Then I realized that, unless we place them in the community in jobs where they were making other contributions than to the camp, we were a failure. We couldn't just raise our campers to carry on in our image. That is like parents insisting that children follow in their footsteps. The youngsters go on to get good jobs in the community. They are doing the things they want to do and doing them well.

"I do not see a cure for diabetes within the immediate future. There will always be psychological problems that accompany it. We still have to teach that ability, not disability, is what counts. Until there is a cure for diabetes there is a need for camp, for its psychological contributions, social contributions, and medical contributions. To get all three in one camp experience is pretty wonderful. It has been a wonderful, most gratifying experience."

RHOADS

Doctor, Scientist, Patient—Three Views of Illness

HERE RHOADS describes his initiation into medical maturity: the operation he performed on his teacher and mentor. A Quaker and pacifist, Rhoads thought his career might end when the Second World War broke out. Instead, his work as a teacher, researcher, and surgeon intensified, because so many men were away. He describes the continuation of his nutrition research during the 1940s. He also talks about developments in anesthesia through that period. He recalls the experimentation on medical students and patients and physicians' attitudes toward it.

On the final day of our interviews together, Dr. Rhoads told me he wanted to talk about the impact his own serious illnesses have had on his life and on his understanding of patients. He feels the story of his life in medicine is incomplete without some discussion of the uncertainty and vulnerability that illness created in his own life. He says those experiences contributed greatly to his empathy for patients and to his understanding of what it is to be a doctor.

"In 1940, the year after I finished the five-year residency, Dr. Ravdin got an acute gallbladder attack himself. He appealed to his friend Dr. Alan Whipple in New York to come down and look at him. I was at his house when this consultation was going on. Dr. Whipple went over him and said he had an acute gallbladder and would have to have it operated on. At that point, his wife, who was also a physician, Dr. Elizabeth Ravdin, came out the bedroom and said, 'Jon, Rav wants you to operate on him.' So I sort of drew a breath and said, 'Well, if he wants me to, I will.'

"Dr. Ravdin came to the hospital and set it up so that Dr. Eliason, the other senior surgeon, and Dr. Whipple assisted me. He made this decision, I think, to put him in a stronger position to tell his patients that if he was busy I could operate on them, because I had operated on him. I had done quite a bit of gallbladder surgery during my residency, so he knew that I could do it. But one doesn't quite expect to be called to operate on his chief when he is less than a year out of his residency. I mention it, not only because of my own pride in his having trusted me to do it, but also as an example of his innovative and perceptive thinking even while he was in a good deal of pain. Of course, he was well covered with these other two senior surgeons there.

"My brother-in-law was in the hospital at the time with bad arthritis. I stopped in to see him and told him I was going over to operate on Dr. Ravdin. He asked, 'You're not going to do that are you? Here you've worked these seven years, and you're going to risk the whole bit on one roll of the dice?' I guess it wasn't quite that bad, but it seemed a little like that at the time.

"Dr. Ravdin was an impatient man. He was also a great believer in spinal anesthesia, which he elected, so he was awake during this procedure. He kept 'kibbitzing' me throughout the procedure. He would say, 'What do you find? What do you find?' All I could do was just work along. Apparently, this pleased Dr. Eliason very much. Word of the operation traveled around the surgical circles a certain amount.

"I can talk about developments in anesthesia almost on the basis of the anesthetics I have had personally. At fourteen, I had nitrous oxide for removal for a large mole and vomited afterwards. At twenty-three, I had mastoid surgery under an avertin anesthesia. It was a rectal anesthesia, a retention enema. I went to sleep and stayed asleep for a number of hours after the operation was over. It's now thought too dangerous to use.

"Later at Hopkins, they thought I ought to have my tonsils out. Most people in that era did tonsils in adults under local anesthetic, because they felt it reduced the risk of inhaling the pus from the tonsils and getting a lung abscess. But they didn't worry about that at Hopkins. They gave me nitrous oxide and I woke up reeking of ether. I vomited every hour on the hour for twelve hours, and then it passed.

"While I was a medical student, I was required to witness a few deliveries. One woman tore her perineum and required suturing. I was given the task of pouring chloroform over her face so that she would be asleep. I told them I would hold the bottle if they would tell me how fast to pour. That was all I knew about it. It went very smoothly. She went to sleep easily, without any excitement phase. It was a very brief anesthetic; that was why they felt confident in using it. That was my only experience with chloroform. I never had it myself.

"About 1942, I had appendicitis and I was given spinal anesthesia. That was a curious experience. I would feel the side of my leg with my fingers, but my leg wouldn't tell me that I was feeling it. I was a little too tall for the amount of spinal I got so that I wasn't completely anesthetized. It hurt somewhat when they were taking the appendix out, but I survived that. In this hospital, I think spinal anesthesia came into use around 1930 or 1932, but it had been used elsewhere earlier. The early advocate of it in this city was Wayne Babcock, who was chairman of the Department of Surgery at Temple University. It came into broader use in the 1930s and 1940s. It was used for deliveries beginning in the 1940s.

"Later, when I had a parotid gland tumor removed, I had an intravenous anesthetic for induction, one of the short-acting barbiturates. Then I had one of the newer gases. I had scopolomine with it so that apparently I woke up and talked for a couple of hours before I could remember that I had been awake.

"Anesthetic deaths were not unknown. In the earlier years, I witnessed a few. They are very rare now, because there is better monitoring and better control of the airway. It has become exceedingly rare, even in very sick people. But there is always a danger of it.

"We rely on our anesthesiologist so completely now, we don't have to keep one eye on the anesthesia. We used to have to keep looking at the patient while we were operating to be sure the nonmedical anesthetist wasn't getting the patient too deep and the patient wasn't getting blue or something. The surgeon had the ultimate, direct responsibility for any anesthetic death. That fact made life in the operating room more tense. We were more anxious to get through faster; it was more important to abbreviate the operation when anesthesia was less safe. Our anesthesiologist took over close to 1940. As he took over the department, he hired only medical anesthetists, recruited residents, and got an approved residency program going. He rapidly took all the nurse anesthetists out of the operating room, though they kept some of the nurse anesthetists in gynecology, because some of the gynecologists liked them very much. Some of the nurses were very skillful, but at that time they didn't do tracheal intubations and they never did the spinals. So, it was about 1940 that the change from nurse to medical anesthetists came here. I suspect it was a little earlier in some other places, but it was a general change.

"When the war broke out, I thought it would mean the end of my career. I was raised a Quaker and a pacifist, and I didn't want to go into the army. But Dr. Ravdin saw it as an opportunity to cover the home service. There had to be some people here to carry on the teaching. So he had me set up as an essential to the teaching program, and I stayed and taught and carried on his service. I did not go out with the group that staffed the 20th General Hospital, which was a very fine group of people. So, I didn't get any war experience. But I got intensified civilian experience. It was agreed that there would be no promotions in the clinical aspects of things while the men were away. In 1944, I was put in charge of the laboratory too. I ran that until Dr. Ravdin got back at the end of 1945, a year and a half.

"In addition to the medical students, we had the graduate school students. We also had a lot of short courses to mount for medical officers, who were sent here for six weeks or eight weeks to hear what we could tell them about antibiotics. This was before penicillin. We had had a good deal of experience with the sulfonamides. The medical officers also wanted to know about plasma and about blood and plasma expanders, so we gave a lot of lectures on this. I remember one day I gave six hours of lectures.

"Then the patients kept flocking in. Some of them were for small operations, some of them were for larger. It was very busy during the war years. I think the service as a whole ran pretty well over a hundred cases a month. I had to supervise the cases I didn't do myself for Dr. Ravdin's service. Dr. Eliason was here carrying a similar patient load. So it was a period of few people, lots of work, lots of experience, and multiple responsibilities between caring for patients, teaching, and research, and trying to keep the laboratory active. That turned out to be a very valuable experience for me. I don't think we had any vacations, more than perhaps three or four days one summer or two. I'm not sure it was a healthy period, but it was a good period in terms of the opportunities to do things.

"During the war, there was a great effort to find out what the nutritional requirements of the postinjured were. In civilian life, that meant postoperative patients. Work was going forward actively on that at a variety of places. I think our emphasis was that if you just put into the bank the amount of money that is spent, you don't build up your bank account. You have to be able to put in substantially more than you take out to either replace a deficit or build up a cushion. I'm not sure how far you can build up a cushion, but Dr. C. Everett Koop got some evidence that you could build up a bit of a cushion. He did this by force feeding a group of patients for about a week before an operation and then giving them just ordinary regimens of intravenous glucose afterwards until they could eat. I think ten of eleven patients were in positive balance for the whole two weeks, the week before and the week after surgery. He built up quite strong positive nitrogen balances in the week before surgery by giving them huge amounts of calories and protein, which he would put in by tube if they couldn't eat it. He was very convincing to his patients and persuaded them to do this.[1]

"We later challenged the idea that you could not get positive nitrogen balances in the early period after an injury. I think Dr. Harry Vars, Dr. Stanley Dudrick, and our group devised a practical method of getting a large number of patients who couldn't eat into positive balance. This took us in various directions. The advantage of giving the solution in the big vein above the heart, the superior vena cava, is that you can give concentrated solutions without causing thrombosis, because as the sugar and amino acid solutions trickle in, they are immediately diluted by a huge volume of blood coming back to the heart. We had experimented a little with central venous administration, putting catheters up from the elbow, but we had done it on patients who were dying of cancer. We examined them at autopsy and found there was quite a bit of clot formation along the catheter. We were afraid we would get pulmonary embolisms, so we backed away from the technique. Later we used either the jugular vein or the subclavian vein as the point of entrance; those are big veins and comparatively short lengths of catheter in the vein were needed to reach the superior vena cava. You get a little clot formation, but it hasn't been much of a problem.

"My wife's father [Otto Folin] had worked on the absorption of split proteins, hydrolyzed proteins, in the cat back around 1910 and 1912, I think.[2] He had shown that some fractions that were larger than amino acids, but smaller than proteins, could be absorbed. So we undertook to repeat this. We used to keep animals for long periods in those days. We had a dog who had a chronic intestinal loop, and we got him out of the vivarium. We ran these studies on him and confirmed the fact that the amino acids would be absorbed and so would some of the polypeptides, and perhaps peptones. We collaborated with a chemist, Dr. Cecilia Riegel, on that. By 1936, a group in St. Louis had shown that split proteins could be given intravenously. Preparations were made in Evansville, Indiana, by the Mead Johnson Company and were given in St. Louis by a surgeon, Dr. Robert Elman. He had shown that you could give this material to patients and that a good deal of it seemed to be absorbed. So we got this material, which was called Amigen. It was made by taking casein, the leading protein in milk, and grinding it up with pig pancreas. Presumably, it was mostly derived from casein, but some of it could be derived from the proteins of the pig pancreas. We found that we could get a good deal of protein into patients with this. I think in 1943–1944, Dr. Isaac Starr of the Department of Medicine and I had a joint grant to study the convalescence of both well-nourished and ill-nourished surgical patients. We fed some of them by this intravenous technique, and others we fed by putting a tube into the jejunum at the time of the operation on the stomach and fed them through that.

"A variety of other experiments were done, and these eventually showed us that we couldn't quite meet the protein requirement of the postsurgical patient whose metabolism tends to be about 50 percent higher than the basal metabolism after an operation such as removing part of the stomach or removing part of a colon. This was a troublesome problem we worked on over a number of years. We thought intravenous fat might be the answer. We were supplementing the protein with sugar, glucose, and then we went on to try fats. But the fats we had available were not very good. The Swedes finally got good emulsified fat preparations for intravenous use, but we didn't have them. So that research effort broke down.

"The problem of giving a patient enough food intravenously not only to meet his requirements but also to replace his deficits got to be somewhat of an obsession. After we had played around with intravenous fats for several years, we still hadn't solved the problem and we didn't really have a way of building up patients who couldn't eat. We see a number of patients who can't eat, and those who can't eat tend to be placed into surgical services for opening up the alimentary tract. We knew from these earlier studies that these patients were not as good risks as patients with normal nutrition.

"One day I had a sudden inspiration. It occurred to me that our medical colleagues were using diuretics with great freedom for the treatment of hypertension. The earlier diuretics had been a little hazardous, but these apparently were not. By using these we could greatly increase the volume of intravenous solutions that it was safe to give. We had been limited to about three liters a day previously. If we gave more, some of the patients got their circulation overloaded and developed pulmonary edema, which is life threatening. If we gave the diuretics, we could perhaps go to five or seven liters a day and in that way carry a much larger volume of nutrients in. The reason you couldn't just load them in by increasing the concentration is that the higher concentrations caused thrombosis of the veins that you stuck needles in. Such increased concentrations would thus stop the flow as well as create a local phlebitis. We started with the diuretics and it worked very well. The main problem was that the patients didn't all react the same, so that one had to watch the patients like a hawk. One of the patients didn't get watched like a hawk, and she developed pulmonary edema but pulled out of that. Her cause was not advanced because of that episode.

"So we then took the problem over to the laboratory. I got my oldest son, who was then a Harvard medical student, to come and spend a summer working on it. The idea was to work on dogs and see which diuretics would upset the dogs' electrolyte patterns least. Dr. Harry Vars, a biochemist, had devised a method of giving a continuous intravenous solution to dogs without their being tied down. He was working with a young surgeon named Martin Rhode. They found they could put a plastic tube down through the jugular vein into the big vein just above the heart. That was connected to the back of the neck where the dog wore a sort of harness. From the back of the neck there was a tube going up outside the cage, and the dog could get up and lie down, because there was a counterweight and the tube would come down to him. The slack would be taken up if he got up, and he could turn around. Dr. Vars got this equipment reorganized, and my son worked with it and did several dogs that summer. They showed that the dogs could take all this intravenous solution and no other food, and they looked lively and were jumpy and eager after several weeks being nourished in this way.

"Then, Dr. Vars and I decided we should do it on puppies. Our rationale was that, if you got a 10 percent weight gain in an adult, someone might argue that you might just have put more water into them and it hadn't come out yet. If you did it with a puppy and the puppy doubled his weight, you wouldn't have to meet that argument. The puppies were fragile and a number of them were lost. Not much was accomplished, except that it was better to wait until they were weaned at twelve weeks and then start them. The second year, Dr. Stanley Dudrick took on the project and made it work. He was a very hard-working, industrious, and perceptive person. He showed that dogs could live on nothing by mouth except water and yet grow, triple their body weight in the course of eight or nine months, during which I think he took no day off. This was a pretty clear demonstration of the effectiveness of the technique.

"Dr. Dudrick then came up with another idea that he borrowed from the literature—to give the nutrients, not through the jugular vein, but through the subclavian vein. You can do it either way. We have done it both ways. We coined the term 'intravenous hyperalimentation' for this, meaning that we would try to give 2,800 to 3,000 calories to a person whose basal requirement might be 1,400 or 1,500 calories and whose postoperative requirement might be 2,100 calories. So patients not only got enough to balance their losses, but also got enough to replace their deficits over a period of a few weeks. This technique has become pretty well standard and accepted.

"So that is the nutrition story. The research reached way back into the time Dr. Ravdin was chairman, indeed, before he was chairman. I think it was clearly the most influential work that came out of the department during the time I was chairman. I would give the major credit for it to Dr. Dudrick. Locally, it enabled us to operate on people that we previously thought were inoperable. And it's been adopted pretty widely. Dr. Dudrick and I jointly received the Goldberger Award of the American Medical Association in 1970. In retrospect, I suppose that Dr. Vars may have been more deserving than either of us. I think it was the first time it had been given to any surgeons. So, we have taken a lot of satisfaction in what the method has done.[3]

"At the end of the war, about 1946, there was a lot of albumin left over, and Dr. Ravdin obtained a supply from the Red Cross. We had a doctor with us who, along with two medical students, undertook to live on a diet with no protein except the albumin. Albumin by mouth is not a very good source of protein; they began to get positive nitrogen balances. They stayed on that regimen for about three weeks, I think. By that time, the doctor was on the verge of congestive heart failure. I think the students were too. They stopped the experiment and had a luncheon for everybody who cared to come, at which they ate meat. And they recovered. That experiment showed some interesting things. The reason they were in positive nitrogen balance was that the albumin was retained as albumin; not much of it was actually being metabolized.

"One of the medical student's mothers was rather upset about the experiment and didn't think it was quite right. People experimenting on themselves is not always good. In the days before informed consent, we used to experiment on medical students also. They were usually boys who were reaching for participation in research; they were very much game for it. They wanted to do it. People at that age are more prone to take risks than people a little bit older. The dean finally called a halt to using medical students. I think he assumed that sooner or later he was going to lose a medical student and have tremendous trouble on his hands.

"The first experiments I ever participated in with patients were with newborns in the nursery during my first medical school summer [1929], when I worked for Dr. Joseph Stokes, Jr., in pediatrics. Dr. Stokes wanted to know how concentrated the acid was in the stomach at birth, and he got a pH-determining device rigged up over in a borrowed lab. Our job was to go to the newborn nursery whenever the nurse called us to say there was a newborn, put a tube down the child's nose into the stomach, aspirate some gastric juice, and run over to the lab to see what the pH was. Dr. Stokes used to say that one of the advantages of pediatrics is that you didn't have to have the consent of the governed. Obviously, you couldn't talk to the newborn, and we didn't talk to the parents. That was a long time ago. Nobody was harmed physically.

"The days of informed consent arrived. I think it is much better to work with informed consent. Apart from the medical and legal constraints, I think it's more ethical. I think we tried very hard to be ethical during my surgical years. I think where we exposed a patient to risk, it was generally a situation in which the patient was already at great risk. We had reason to believe that what we were doing might help the patient and might diminish the overall risk. I think in general, people felt that they wouldn't do anything to others that they hadn't tried on themselves first.[4]

"I think it is of some interest to talk about my own illnesses, in that I think to be sick yourself enlarges your perspective a great deal as a doctor. After the upper respiratory infection and the mastoid operation when I was a medical student, the next threatening experience was tuberculosis. In a way, I learned more from that than anything else. I was then thirty-nine [1946]. Perhaps it was just before my thirty-ninth birthday that I picked this up. I was not sick and was planning to go to Poland for the United Nations, one of those postwar programs to help update medicine in some of the countries that had been deprived. They sent me down to the U.S. Public Health station in the city for a chest X–ray. They called me up the next day and said, 'Did you know you had moderately advanced pulmonary tuberculosis?' I said, 'I didn't know anything about that.' I came over to the hospital and got another film, which confirmed it. I went to the man who was our senior TB consultant here,

Dr. David Cooper, who was not an alarmist about it. He had me slow up and then, in a few weeks, stop working.

"In the meantime, my wife was pregnant for the last time. She had gotten her chest X-rayed before we decided on this last pregnancy, but I hadn't had one. I hadn't had a chest X–ray for about ten years. She was having the twins, though we didn't know that yet. She developed a breast lump which had to be biopsied. We were very worried about that, because breast cancer during pregnancy usually ends fatally. When that turned out to be benign, we decided tuberculosis wasn't too bad. I think mortality then was down to 7 percent. My wife took the rather cheerful point of view that, if I had survived the working hours I had been putting in, I ought to come around if I rested.

"I went out and rested on the farm with my mother for a while and then went out to New Hampshire to my wife's family's place and continued to do a lot of resting. I came back in midsummer. They checked me out again. There wasn't much change in the chest film. By September we knew I still had active bacilli. Dr. Cooper put me in the hospital so he wouldn't have to worry about me. Streptomycin had just been shown to be of some use against the disease. We were able to get some streptomycin from the Merck Company. We didn't know what the dosage should be, so they gave me close to twice the current dosage, and I developed a lot of trouble with my eighth nerve and my vestibular apparatus. I lost my balance very completely. I never got it back entirely, but it didn't really matter very much. My tuberculosis got better, and I went out and completed my convalescence in New Mexico the first three months of 1947. I came back to part-time work in the laboratory, and by the next fall I was pretty well back to full-time work, or nearly full-time work. I guess I lost about a year.

"Regarding the psychological implications, I had a fair amount of time wondering whether I would get better, and there was no way to know that really. I had had two friends in medical school who had gotten fatal complications of tuberculosis. We were also not in a very sound financial position, in that we had four children already plus whatever emerged from this last pregnancy. That was a rather interesting episode too. Our obstetrician was a very distinguished man named Robert Kimbrough. He had been called on to deliver one of Franklin Roosevelt's grandchildren. I was in the hospital when my wife went into labor about five weeks early. I asked if the fetus was large enough to survive, and he thought it certainly was. He called me about suppertime and said I had a boy. Then he called back about two hours later and said we had still another. He missed the fact that she had twins! It made the problem a little stickier. If I had had a very long illness, or if I didn't get better, how would they be provided for? Thinking about all of that gave me quite a different perspective on illness.

"The year with tuberculosis also gave me a break of continuity. It is not always such a bad thing to have some sort of break of activity. I didn't work and I took a great deal of time to read and think. I read thirty or forty books I suppose. I thought it was a good time to inquire a little into what people who studied education were learning. I thought that, since we were teachers at the medical school, we ought to know what was going on in the profession of teaching. So I wrote around to see what the offerings were in correspondence schools, and I found that education rested on three pillars: (1) the history of education, (2) the philosophy of education, and (3) educational psychology. I did the course from the University of New Mexico on the history and philosophy of American education, which I passed. And I took the one from the University of Indiana in advanced educational psychology, which I passed. With that much training in education I concluded that it was not something I wanted to see integrated into the medical curriculum or as a requirement for teachers in medicine.

"In 1961 I developed a tumor under the jaw which grew to be a parotid gland tumor. My wife's father had had one of these back in the early part of the century and had had it removed at the sacrifice of his facial nerve. The facial nerve usually goes through that gland. Now, the nerve usually can be saved. I didn't know whether I had a benign or malignant lesion, but it was benign. I mention these details because I think it is in some ways a good thing for a physician to have been sufficiently sick himself so that he is not sure he is going to get well. It gives you a little deeper empathy with patients, so many of whom don't know whether they will get well. You don't know for sure either. Personally, I've been fortunate on a number of occasions."

HODGKINSON

Breasts, Babies, Science, and Idealism

WHEN HIS RESIDENCY in obstetrics and gynecology at Henry Ford Hospital ended in 1942, Hodgkinson entered the service as an army doctor. He spent the remainder of the war years treating women and children and performing general surgery at an army hospital in Denver, Colorado. His experiences there reveal a little-known side of the armed services.

He continues to describe specific obstetric and gynecological cases in order to illustrate the medical problems he faced, the limits of his abilities, and the tragedy of premature death. Through recollection of individual patients, he is able to characterize his life's work as intimate relationships with many suffering people as well as the accumulation and application of scientific knowledge and surgical technique.

"In August 1942, we bought a second-hand Ford and drove out to Denver. I was assigned by the army to be head of the Women's Surgical Department at Fitzsimmons General Hospital in Denver, Colorado. I stayed at Fitzsimmons for the remainder of the war. I had a wonderful service there. I had to do more than gynecology, because in the army, women's surgery consists of any operation in women and in children up to the age of twelve. So I had pediatric surgery and general women's surgery. From the surgical standpoint, it was one of the greatest experiences of my life. We did a tremendous amount of surgery. We used to operate three days a week. Often we would start at 7:30 A.M and would finish up about 7:30 P.M. It was an invaluable experience. I did a little bit of everything while I was there.

"The medical departments of the army and navy made some big mistakes when they started to recruit women. The army doctors didn't like to examine women. They didn't want to have anything to do with women. We had two companies of WACs at Fitzsimmons General Hospital. I think there were eighty-five to each company. They were admitted to the army without any kind of complete pelvic examination, and

often their breasts were not examined. Some of these women had carcinoma of the breast when they came into the service. They were very
patriotic women who hid their problems. I remember one captain, from
Boston, who had cancer of the breast when she went into the service.
When I examined her at Fitzsimmons, she had a great big cancer. I asked
her, 'How in the world did you hide this?' She said, 'It was easy. In the
first place, these guys didn't want to examine me. In the second place, I
just acted real modest and they wouldn't even touch me. I got away with
that for two years.' By the time she got to Fitzsimmons, she was hopeless. I was very fond of her. When she was discharged from the service, a
medical officer had to accompany her back home, because she was still a
patient. By that time she was in terrible shape; she couldn't walk. I was
the officer assigned to take her back to Boston. We went by train. We put
her in a bed. I'm sure she died not very long afterward.

"With that terrible experience the army then overreacted. The general decided that I should examine all the women every four months. He
would send me a note: 'You will examine Company C, WACs, at 2:00
Tuesday.' Me! I was the only doctor there with eighty-five women to
examine in two hours. I worked out a system with the sergeant and two
nurses. The women took off all their clothes except a khaki nylon slip.
They wrote their name, serial number, the date of their last menstrual
period, and any complaints they had on a piece of paper. The nurses
would bring them into me. I didn't have time to say anything to them.
I'd just look at the piece of paper and stick it in my pocket if there was a
problem. I always found two or three who were pregnant. I'd do a pelvic
examination and a Pap smear and examine their breasts. To save time, I'd
examine the breasts through this nylon slip.

"One time, I examined a woman's breasts through the nylon slip and
felt a lump. I didn't say anything to her. But after I had examined all the
women in the two hours I was allotted, I told the sergeant I had to see
that woman again. This time, I examined the breast like I should have
examined it in the first place, without the slip. Well, I couldn't feel any
tumor. I was sure that I could feel a tumor before. She put the slip back
on, and we sat there and talked about various things; by that time we had
plenty of time. She was an X-ray technician from Omaha, a very fine
woman. She had several children. She was very patriotic, there to do her
duty for the war effort. I said, 'I just can't believe it; I know I felt
something in your breast.' I went back and examined it through the slip,
and there it was. When I examined it through the slip, I could feel it.

When I took the slip away, I couldn't feel it. So I called the surgeon-in-chief and asked him to examine this girl's breasts. He said he couldn't feel anything. Then I asked him to examine her through the slip. He said, 'Yes, I can feel something there.' That changed my practice. After that, I always examined breasts through a piece of cloth; usually I would use a hospital towel, which is smooth. I always examined the breasts through a towel and then examined the breasts without the towel. When I came back to Ford Hospital, this became known as the towel trick. My residents were taught to examine the breasts through a towel. I think a lot of them are still doing it. I was able to pick up some very small breast tumors that I couldn't feel without the towel, because little bumps accentuate themselves through the towel.

"For several years after I graduated from medical school, there was no such thing as antibiotics. Sulfanilamide was developed first in Germany, and rapidly spread over the world. We used it a great deal. Then penicillin was discovered, and that rapidly changed the practice of obstetrics and gynecology. Many of the infections that were thought to be incurable, such as syphilis and gonorrhea, all of a sudden became curable. We would bring a patient with gonorrhea into the hospital and put her on an IV drip with penicillin for two days; that was all there was to it. She was cured. Nowadays you seldom hear of anybody dying postoperatively because of infection. But before the advent of sulfa and antibiotics, it was not at all uncommon to lose patients from infection, particularly after cesarean sections. It was a serious operation then.

"I was one of the first to use penicillin, because I was in the service, and all the penicillin went to the service initially. I became very interested in the prevention of breast abscesses. Until penicillin, if a woman got a breast infection after delivery, it usually ended up as an abscess, and you would have to incise the breast and allow it to drain for a long time until it was finally cured. At Fitzsimmons, we had a large obstetrical practice, and for some reason we had a lot of breast infections. I got permission from the surgeon in chief to use penicillin to prevent abscesses. Over a couple of years I collected about fifty cases. I was able to prevent the development of abscess formation with the use of penicillin. I think I wrote the first report ever on breast infections treated with penicillin.[1] It was simply because we had the drug and the civilians didn't. We gave it by intravenous drip. It was a very crude product at first, an impure substance, and a lot of people became sensitive to it. We would see a lot of allergic reactions, but it cured breast infections remarkably well.

"Our second child, a girl, was born in 1940. In retrospect, I probably wasn't a very good father, because I was working so hard at the hospital. I probably didn't spend as much time with the children as I should have. I think our closest relationship with the kids was when I was in Denver. We lived on the post at Fitzsimmons General Hospital. That's really a choice life for kids. The kids of the officers are treated very well. We had a very close family relationship then. We would go fishing and hiking and that sort of thing.

"When the war ended, we drove back to Detroit. I had been offered a place on the staff of Ford Hospital and the magnanimous salary of ten thousand dollars a year. That wasn't much, but in those days you couldn't dictate too much. I had, and still have, a very idealistic attitude toward medicine. But the result was that I neglected the financial part of medicine by going into Ford Hospital on a salary. If I had been in private practice doing what I did, I'd be a rich man today, but I wasn't interested in that. I was interested in science, basic facts.

"It hurts me to see some of the conflicts that are going on now. A lot of controversy and difficulties that arise in medicine are mercenary. I never had a problem, because I didn't have anything to do with the finances of the institution. At Ford Hospital, the patients didn't pay me. My private practice was all through the hospital. So, it's been very easy for me to have good relationships with my colleagues, with everybody.

"I worked in the Department of Obstetrics and Gynecology and developed a tremendous practice and a tremendous number of obstetrical cases. I used to do fifty and sixty deliveries a month. I did that for year after year and I enjoyed it. It was really the most pleasant part of my practice.

"The most remarkable case I have ever seen obstetrically occurred a few years after the war. A young GI and his pregnant wife came in. She came to the time of delivery and started to have contractions. Everyone thought it was labor. Well, I examined her and it wasn't labor. It was an intestinal obstruction. She was having contractions of her intestines. I had to operate on her. I resected a gangrenous portion of her intestine. She had peritonitis at the time of the operation, but we gave her a lot of antibiotics, which we had then. After the operation, we put tubes down her throat to drain off the gas. The operation was successful. Then she went into labor on her own and delivered this fine little boy. Everything was just great. She got through the operation and got through the delivery just fine.

204 Part III   Generalists, Scientists and Curers: 1930s and 1940s

"Because of the intestinal obstruction and the anastamosis to put her bowel back together, we kept tubes down her for quite a while. In those days, we kept patients in the hospital longer than we do now. Well, those kids didn't have any insurance and their hospital bill was getting to be sky high. I think it had gone up to about twenty-five hundred dollars. They didn't have the money. The operation and the delivery became quite an event in the hospital, and word of it spread through the grapevine. At the time, I had a patient with inoperable cancer of the ovary. She and her husband were very rich. They heard about this case and heard that the young man was a GI and just out of the service, and heard about how worried they were that they couldn't pay their hospital bill. So one day, they walked into the front office and paid the couple's hospital bill.

"That was three weeks after the operation, and the patient was just about ready to go home. I went down to make rounds, and she was crying and laughing at the same time. She was just so excited that somebody had done this for them. She and her husband went crazy being so grateful. About 3:00 that morning, the nurse called me to say that she had a serious convulsion and was in a coma. Well, she died. In the weeks after the operation and delivery her blood pressure was perfectly normal. We went back over her chart. Now, a convulsion in pregnancy is usually thought to be eclampsia. But this was three weeks after her pregnancy was over. I don't know why she had the convulsion. Her husband came and took the baby home, and that was the last I ever saw of him. I don't know whether the great excitement about her bill being paid caused an emotional reaction that shot up her blood pressure. She must have had a hemorrhage in her brain, after we had worked so hard to save her life from the intestinal obstruction. I'll never forget that. You can't walk away from obstetrics. It is probably the most interesting specialty in medicine. You see all ranges of emotional reactions to the pregnancy. Some are good and some are bad.

"I did a few abortions at Ford Hospital after they became legal, but not very many of them. My patients just didn't have that kind of a problem. We had some abortionists here in Detroit, doctors who did abortions long before they were legal. They would get arrested occasionally, but they wouldn't stay arrested very long. They did a good job; the women didn't die. Being in an institution like Ford Hospital, I couldn't afford to do that kind of thing before it was legal. In those days, it was the publicity that was a worry. It wasn't a malpractice worry. I do think that abortion is a woman's right, and I think it ought to stay that way.

"After the war, there began to be a marked changed in the philosophy of using drugs in labor and delivery. Women were counseled so that they would tolerate labor better, so they could go through labor without any medication. I think less drugs was a good thing. I think it has been carried a little bit too far. I think that some poor obstetrics has resulted because of that philosophy. Rooming-in also became more prevalent. The idea of having the husband in the delivery room is all right if things are well-controlled. But every now and then an emergency happens at the time of delivery, and that is a bad time to have a husband present, especially some husbands. If everything is well and good, that's okay. But if an emergency comes up, it's not so good.

"I think women are not getting as good care perhaps. For instance, a lot of people talk about having babies without an episiotomy and without forceps. Well, there is an indication for forceps and there is an indication for episiotomy. A woman I know had a baby vaginally and tore the perineum into the rectum. She hadn't been put up in stirrups, and the doctor was faced with repairing this laceration without any preparation. He put in some stitches, but they became infected and the whole thing broke down. She had an opening right into the rectum. This wouldn't have happened if the patient had been properly prepared and delivered in stirrups, where the doctor could see. You can't see the perineum if the patient is thrashing around in bed. Six months later, she had to go to a proctologist and have the laceration repaired. The next baby had to be delivered by cesarean section. I think that is very poor obstetrics. If that patient had been properly prepared and put up in stirrups for delivery, and if the doctor had done an appropriate episiotomy at the time, chances are it wouldn't have ruptured into the rectum. Even if it had ruptured into the rectum, it could have been adequately repaired at the time, and it would have healed. She wouldn't have had this secondary operation by a proctologist.

"I think to some extent obstetricians have abrogated their responsibility to the patient by simply saying, 'This is her choice.' Well, certain things shouldn't be her choice; they should be the doctor's choice. The doctor knows whether or not she needs an episiotomy. How does she know? She can't even see it. You don't know how big the baby's head is going to be. Women don't really know what they are getting into. The doctor has let the patient make the obstetrical judgment that he should be making. I think that now the patient influences the obstetrician an awful lot.

"Most of my patients left their obstetrical care under my judgment. In certain circumstances I didn't give any options. For example, there are quite a few Jehovah's Witnesses in Detroit, and some of them are very adamant about refusing blood transfusions. A couple came into my office. The wife was pregnant. The husband said, 'I want you to take care of my wife, but I also want you to promise me that under no circumstance, emergency or otherwise, would you give my wife blood.' I thought and thought about it and didn't give them an option. I told them, 'I'm sorry, I think you are going to have to look for another obstetrician. I won't make that kind of promise, because I've got no way of foretelling the risk of complications. It's possible that she would get into a situation where she would bleed to death right under my very eyes. I'm not going to be responsible for somebody's death. If you forbid me to save a life by giving a transfusion, you ought to get another obstetrician.' And they did.

"One of the most pressing cases occurred later when I was department chairman. It was a resident's case. The patient had delivered, and then she started to bleed, and she bled and bled, and they couldn't stop it in the delivery room. Her religion would not allow her to take blood. She was comatose and practically dead. The resident called me in the middle of the night and said, 'What am I going to do? She is going to die if I don't give her blood. I can't get in touch with any member of her family.' I said, 'Give her blood.'

"The next day, all hell broke loose. Her husband came in along with a lawyer and a minister and a couple of other relatives. I assumed the blame completely, and I was about to be hung up and quartered because of my decision. I told the husband, 'Yes, I authorized the use of blood here. Your wife is alive now, and she wouldn't have been otherwise.' He thought it over a little bit and left. That was the last I ever saw of him.

"I had a gynecologic patient who had cancer of the uterus. She had to have her uterus removed. That can be a formidable operation, and sometimes there is considerable blood loss. She wanted me to promise not to give her blood. I told her my attitude: 'I promise you I won't give you blood except under an extreme emergency where I know I have to give it to you to save your life. Then I will give it to you, and I won't ask you, because you probably won't be in a position to make decisions.' Most Jehovah's Witnesses accepted that. The few who wouldn't accept it went someplace else.

"Dr. Pratt was getting up in years. In 1952, when he was seventy-two, he very reluctantly gave up the head of the department and retired. I was appointed chief of the Department of Obstetrics and Gynecology, and held that position until 1976—twenty-four years. Ford Hospital afforded a unique opportunity, because there was actually no limit on what one could do."

ROMANO

"One Song to Sing"—Education of the Medical Student

ROMANO REPEATEDLY told me how lucky he was to have had such marvelous training opportunities during the 1930s, when psychiatry was in its infancy as a modern medical field. He characterizes his experiences at Yale, Colorado, and Boston as "truly great"; they were chances for him to be on the cutting edge of his specialty. For aside from a few prestigious university centers and psychoanalytic institutes, psychiatry in the United States in the 1930s consisted of custodial care for the chronically mentally ill in state-run institutions.

Romano's teaching career really began in 1939 at the Peter Bent Brigham Hospital, where Soma Weiss appointed him to the Harvard faculty of the Department of Medicine—a first for a psychiatrist. Romano treated neurological and psychiatric patients and worked closely with physicians, medical students, and interns in medicine, neurology, and psychiatry. His research activities expanded. Here he discusses attitudes toward self-experimentation and the use of patients as subjects in research.

In 1941 he had the opportunity to chair the Department of Psychiatry at the University of Cincinnati College of Medicine. He instituted preclinical courses in psychological development and psychopathology and developed a full psychiatric curriculum for the four years of undergraduate medical education. His desire to train medical students to understand and appreciate the psychological and emotional problems of patients became his central interest during these years, and it remained so throughout his career.

Romano spent the years of the Second World War in Cincinnati, where he was deeply involved as a consultant to community agencies, advising them about the range of psychological problems that emerged on the home front during the war years. He conducted experimental research for the government. He was one of five psychiatrists selected by the State Department to study the emotional and psychiatric problems of combat in the European theater. The range of psychological problems

208

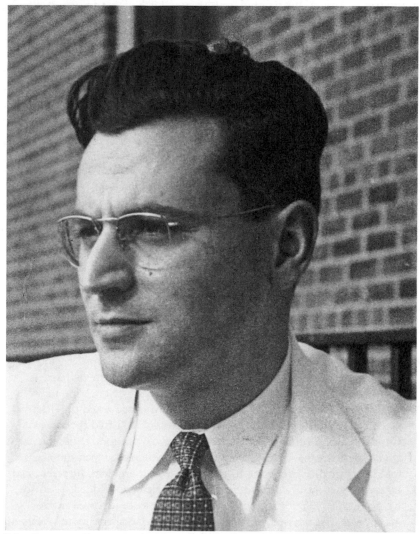

John Romano, Instructor in Neurology and Psychiatry, Peter Bent Brigham Hospital, Boston, 1939.

caused by the war made it evident to the military, to medicine, and to the public that psychiatry was no longer an occupation relegated to the back wards; it was now a specialty field relevant to many people's lives in a changing world.

When I submitted an early draft of the manuscript to Dr. Romano to check for accuracy, he deleted comments he had made about Soma Weiss's refusal to hire Jews on the medical staff of the Peter Bent Brigham Hospital in 1938–1940. He told me that remarks about Weiss could potentially hurt members of his family. I asked him to reconsider and suggested that his recollections of Soma Weiss, a Jew himself, are important historically. He agreed to retain the paragraph and wrote me a letter containing the following additional comments on his experiences with discrimination in medicine:

> Speaking of discrimination, I remember vividly an event which I considered outrageous. A black woman intern, the first to be appointed at Cincinnati, soon after her arrival walked into the house officers' dining room, where a number of interns of southern heritage threw chicken bones at her and left the room.
>
> I became most aware of antisemitism when I came to Rochester. If you have not read the recent biography of Arthur Kornberg, entitled *For the Love of Enzymes* [Harvard University Press, 1989], do so. He received his M.D. in Rochester in 1941. You will remember that he was the corecipient of the Nobel Prize in medicine in 1959. In his biography, he draws attention to the antisemitism at Rochester, particularly the attitude of the dean. Perhaps I became more aware of discrimination because of my role as a department chairman, meeting in regular sessions with other department chairmen. I had not done this at Cincinnati. On one occasion, one of the department chairmen wondered whether we (Rochester) were admitting too many "New York arabs" (which meant Jewish students). When I heard this, I asked the dean whether I could make a remark, which he allowed. I told the story of Christian X of Denmark, who told the Nazis, when they came, that he would wear the first Star of David on his sleeve. And when the Nazis told him that they had come to settle his Jewish problem, he responded by saying that the Danes had no Jewish problem, and added, "You see, we do not feel inferior to the Jews." A deep silence followed my remarks, and I am pleased to say that in the following twenty-five years of meetings of the Advisory Board (chairmen of preclinical and clinical departments, the dean, and occasionally the provost or president of the university), I never heard one public remark about Jews.

Romano was a pivotal figure in the creation of modern psychiatry, and he worked in several ways at once. He was among the first handful of psychiatrists to integrate psychiatric and related subjects into the medical curricula. He conducted scientific research for the government. He worked with local agencies, the military, and the public to treat mental disorders and to provide social services that would ease psychological problems. Through these endeavors he began to take psychiatry beyond the walls of the university and hospital setting and into the national community.

"I met Soma Weiss while I was at Boston City Hospital. He saw me working with patients. His house staff would talk about me. I remember seeing a couple of patients who were great problems. One was a young girl who had some strange, perverse behavior, and I helped her somewhat and that impressed one house officer, and he told Weiss. Weiss would make Tuesday night rounds for the whole City Hospital. I presented to him on a couple of occasions. So then he called me in. He asked me to come to the Peter Bent Brigham Hospital, along with Eugene Stead [general medicine] and Charles Janeway [infectious disease], to start the new Department of Medicine. He said, 'Will you become one of our three young men?' It was very exciting. I thought it would be a great opportunity. Stead later became professor at Emory and then professor of medicine at Duke, a very outstanding man. Charles Janeway was from the famous Janeway family, which goes back maybe a hundred years or so to nineteenth-century New York: Theodore Janeway was a professor of medicine at Hopkins after Osler. Charlie was professor of pediatrics later. We were the three young men that Weiss appointed to the full-time faculty.

"Soma Weiss was a very enthusiastic, charismatic man. He came here as an immigrant. He came to Boston and was put in the research unit, Thorndike Memorial Laboratory, at the Boston City Hospital. He did some very interesting work on hypertension, syncope [fainting], and kidney disease. He was chosen to become the Hersey professor in the theory and practice of physick, the oldest and most prestigious medical chair at Harvard. I remember some not very loud but distinct rumblings and questions about a Jew being chosen for this chair. Soon after we started at the Brigham, I proposed the name of someone who could assist me in my new appointment, and Soma Weiss gently, but firmly, rejected his name. The candidate I had in mind was Jewish, and I have forgotten exactly what Soma Weiss said, but something to the effect that he was not quite ready to make such an appointment. As I look back on it, he probably had been warned by others not to make many Jewish appointments at the beginning. Remember, this was 1938, 1939, 1940. Later on, as his confidence grew in his job, he made several appointments of Jewish persons.

"I will never forget the day we started, September 1, 1939, the day that Hitler bombed Warsaw. Soma Weiss got together the oldtimers, Samuel A. Levine, James P. O'Hare, Marshall Fulton, Russell Monroe. I'll never forget what Weiss said: 'These are my three young men, Stead, Romano, and Janeway. I hope you will give them the opportunity to earn your respect.' So they took me on rounds immediately, because I was the one whose throat they were ready to cut, being the psychiatrist. They showed me a patient, a beautiful young woman. She looked very much like Botticelli's 'Venus on the half shell.' They said she had periarteritis nodosa.[1] Among other findings, they said she had involvement of the median nerve. I saw her and saw a huge hematoma from a venipuncture. I thought maybe that had affected the median nerve. So I challenged the diagnosis, and guess what, I was right. After that, they said that Romano even knows where the median nerve is. The gossip from that traveled around the hospital. So that helped a great deal, just that one incident, just plain good luck.

"Then I worked very hard and saw patient after patient on the medical and surgical floors with the house officers without having a psychiatric service. I developed a new liaison service in medicine, neurology, and psychiatry. I had responsibility for both neurologic and psychiatric patients. The house officers were assigned to me for four months during the famous two-year Brigham internship. We would see every kind of neurological or psychiatric problem in the hospital. I was very busy as a clinician, seeing many, many patients of all kinds—neurologic, psychiatric, neurotic, psychotic, delirious, brain diseased, the whole repertoire. I saw everything. It was very broad.

"I took part in the teaching of neuroanatomy. I'd be called upon to present to the first-year students at Harvard examples of patients with lesions of the spinal cord, cerebellum, cortex, peripheral nerve, and so on. I was pleased to do that. I had a tremendous group of patients with all these lesions. This was to teach students very directly what happens if you have a stroke and how it would affect the body or affect the person with aphasia. I would present the case history of the patient, and the patient would come in. Then the patient would be dismissed or excused to go into another room, and we would discuss the implications of the case.

"In addition, I was involved in research along with Eugene Stead, James Warren, Max Michael, and others. We did research on neurological disease.[2] Also, I did a study of patients' reactions to ward rounds teaching. I studied them before, during, and after ward rounds.[3]

"In 1941, George Engel came to the Brigham, and we began our studies of delirious patients and of fainting. We would study the clinical course; we studied the person during his delirium—delirious with fever, delirious with infection, delirious with brain injury. We did psychological studies of attention, vigilance, memory. We did brain wave [EEG] studies. We would take blood from time to time and do blood chemistry studies. We would at times provoke fainting. For example, there was one man who could not stand; he would faint if he stood. He was all right when he was horizontal, but as soon as you raised the tilt table a certain degree, he would begin to faint. We found that he could postpone the fainting by mental effort. I had him do serial subtractions, three from one hundred, seven from one hundred, and so on. Or count from twenty backwards. Even though he was supposed to be fainting, he wasn't because of the mental effort. We did things like that.

"We studied patients with ulcerative colitis. We used a water balloon in the rectum to see whether or nor discussing emotional things would cause contractions. We didn't get positive results, because I learned later that timing is a problem; there isn't a point-to-point relationship between the discussion and the contractions. Once in a while we put air balloons in the stomach to provoke fainting. We did these things on ourselves first. It was open and voluntary. We continued those studies in Cincinnati and in Rochester.[4]

"As I look back on it, we never hurt anybody. We always had patients' oral permission and the permission of their doctors. One time one of the doctors sort of scolded me and said, 'I think you had Mrs. So-and-So down in the lab too long. I think she got fatigued.' I said, 'I think you are right, we were too long, we were wrong about that.' I remember that. But I don't remember any other comment of that kind. No one ever signed anything. You see, we knew these patients. They weren't strangers to us. We cared for them; we were their doctors and they trusted us. We trusted them and they trusted us. That was how it was.

"Everything was very modest in those days. My salary at the Brigham was four thousand dollars, with the opportunity on the Harvard plan to match it with more income from private care. But I didn't have much time for private care. The Commonwealth Fund contributed to our research program and wanted me to stay there permanently.

"In 1939, I was offered a Sigmund Freud Fellowship in psychoanalysis [1939–1942]. I was in a five-day-a-week analysis for almost three years. My analyst was John Murray. I learned something about myself. I experienced no major change. However, I was interested. I wanted to be as prepared as possible to be a psychiatrist. I didn't want to be a psychoanalyst. There were some very able people at the time at the Boston Psychoanalytic Institute. My closest friend there, Charles Brenner, another fellow, became a very distinguished psychoanalytic scholar. I attended the seminars at night. The claims made about psychoanalysis, the statements made at the time without any kind of support, any kind of validation, puzzled and troubled me.

"The breaks that I had—Yale, then the Commonwealth Fund in Colorado, and then the Rockefeller Fellowship at Boston and Harvard, then the Peter Bent Brigham job—all were major, truly great things that happened to me. I was lucky. Through all this, my interest in teaching was beginning: How can I help young doctors to be more aware of psychological problems? How can I help them understand something of their relationship to patients and their families? Someone once said, in one's life a man or woman has but one song to sing. If that is true, I think mine would be my interest in undergraduate medical student teaching more than graduate teaching or other matters. Intimately interwoven with this interest were the research activities and the continuing care of patients. My interest in teaching and in affecting the lives of others through teaching was the red thread woven into the whole fabric over the years. I don't think I can overemphasize that point.

"The dean at the University of Cincinnati College of Medicine was looking me over for the post of department chairman. It was a very modest department, just one or maybe two full-time people. They had a central clinic supported by the community chest. The university contributed about ten thousand to fifteen thousand dollars to it. There were a number of people whom I liked very much. Charles Aring was a prominent neurologist, and I'd known him for some time. I had known Milton Rosenbaum in Boston. He had gone back to his home in Cincinnati. So it looked interesting to me. I saw a broad opportunity at Cincinnati in terms of research, clinical teaching, a residency program for psychiatrists, and community service. So I made the decision to go. But it was not an easy decision. I went there as chairman in November 1941. Pearl

Harbor took place a month later, December 7. I was in the Harvard medical unit to go abroad, but Cincinnati asked for me: Could they excuse me to come and chair the department during the war years? I was taken out of the Harvard unit and allowed to go to Cincinnati. I finished all my research work and other things in Boston and left. One of my associates, George Engel, came with me.

"In Cincinnati, we were involved in war work. I chaired the department, taught medical students, and ran a ninety-bed unit. When I came to Cincinnati, they didn't have preclinical courses in psychiatry. I started those. In the first year, I tried to teach them something about growth and development, about the problems people have at certain stages in life, something of the psychology of illness, of convalescence, of disability, something of bereavement, grieving, something of the nature of the doctor and his patient and the relationship between them, and the nature of the patient and the patient's family. The second year, I taught psychopathology, including disturbances of attention, like delirium, dementia, and memory. There are disturbances of emotion, and I talked about mania, hypomania, the various kinds of depression, schizophrenia, and mental retardation. The third year, there was a four-week clinical clerkship on the psychiatric floors of the hospital—two floors for men, two for women. As a department chairman I was active in other affairs in the university, too.

"I really plunged into community affairs. I became a consultant to the Red Cross and would meet with their counselors. We would go over methods of counseling and advising. I'd give them some lectures on neuroses and psychoses and bereavement and grief and all kinds of other things. We were invited to the Wright Aeronautical factory, where thousands of people were making the motors for planes. Milt Rosenbaum and I conducted a teaching-counseling series for high school graduates who became counselors of employees. We persuaded the community to start movies early in the morning for people getting off the night shift, because you can't go to sleep right after you finish work. You have to eat and have some recreation. I would take the streetcar down to the juvenile court and meet with Judge Hoffman about problems of children. Then I would take the streetcar back and make rounds at the hospital. In the meantime, I was teaching medical students and running a department in a large city hospital, Cincinnati General Hospital, a huge, sprawling hospital.

"There was splendid harmony during the war years between the public and private health agencies. We had to work with many of the agencies, and I really learned through that experience how the community resources worked. Some of those agencies went back to the late nineteenth century. I was chosen to be the first professional member of the board of the Family Service Society in Cincinnati. Mostly, the board members were descendants of old families of wealth, but the membership became increasingly professional. I served on that board. I saw something that few psychiatrists at that time had an opportunity to see, something of the inner workings of an agency—its past, its present, where it is going. So those things were happening during the war years.

"I was one of the principal investigators in the war research we conducted for the Office of Scientific Research and Development.[5] We had a decompression chamber. I helped run the chamber, and I was also a subject in the chamber. I would go between thirty-five thousand and thirty-eight thousand feet in the chamber with oxygen while we studied bends. We were the first to show bubbles in tendon sheaths. We studied bends, decompression sickness, choking, fatigue. We wrote many papers on fatigue and on our other experiences with decompression.[6]

"We did a number of studies using the EEG machine to measure brain waves. At one time, the air force wanted to put freon into cockpits of combat planes as a fire preventive. We did one experiment with one human being using only 10 percent of the amount of gas that was to be introduced into a cockpit and found the man became delirious. George Engel and I had worked on delirium for a long time in Boston. So, the freon was out. The air force had worked it through experimentally with monkeys and chimps. But chimps don't fly planes. We were able to tell the air force immediately that you can't use freon.

"Then we were asked to study Atabrine. The Japanese had sunk the quinine ships; malaria was rampant. Atabrine was being used instead of quinine. It had been a drug that the Germans had introduced late in the nineteenth century. It had not been used very much and we had it, so we began to use it. However, there were troubles with it. Sometimes people got wacky with it or developed skin problems. Four of us took ten times the therapeutic dose of Atabrine for about ten days. Well, here I was, chairman of the department, and I was getting yellow, because it's a poison in a sense, like a dye. I became very yellow. Not only was I yellow, but my urine was yellow, perspiration was yellow, I even had yellow sclera. People would stop me in the street and ask if they could do something for me. I became restless, sleepless, and had frightening dreams. My wife and I used to drive to the hospital, I'd drive and she'd drive home again. She said she'd better drive, because I was making some mistakes. Atabrine was a cortical stimulant. My brain waves showed an increase in frequencies. It was causing similar behavior with the troops. One of our co-investigators on that project became acutely psychotic with this experience. It scared the hell out of us. We hospitalized him. We put a lot of glucose and salt through his veins. His manic psychosis lasted about two days. We were scared to death about him.[7]

"I look back on it now, the things I did and the things I had done to me: a balloon in my rectum, a balloon in my stomach, fainting with arterial punctures, puncturing the radial artery and the femoral artery in the groin. Even with an anesthetic a puncture of an artery is very painful. We did all these things in good faith. We never did anything on anybody before doing it on ourselves. One day at the Brigham we were studying blood volume with the dye, and I had two legs and one arm sealed off with tourniquets to pool the blood from circulation. I was horizontal but still fainting. I'll never forget the pain that came when the tourniquets were released. It's a pain like testicular pain. You feel nauseated; it's a terrible pain. That lasted maybe twenty or thirty minutes, that was all. We did all these things because we thought it was the right thing to do, to conduct that research. We couldn't ask anybody else to do it if we wouldn't volunteer to do it.

"Milton Rosenbaum was a tremendous help to me, more than anyone I can think of. There were only a few of us [full-time faculty] in Cincinnati, and we knew each other very well. There was a camaraderie and friendship, and we laughed at ourselves. There was humor. Milt would come out at the end of the day and say, 'There must be a better way to earn a living.' There was humor and a good feeling, even though we were working like hell with all those community things going on.

"Toward the end of the war, the State Department and the Department of the Army appointed five of us—Karl Menninger, Leo Bartemeier, John Whitehorn, Lawrence Kubie, and myself—to study the psychiatric problems, the combat problems, of our troops in the European theater. We were commissioned in uniform with a scientific consultant patch, and we were sent abroad. It was the last week of the war, almost too late in a way. We were sent to Paris and briefed there by General Paul R. Hawley, who was in charge of medicine for the European theater. He had been a Cincinnati graduate, and later on Cincinnati gave him an honorary degree. The five of us were sent in a command reconnaissance car to the Ninth Army, the First Army, the Third and the Seventh Army, and then back to Paris. On V-E Day—May 8, 1945—we were in a little town called Sušice—Schuttenhofen is the German name for it—in Czechoslovakia, not far from Pilsen. The military doctor in the battalion aid station had been a student of mine at Harvard. From the radio in the battalion aid station we heard Churchill's victory speech in London.

"We studied the problems of our troops at the battalion aid station. We had a chance to see some of the acute combat problems and also the problems as they emerged later on, which were different.[8] We studied patients in the rear of the front lines, in camps and hospitals in France and later in England. We went to Buchenwald shortly after it was opened up. Even though I had been a physician and psychiatrist for some time, the shock of Buchenwald made tears come to my eyes. I was shocked and saddened and thought, 'My God. Human beings did this. I, too, am a human being.'

"The military and the war experience emphasized the significance of psychiatry in relation to medicine and in relation to soldiers' morale. Many people pointed out that there was a higher incidence of combat fatigue in World War II than there had been for what was called shell shock during World War I. The war experience made it clearly evident that psychiatric problems were significant in terms of the selection of soldiers, recruitment, and induction.

"In 1945 I was invited to come to Rochester to give a lecture. The thing that impressed me most about Rochester was that I could have a better opportunity to teach medical students than I had in Cincinnati. I was well liked by the community in Cincinnati and by the university, but it didn't have the promise that Rochester had. I sensed that at Rochester the tradition of teaching medical students was of paramount importance. It was not easy to leave Cincinnati. The university, the medical school and the hospital, and the community were more than generous to us. Our friendships have survived these years."

A MORAL-TECHNICAL PROFESSION

MEDICINE DOES NOT stand outside or beyond morality. Medicine is a "moral-technical" profession as Eric Cassell, M.D., suggests, precisely because its goal is the welfare of others.[1] Morality in medicine includes a set of notions (albeit changing notions) about respect, responsibility, empathy, individuality, obligation, and dignity. It is concerned both with standards which guide action—what is right to do—and with a vision of what is good in society.

What is "right," of course, changed over time as medicine embraced science, became centered in the hospital, became committed to technology use, acquired potent drugs, and cured more and more diseases. Shields, in Part I, best articulates how "the right thing to do" therapeutically has changed so dramatically since his father practiced medicine. In this section, the doctors' narratives illustrate how the right thing to do has changed in other areas of medicine as well. The narratives reveal how standards of appropriate action and a vision of the good have evolved over the past decades with regard to experimentation on patients, house calls, and the physician's responsibility.

EXPERIMENTATION ON PATIENTS

The popular image of the physician during the 1920s, 1930s, and 1940s was of an empathetic caregiver primarily concerned with the welfare of the patient; that of the scientist was of an objective, detached experimenter and observer in pursuit of knowledge about the natural world. From a contemporary perspective, it is surprising that decades went by before the two roles—when combined together in one individual—were thought to clash. At the time these individuals were becoming physician-scientists, relatively little research on human beings had been conducted anywhere in the United States.[2]

Physician-scientists did not consider their subjects as free-choosing,

219

autonomous human beings for at least three reasons, as Beeson notes. Research subjects/patients were very ill, and many hopelessly so. Subjects were mostly drawn from charity hospitals, where their nonpaying status somehow made them grateful in physicians' eyes for medical attention and justified their use as subjects. Doctors did not identify with their study subjects, because they were different from them ethnically and socioeconomically. Taken together, study subjects' race, class, and patient status far outweighed their individual autonomy.

Only after the Second World War, when research efforts in general expanded rapidly, did the traditional role of the physician (empathetic caregiver) begin to challenge the newer role of the scientist (objective experimenter) over the issue of experimentation on human beings: How could one foster the best interests of the patient/subject while designing and carrying out systematic and rigorous research that would answer pressing medical and scientific questions? Today, patients and potential subjects have the right to decide whether or not to participate in research on the basis of as much information as they can possibly be given about the project's specific risks, discomforts, and direct benefits to them. They are free to withdraw from participation in experiments at any time. The process of gaining subjects' informed consent has been legally required for all federally funded research since 1966. It is from today's perspective that the doctors talk about the values that determined the relationship with the research subject and the entire research climate of the 1940s.

Beeson, Rhoads, and Romano comment that experimentation—on patients, medical students, or colleagues—was not fraught with perceived ethical dilemmas. There are at least two explanations for this. First, interests surrounding human experimentation that we now take for granted as potentially conflicting—medical, scientific, ethical, and legal—were not distinguished at all. Thus they could not be conceived as problematic during that era. Nor could they be evaluated by a public forum. The physiological or psychological risks of participating in a study were not weighed against the benefits of such participation. Such considerations were not even publicly formulated, let alone examined. Patient choice, autonomy, and education did not exist as values. Legal ramifications were rare or minimal.

Second, early research programs such as those described here were infused with a moral certainty that transcended potential ethical problems in the use of human subjects. The doctors did not question the value of their research endeavors, nor did their peers or superiors. Risks of participation—even those risks which had potential to be life-threatening—were in service to the knowledge gained by the research findings. Moral certainty legitimized human experimentation and helped keep any moral conflicts from surfacing.

Beeson reminds us of the social distance that separated doctors from most patients and the fact that patients seemed glad to be receiving care and attention, regardless of personal discomfort or risk to themselves. Patients were told they would be in a study; they were not asked to volunteer. They never questioned the importance of the research, asked for more information regarding risks or benefits to themselves, or refused to participate. Rhoads discusses experimentation on medical students, who, more than very ill patients, understood risks of participation in research yet were willing and eager to take part.

Both Romano and Rhoads inform us that in their experience invasive experiments were first performed on doctors who volunteered before they were tried on research populations. They explain that during this period, self-experimentation seemed justification enough for experimenting on others. The fact that the investigator personally experienced the risks and discomforts meant that others could be asked—and be expected—to face the same procedures. Romano notes that patients who served as subjects in his research did give their verbal permission to participate. They agreed on the basis of trust, *not on the basis of informed consent:* patients trusted their physicians not to harm them, to do something positive for them, and to act in their best interests.

Though it was not articulated, physicians also trusted their patients to be compliant research subjects and not to challenge the legitimacy of their projects. Assumptions that trust between doctor and patient was reason enough to experiment, that knowledge gained would outweigh any negative outcomes, and that authority and charity could command patient participation were not shattered until 1966. That year physician Henry Beecher published a report which disclosed how various investigators failed to protect the rights and interests of research subjects in a number of large studies.[3]

His work called into question assumptions about using research subjects without their informed consent. A cultural consciousness about subjects' rights to information, to volunteer or not, and to ask questions freely about risks and benefits emerged from the information Beecher published. As a result, federal guidelines and regulations about the protection of human subjects were instituted and physician-scientists could no longer carry out experimental research without institutional and federal approval.[4] The conscience of experimental medical science became constrained by the rights of its subjects.

THE HOUSE CALL

For Shields, Jarcho, and Olney, the house call both extended the physician's work into the community and symbolized the breadth of the physician's responsibility. The home setting was valued, because in it the doctor could know more about the patient. Shields talks extensively about the importance of the house call. He told me: "When I enter the house, I learn about the economic status of the patient's family. I become familiar with the interrelationships of family members, their emotional problems, something about the capabilities of each individual, and their strengths and weaknesses. In other words, I learn about the many factors that impact on the patient." Similarly, Jarcho and Olney comment that getting to know patients' families and working with social workers "to solve problems with the family" were invaluable aspects of their education and practice, enriching their ability to understand the full range of patients' illnesses and then treat them more effectively.

The house call diminished in importance following the Second World War. When medical care became centered in the hospital and clinic, physicians came to rely more on objective laboratory and technological criteria for diagnosing and understanding diseases and less on the psychological and social features of the person who was ill. "Hard" laboratory results were becoming the key to curing diseases. Knowledge about the patient's life, useful and important in care plans when cures did not exist, came to be seen as relatively useless, irrelevant, and unnecessarily time-consuming in the practice of scientific medicine. In addition, the more intimate personal relationship with the patient fostered by the house call came to be devalued.

"Home care" clerkships exist today in medical school training, and those training experiences may be the only time some doctors make house calls. With the use of technology so dominant, some medical students become deeply troubled or uncomfortable interacting with patients in the home, where most technology is absent. In a recent study of one home care program clerkship, anthropologist Andrea Sankar found that medical students were overwhelmed by the amount of nonbiological information they encountered in the home setting. Those students felt "out of control" when they could not direct conversation and activity as smoothly or authoritatively as they could in the clinic. They were extremely ill at ease managing the emotional intimacy with patients that the home setting engendered.[5] Such negative responses to being in patients' homes are a relatively new development in medicine. Unfortunately, federal and private insurance reimbursement policies reflect negative attitudes toward house calls, thus adding fuel to the fire: It is simply not cost-effective for doctors to make house calls today, even if they want to.

RESPONSIBILITY

The lines between organic disease, psychosomatic illness, and nonmedical personal problems have never been clearly drawn, and today problems such as stress, chronic fatigue syndrome, disabling allergies of unknown origin, and depression still confront physicians with how little is known about relationships among mind, body, and emotions. In patient care before the Second World War, patients whose illnesses had a psychological component generally were not referred to the relatively few psychiatrists in community practice. Rather, doctors attempted to treat whatever patients presented to them. Both Shields and Jarcho, the community-based doctors, note that much of what they treated was "psychic trouble," "emotional trouble." Shields states that 80 percent of the illnesses he saw in his early years of practice were psychosomatic in nature. Both men treated nonorganic illness with talk and felt it was their responsibility to do so; however, Shields specifically discusses the problems of the internist whose sense of obligation encompassed more features of the patient than he was trained to deal with.

Perhaps Olney defines the doctor's responsibility most broadly among these individuals, delineating her role as one of nurturing the self-image of children and youth who had more than strictly physiological problems resulting from their diabetes. The camp she created and directed for fifty years enabled her to treat psychological and social problems as well as biological aspects of disease. Olney's goal was to give children the self-esteem and interpersonal skills that would enable them to go into the world and lead productive, full lives not dominated by what was once an extremely debilitating and ultimately fatal illness. At the same time, camp provided an environment in which Olney could learn about the nature and management of the physiologic disease process itself.

Outside of pediatrics, nonorganic aspects of illness became more and more problematic for medicine when medicine embraced science. Because those aspects were less likely to be cured or treated by technological means, they came to be considered peripheral to medicine's purpose—the cure and management of disease. The nonorganic was pushed outside the realm of the new biomedicine. This has been continually difficult for psychiatry, the specialty that treats organic and nonorganic illness with both "scientific" drug therapies and "nonscientific" talk therapies.[6] And during the 1940s, it was problematic, as Shields describes, for internists whose sense of responsibility included treatment of the nonorganic.

Even within the realm of organic disease, there were mixed opinions about limits to a physician's responsibility. Hodgkinson's sense of responsibility extended to women's breasts, which had been previously excluded from gynecologists' care for monetary and turf reasons. The consequences of army doctors who failed to fully examine women in the armed services were sometimes tragic, as he reports. His personal obligation to discover and treat breast diseases led him to conduct prophylactic breast examinations and to use the new drug, penicillin, to treat breast infections and prevent breast abcesses in postpartum women.

Hodgkinson also describes how the physician's responsibility extends to the issue of control over choices in treatment: the surgeon must be free to make decisions about blood transfusions, and the obstetrician is obliged to control the birth process. He argues that professional knowledge and technology, when used appropriately, benefit women and their babies and that physicians' assumptions of authority are for the welfare of the patient. Recent critics of obstetrics' power argue that physicians' control and the increased use of technology are detrimental to women's and families' experiences of the birth process as a profound and wonderful life-cycle event.[7] For Hodgkinson, lack of appropriate intervention in the diagnosis of disease, prevention of infection, promotion of complication-free deliveries, and saving of lives constitutes moral-technical failure.

The debate about physician versus patient responsibility and authority has been perhaps most vocally illustrated in the field of obstetrics since the 1960s with women's growing desire for more control over their pregnancies and births. They have wanted to be free to choose whether or not to have drugs, hospital or home births, and friends attending them during their births. The mastery women desire over pregnancy and birth can be seen as a paradigmatic case for the responsibility-in-medicine debate in general. But the demand for access to therapeutic choices, medical information, and experimental drugs, and the desire for control in carrying out treatment plans were not yet features of the doctor-patient relationship during the 1940s.

PART IV

Power and Influence: 1946–1970s

Biomedical technology is rapidly approaching a state of development that will make it possible to modify several aspects of man's nature. The transplantation of organs and the use of mechanical prostheses may soon become commonplace. Personality will be increasingly modifiable through physiological and embryological manipulations. Even the genetic make-up of man may become amenable to willful alteration. Since most of what we try to do will probably come to pass, we must give thought to the long-range implications of our scientific programs; we must try to evaluate prospectively the potential effects of manipulating the human body and mind, lest there be analogues of the nuclear bomb in the medical future of mankind! Unfortunately, while the scientific method is immensely effective for dealing with the technical aspects of biomedical problems, it provides no philosophical basis or ethical guidance for relating technical solutions to the fundamental needs or aspirations of man.

—*René Dubos,*
  Man Adapting, 1965

IDEALISM AND CONFLICT
IN THE GOLDEN AGE

THE YEARS OF unprecedented growth in university medical centers, medical school departments, and biomedical research programs have been referred to as medicine's Golden Age. Those years of expansion, approximately 1945–1965, also represent the period of medicine's greatest prestige and political influence in American society.[1] The seven doctors' mature years of practice coincided with medicine's Golden Age. I wanted to know how they defined their goals, responsibilities, and constraints during those years. I asked them to describe the period they consider to be the height of their careers. I also asked when and how they knew they were becoming role models for others.

When they described the height of their careers, the physicians spoke about their roles in medical, community, and government organizations. Their discussions emphasize both their views of medicine's responsibilities to a wider society and their personal commitments to widely conceived public service. The doctors were called on and were willing to broaden the scope of their medical activities beyond direct patient care, teaching, and clinical research to include: work for medical organizations (Shields and Hodgkinson), universitywide service (Rhoads and Romano), government service (Jarcho, Rhoads, and Romano), work for philanthropic organizations (Rhoads), the creation of state and county insurance plans (Romano), and participation in community education programs (Olney). They each felt that their perspective, as physicians, could contribute in some way to a larger social good.

But reflections on their idealism were tempered when they also recalled the emerging tension created by the proliferation of information and technology and a rapidly changing health care delivery system. When they talked about the more recent past, Shields and Rhoads discussed conflicts over how doctors were paid. The tension between predetermined salary versus fee-for-service reimbursement concerned Shields as a community practitioner and Rhoads as an academic surgeon. Those conflicts reflected a clash of values between the desire for equality among

229

colleagues in order to promote institutional democracy and cohesion and the desire to be paid according to one's individual efforts, stature, and seniority.

Tensions developed also between old medical ideals, such as the responsibility for making house calls and doing charity work, and new priorities created by an increasingly complex health care bureaucracy. For example, the need for patients to have "diagnoses" covered by insurance plans, the trend of seeing patients only in offices and hospitals, where diagnostic tools are located, and the rising cost of malpractice insurance, all forced older physicians to rethink their established routines and led younger doctors into patterns of work that differed dramatically from that of their predecessors. Shields and Jarcho discuss the ideals of medical practice as being potentially and actually threatened by the monetary interests of the solo practitioner. Jarcho echoes Hodgkinson's deep concern about threats of lawsuits brought by litigious patients and their families.

The postwar decades were a period of rapid and extensive subspecialization with the proliferation of scientific knowledge and diagnostic and therapeutic capabilities. Specialists were constantly redefining their areas of expertise. Shields and Jarcho took the board examinations for internal medicine. Though they continued to practice general medicine during the early postwar years, their mutual goal was to be regarded by patients and colleagues alike as specialists in internal medicine. Olney recalls that, when cardiology became more of a surgical specialty and surgeons could more frequently correct the cardiac problems of children, she was less often called on to treat problems in that field. As a result, diabetes came more to the forefront of her work.

With subspecialization came increasing fragmentation in the delivery of medical care. These physicians fought and resisted that fragmentation as best they could. Shields and Jarcho remained broadly based community internists. Beeson began reflecting on and writing about problems in medical care created by too many specialists.[2] Olney, who became a cardiac and diabetes specialist, emphasized the emotional and social as well as physical treatment of the child throughout her career. Her ability to bring together a variety of approaches to treatment, care, and healing in the diabetes camp is a testament to her integrative capacities and her vision of the whole child. Hodgkinson worked for years to create general surgical training for his obstetrics and gynecology residents in order to broaden their fields of knowledge and expertise. He strongly believed that gynecological surgeons should be able to handle any surgical problem they confronted, and that they could be prepared to do so only if they were trained as general surgeons, as he had been. Romano understood that psychiatrists were physicians first and foremost. He created a two-year internship program that thoroughly integrated psychiatry with other medical fields. And he educated countless numbers of medical students to incorporate principles of psychiatry into their work—regardless of their specialty field.

SHIELDS

"Medicine Was Glorious Fun"

IMMEDIATELY AFTER THE Second World War, Shields got his chance to specialize in internal medicine. Here, he talks about the first uses of penicillin and the antibiotic streptomycin, and how miraculous and dramatic they were. He recalls the introduction of new laboratory equipment which enabled him to make more precise diagnoses. He was the first person in his area of the state to specialize in pulmonary diseases, and he talks about his treatments of tuberculosis, emphysema, and polio, and his establishment of the respiratory therapy department at Concord Hospital.

Of all his accomplishments, Shields is most proud of his group practice—a partnership of three internists during the 1950s. He describes their arrangement, though short-lived, as idyllic and extremely unusual. Their earnings were pooled and divided equally among themselves. Each doctor in the partnership saw every patient and they consulted on each one as a team, thus giving their patients maximum attention. They learned medicine from one another by discussing cases and reviewing the medical literature. They created a community in which the common good had the highest value. When the practice expanded to include other physicians, it became more efficient. As a result, the partners stopped sharing information in conferences. And they no longer divided their earnings equally. In retrospect, Shields regrets the loss of that ideal community and feels that its breakdown is his greatest failure.

Shields wanted me to know throughout our interviews that his wife was an essential part of his career. He is the only one of these physicians who expressed such a view. He told me that she helped him expand his practice and attain positions of leadership in medical organizations through her ability to meet people easily—a trait he claims he has never had.

"Beginning immediately after the war, I became the medical consultant to the VA hospital which is in Manchester, New Hampshire. That

232

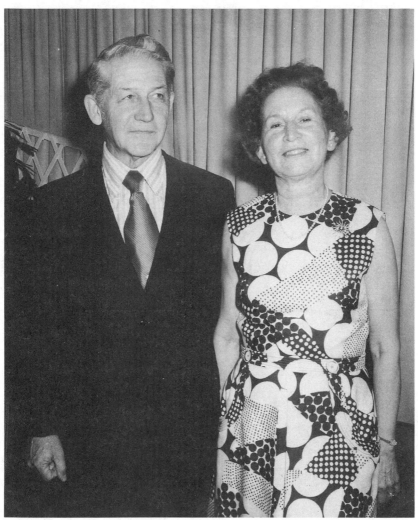

Dr. and Mrs. J. Dunbar Shields, 1968, the year he was president of the New Hampshire Medical Society and she was president of the Women's Auxiliary of the Medical Society. At the time, they were the only doctor and wife in the U.S. holding such positions in state medical society/auxiliary affairs. Courtesy John P. Bowler, MD Memorial Library, New Hampshire Medical Society.

allowed me to do some teaching. We had students, first from Boston University School of Medicine, and then from Harvard. I went down twice a week and made rounds with the staff or the students. I occasionally gave a talk. I usually spent about three hours there. The chiefs of medicine that I worked with were very fine people. The staff was interesting and good. I saw their tough cases. That work gave me some experience in government medicine: What input should the government have here? It was an interesting part of my medical career and I continued that after I retired.

"The war was a terrible hiatus as far as my own practice was concerned. When I came back, I found that some other doctors had gotten fat on my practice. Some of my patients were so loyal to the people who had taken care of them when doctors were so scarce, they felt they couldn't just leave them. But that was not true of my referral doctors. So I actually concentrated more on hospital work and on seeing patients that were referred to our office largely for diagnosis and for suggestions for treatment. A lot of my work was in the hospital. At one time I had 85–90 percent of the medical patients in the hospital.

"Penicillin became available very quickly after the war. That changed my practice. With pneumonia, we just threw the antitoxin serum away. We now could do such wonders. We stopped losing the forty-year-old men with pneumonia. And it completely changed the course of venereal disease. But penicillin was restricted to the coccal organisms. We began to get more of the bacillary infections it seemed. Those became a big problem.

"I had a very dramatic introduction to the antibiotic streptomycin. My daughter, Eve, had idiopathic peritonitis when she was eight years old. She did not have a ruptured appendix or an obvious cause of this. She just got desperately ill and looked as though she were going to die. Of course sulfonamides didn't help, and penicillin was useless. I had heard of streptomycin, and I knew Dr. Chester Keefer. He was a Boston man and the infectious disease man in America. He had control of streptomycin as an experimental drug. I also knew that, in order to use streptomycin in the experimental program that was conducted in teaching institutions, one had to have a proven culture. That was reasonable, but my daughter was dying. If she had had a ruptured appendix, we would have been able to isolate the organism. But all of her symptoms said peritonitis. It wasn't pneumococci, because penicillin didn't do any good. We thought it was probably colon bacillus, although we couldn't prove it. So I went to see him, armed with nothing. Chester Keefer was the most compassionate individual that ever lived in the history of civilization. He broke all the rules and gave me streptomycin. I gave it to my daughter, and she was better in the expected period, about two days. That tells you what antibiotics did. After streptomycin, the antibiotics just piled up, one after another, and from that time we were able to do so much for anything that was caused by a bug.

"The other thing that changed my practice after the war was the laboratory. One of the people that influenced my practice was our pathologist, Jim Parks. He was the closest friend I've ever had in my life. He was a brilliant man, even though he worked just in this small hospital. He was a mathematician. He loved to do math so much that he did intricate analytic geometry or algebra problems for pleasure. He was a great pathologist. I went to almost every autopsy he did, because I learned so much from him. Back in those days, we learned from autopsies.

"I got Jim Parks to get a flame photometer [for blood sodium and potassium determinations] so we could do blood chemistries. Prior to that we could only do blood sugars and blood ureas, but then we got into the elements: sodium, potassium, chloride, and carbon dioxide. We learned the importance of sodium depletion, potassium depletion. We used to estimate potassium by taking electrocardiograms to see what the ECG looked like. That was the biggest early diagnostic advance as far as I was concerned. We learned to do arterial punctures. We were finally getting a little more sophisticated. Following that were the tecniques in radiology and the injection of blood vessels. And later came the CAT scan.

"I took the internal medicine boards in 1947. That was not required at the time. I was one of the first people in New Hampshire to take the boards, and I'm rather proud of that. I didn't get in on the grandfather clause as a lot of people did. Some of the professors of medicine were certified by the grandfather clause. For example, somebody who was the head of a medical department at Dartmouth would be given certification. None of my contemporaries took the boards at that time. But I felt it was something that should be done. If I really was going to be an internist, I didn't want to go under any false colors. The only way to be a real internist was to take the boards to prove you were. I really studied for the exam. My wife and I went out to Chicago. I spent about a week before the boards in the hotel room cramming to the last degree. And then I took them at the Cook County Hospital.

"My sponsor for the boards was a great influence in my life after coming to New Hampshire—Paul Dudley White. He was my ideal. Until I moved here, I didn't know much about him. He was not as well-known in the South. But when I came here I took a course in cardiology in Boston, and he ran the course. I got to know him slightly then. He was very, very kind to me after that and took an interest in my taking the boards. He wrote to the boards and recommended me. Later I had some cases I wanted seen on consultation, and I sent people down to him. Then I got to know him quite well. Dr. White was one of the great pioneers in medicine. He is known now as one of the two or three greatest contributors to the knowledge of cardiovascular disease. He also was an outstanding clinician, and in addition, he was an extremely compassionate person who loved his fellow man. My relationship to him included not only "sitting at his feet" but also sharing with him in the care of patients.

"I was seeing a lot of people with lung disease. I became particularly interested in tuberculosis, because it was such a widespread disease. It had a great impact on our health care. So many people had tuberculosis, and we could do so little for it. But we were trying to do things for it. So much of our medical resources prior to the advent of antibiotics was used in the investigation, research, and care of tuberculosis. One of the main things we were trying to do was keep the lung at rest as well as the body. In order to do that, we collapsed the lung. We collapsed the affected area by doing what we called pneumothorax. We put air into the space between the lung and the chest wall and pushed the lung down, deflating it by putting air into that cavity. The lung acts as a bellows. When we couldn't do that we did various things to the diaphragm, because the diaphragm is a big muscle between the abdomen and the lung and is most responsible for breathing. We would collapse the diaphragm on one side by crushing the phrenic nerve, which is found in the neck. It energizes the diaphragm. We used a combination of pneumothorax and phrenic crush. Thoricoplasty was another treatment. The surgeons would take out pieces of ribs, maybe five or six ribs, which would crush in the chest. That was a more defacing job of course. But in those days, when we couldn't do anything else, we just had to try to stop the course of that horrible disease. Those methods of therapy were perhaps not as gruesome as they sound, and they represented the choice of the lesser of two evils. The patient was very ill, suffering, and without intervention could only look forward to a slow death. Those methods were resorted to only in extreme cases. Many people with the disease got well with rest and supportive treatment. When definitive treatment became available in the early 1950s, those extreme measures were no longer needed.

"I became interested in doing pneumothoraces and got a machine and learned how to do them. The air that we put in was gradually absorbed. So about every ten days or two weeks, we'd have to do a refill of either the chest or the abdomen. I started doing that on a couple of patients. Then I decided that I wanted to do it for the state. I got in touch with Dr. Robert Kerr, who was an authority on tuberculosis and who headed the two TB hospitals in New Hampshire. One was here near Concord and the other was up in the mountains. Dr. Kerr thought there was no reason why TB patients had to go to hospitals anymore for pneumos. He would send them to my office. So I did a lot of pneumothoraces for people all over the state.

"The next thing I became interested in was emphysema, because we knew so little about it. I sent patients up to Hanover. But at that time, that particular clinic didn't have anybody that knew anything about emphysema. The people there didn't know as much about it as I did. But there was a Dr. Maurice Segal in Boston who knew something about it. He came up to see a patient in consultation with me and brought up the first positive breathing machine that I'd ever seen. We used that machine in the early treatment of emphysema. Dr. Segal helped me a great deal. I talked with him a lot, he told me what to read, and I watched what he did with my patients. I became more and more interested. I joined the American College of Pulmonary Physicians and went to college meetings. They had excellent clinical sessions.

"Then I got interested in respiratory therapy. Pulmonary emphysema and chronic bronchitis are almost the same thing. As a matter of fact, in England they call pulmonary emphysema chronic bronchitis. One of the treatments was to get the bronchi dilated and clean the bronchial tree. So respiratory therapy was an extremely important part of the treatment for emphysema. I established a respiratory therapy department at the Concord Hospital. It has become the most lucrative department they've ever had in the hospital and is used now for many conditions. The respiratory therapist comes to see almost everybody who has an operation.

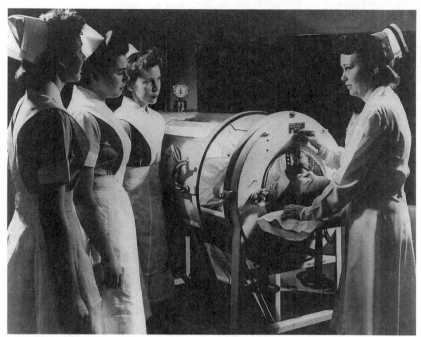

Student nurses learning about the iron lung, late 1940s. Courtesy Concord Hospital Archives.

"I was the first person in this part of the state who did any work with pulmonary diseases, and therefore I did a lot of it. I liked it. On the other hand, I didn't like it because we still can do so little for emphysema.

"I also became interested early in polio. We had a terrible epidemic of polio here in 1952. And we had a lot of bulbar polio, where it affects the brain, particularly the respiratory center. We had such a big epidemic that we turned one floor of the Concord Hospital over to taking care of polio. I did a lot of polio work. I had this wonderful physiotherapist, Lucia [Tookey] Ryan, who later became my nurse and one of the best friends we ever had in our lives. She had some experience with the work in polio. In those days, we treated patients with hot packs; they were wrapped in hot packs. It did a lot of good, because it reduced some of the spasms of the peripheral muscles. But the bulbar polio had to be treated with respirators. That was before the kind of respirators we have now. We didn't do intratracheal tubes and hitch them up to the respirator. That is a more simple procedure and is much more sophisticated and effective. All we had was the old iron lung. We had six iron lungs in Concord Hospital. We had to send all over New England to get six iron lungs. And we had six people in those iron lungs all the time. Tookey was in charge of that aspect of it, along with me. We didn't have a respiratory therapist. We didn't have blood gases. We had to guess by God to run those iron lungs. We did the best we could. We lost a few people. I got interested in respiratory therapy through that experience also.

"My group practice is the thing that I have done in the medical world that I'm most proud of. I'd like to talk about my office organization, because it illustrates some of the problems of group medicine. A group of physicians at that time was somewhat rare; a group of internists was unheard of. I started out after the war being so busy that I needed help. First, I had some young doctors that I hired as assistants. It worked out quite well. I had one young man from Concord who worked with me for a while. He was really a very good guy, a very big help. He worked out of my office and took over for me at times when I wanted to go away. It was a time when my son was up to his ears in athletics, and I had to get to those games. I had three separate assistants, each one of them being a little bit more sophisticated than the last. All of them worked out reasonably well.

"Then I had the idea of having a communal group practice. I wanted to eliminate from medicine as much of the profit element as I could. I wanted to be able to practice medicine, pool our knowledge, and not be worried about who was making more than whom. I started with Dr. Paul Lena. That was about 1953. We practiced together and split what we made. We had an office manager. Paul's first medical interest was hematology and oncology. My son helped us out on a couple of occasions—one summer as an intern and one summer after his residency at the New York Hospital. We never could get him to come with us. In a way, that is a sore spot. But in a way I'm proud of him, because he wanted to do just what I did, but he wanted to do it on his own. He now has a six-man group in Macon, Georgia.

"Then I got Dr. David Underwood. David had had extensive training in gastroenterology at New York Hospital and in London. He also knew a lot of neurology and a lot of cardiology. But he also knew something about everything, just as Paul did. He was top-notch. He was considered the best chief resident that New York Hospital had had in years. Nobody knew how I talked him into coming in with us.

"It was an ideal partnership with the three of us, an idyllic time.

When I told the really big shots that I met at college meetings about how our partnership worked, they just watered at the mouth. There was no money angle with the way we did it. What money we made was split into three equal parts. We had an office manager, and we never looked at the books.

"We had a practice routine. We met at the hospital at 7:00 A.M. From 7:00 to 7:30 we sat and briefed each other on every patient we had on our service. If I had a patient in the hospital who had a GI problem, David would see him. The next day we would talk about that problem. We talked about all the patients every day. We had a free interchange of ideas about the patients, so we were learning all the time. After talking about every patient, we saw every patient as a group. Then we went back and saw a particular problem, someone who was unusually sick or something. If I was away and something happened to a patient and Dave was on call, he knew absolutely everything about that patient. The patients got a lot of attention and the benefit of three brains. And we had the benefit of consultation among ourselves.

"It was a complete community among the three of us. We spent most all of the mornings at the hospital, because there was so much to do. In the afternoons we would see patients in the office. Once a week we had lunch together. That was a full hour of literature. One person would be commissioned to present the current literature on some subject that day. If he had been to a meeting, he would tell us what he had learned there. We arranged it so we went to a lot of meetings and courses. I learned a tremendous amount of medicine from Paul Lena and David Underwood. When you're practicing good medicine, you're learning medicine. Medicine was glorious fun.

"But then we got to be big shots. We were going to have a bigger group to be able to have more time off. It wasn't because of money. It was because we wanted more leisure time. About four or five years into our group practice, we brought in a fourth man. His interest was cardiology. It wasn't very long after he came aboard that he said we were wasting too much time at the hospital. He felt the conferences were unnecessary. He harped on that more and more. Then he said that the business of splitting the money was not right, because he was doing more procedures. That is the big word in medicine today—'procedures.' He was doing more cardiac procedures. He was making more money, so he wanted more money. So we changed our arrangement.

"Now, why didn't I stop this guy? I think that is one of my failures in life. It was lack of proper leadership. That man was very quiet in his movements. It took him quite a long time to make those changes. He was surreptitious. He just worked these things into our meetings, gradually. He had an equal voice, and he was able to convince Paul and David that that was the right thing to do. He changed our method of payment. Each of the four of us was paid according to how much business we brought in. In other words, we got paid according to what money we made. That is the way it is done everywhere. The ideal system that we had before was done nowhere else. Then we took on a fifth and sixth person. And the situation got worse and worse. Around that time I had my first coronary infarct. So I slackened the reins of leadership a little more. And it was a democratic organization. The decision to take on more people was not my decision; it was a group decision.

"I didn't have anything to do with organized medicine for many years. I was too busy, and I looked down on it. But later in my career, I began to think about medicine's problems as they related to society. And I began to think I wanted to find out something about them. I started out as a delegate in the state medical society, doing this and that job. I just became more interested and more involved as I went along. My wife was most helpful during that part of my career. She meets people and is so interested in people and can meet them so well. She would come with me to meetings and get me involved with people. In 1966 I became president of the New Hampshire Medical Society. My wife was president of the medical auxiliary when I was president of the medical society.

"That was also the year I was head of the state chapter of the American College of Physicians. It was the year that Medicare and Medicaid were getting started. Medicare raised its ugly head just about the time I was beginning to get seriously interested in medical politics. It was just about the time I was speaker of the house in the state medical society. So I watched it come. Of course at first, organized medicine was very much against it and fought it. Yet some of us knew that it was inevitable. It has had some of the advantages that we hoped it would have. It has taken care of some people who probably were not getting good medical care. But it has had some disadvantages too. It has ruined the doctor from an ethical standpoint, I think. First, it has taught the doctor to do so much medical padding. When a doctor goes to a nursing home to see one patient, he gets a certain fee. If he's got five patients in there, he walks in and says hello to all five of them. And he gets paid for all five. Second, there's no more charity work done. Doctors now collect anywhere from

96 to 99 percent of their bills. Of course they complain that they are not paid enough by Medicare. And indeed they probably are not. But Medicare has taken out of medicine the pleasure that doctors had in doing work for nothing. And it has made everybody more money-minded. We are undoubtedly a more avaricious society regarding medical fees than we were prior to government control."

JARCHO

Diagnosis, Treatment, and the Conditions of Life

HERE JARCHO TALKS about some of medicine's postwar changes—
to the profession's detriment. He describes the demise of anatomical
pathology as a loss of knowledge, and the obsolescence of the house call
as the neglect of social responsibility. He views the more recent rise of
malpractice suits and general litigiousness in society as terribly problematic for the practice of medicine. He remains keenly aware of the relationship between disease and the cultural background of the patient including language, religion, migration patterns, and behavior. Younger
doctors who lack sensitivity to that relationship trouble him. When he
was still in practice, he continued to conduct research on problems that
piqued his interest in tropical medicine and cartography. His work in the
history of medicine grew.

"One of the first things I did in 1946 was to see about my job in
the Department of Pathology at Columbia. When I was an instructor
and then an associate before the war, we had marvelous anatomical
collections—slides, specimens carefully described, and photographs—
all carefully indexed. This had taken years and years of dedicated
effort. It was a treasury of knowledge. After all, the basis of anatomical pathology was really in those specimens and in one's understanding of them. In 1946, I found that the new professor was throwing
out the specimens. You could have stabbed me and it would have hurt
less. It was knowledge going down the drain. The morgue-keeper was
still there, an old-fashioned, meticulous German. He called me aside
and said, 'Dr. Jarcho, they are throwing away the specimens. I saved
the three jars that you brought in and have hidden them.' He gave
them to me. They contained material about schistosomiasis, which I
had obtained from Egypt through the help of my father, who was the
friend of a professor in Cairo. I took these jars in my arms and carried
them in a taxi to Mount Sinai, where the assistant pathologist, a
Japanese, practically kowtowed in front of me. In the classroom at

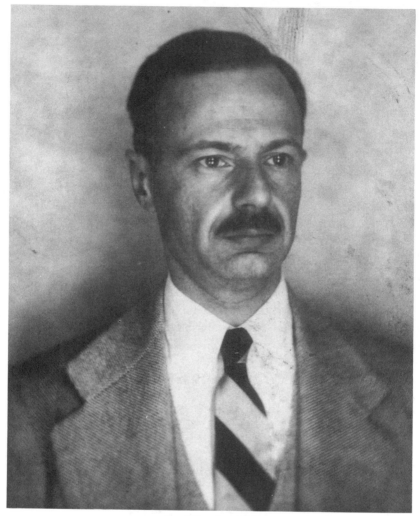

Saul Jarcho, 1948.

Columbia, I saw that instead of teaching the students by means of microscope slides, they were using photographs, a step away from reality. I emerged hurt by the fact that it is possible to destroy a wonderful organization so very quickly, and I immediately decided not to accept reappointment.

"I resumed work at Mount Sinai Hospital. For five years I worked there full time as assistant in charge of research in the Department of

Medicine. It was not then a formally academic institution. I was also active there as a visiting physician for about six years, from 1946. At the same time I was reestablishing my practice. I saw my private patients in the morning and made ward rounds at Mount Sinai in the afternoon. I made house calls whenever I had to. My absence of four years had caused me to lose a great part of the practice, a measurable part of my small income, a girlfriend, and probably some miscellaneous components that I have forgotten.

"After the war the trend toward medical specialization increased. Almost everybody had taken the board examinations in some specialty. I took the internal medicine boards in 1950. There were comparatively few doctors left who were known as general practitioners, but we internists did general practice. House calls almost disappeared.

"I continued to make house calls. I made them willingly, knowing that they were a financial loss. You can hardly make a house call and get back to your office in under an hour. Suppose someone has a respiratory infection and you need to make a few visits. The patient can't pay you for three or four hours. They don't see that as fair. I felt that I was obligated to see patients day or night, whether I wanted to or not, although I knew I was losing money. One night about 3:00 A.M. I was called to see a sick woman. It was raining very, very heavily. The street lights had disappeared. The wind took my hat and blew it under an automobile. My clothes were soaked. I saw the woman and did what I could for her. There was no discernible gratitude. That sort of thing happened with numerous variations. I am often told that I was one of the last physicians in New York to make house calls. I think that is an exaggeration, but I made house calls up until about one year before I retired, in 1980.

"I lost some of the allegiance of my loyal older son because of a certain man who had heart failure and phoned me in the middle of the night nine times in ten nights or eleven times in ten nights, and my little son was always awakened. It was at that time that he decided not to become a physician.

"I was little interested in money. Although not wealthy, I managed. Over the years, I took a beating financially from numbers of patients. Nonpayers. But, as far as I can judge, I remained idealistic throughout my years of medical practice.

"It was wonderful, incredible, when antibiotics came in. We had to be sure we weren't fooling ourselves. We'd have a patient who could be expected to be suffering from high fever and chills. We've given this new medicine, and look, he was sitting up and paying attention—incredible. For many years before this, we had knocked ourselves out. We were even giving mercurial compounds intravenously to try to stop bacterial endocarditis. Look at what antibiotics did to gonorrhea and syphilis, for example. We were in a world that was unbelievable. The newspapers of course made these things into miracle drugs, and in a sense they were right. But they were miracles that happened through well-known scientific methods of observation and putting the facts on their inference— just what Professor Lowes had taught me in 1922 about Elizabethan literature.

"I had a predominantly Jewish practice, but I had a large minority of Christians. I had a great many patients sent to me from Columbia, probably because it became known that I can speak Spanish. I also had certain interesting foreign patients referred to me by the State Department and by other federal government agencies, because I had become known in Washington.

"I was always interested in both diagnosis and treatment, but I was also interested in the conditions of life which could have been an influence either in causing or modifying the ailment. One day I came on the ward to make rounds, and the first patient I saw was a thin, middle-aged man, with heavily furrowed brows, sitting erect, very stiffly and grimly, in bed. I said, 'Sir, what is your name?' He replied, 'Alexander MacTavish.' I asked, 'What is your occupation?' He said, 'Marine engineer.' He had duodenal ulcer. He was having a good deal of pain, a good deal of misery, and probably apprehension regarding his job or other personal factors. After speaking with him, I took the intern aside and asked him, 'Where is the patient from?' knowing that the man could only be a Scot. The intern said, 'He's an Irishman.' I asked, 'Does it matter whether he is a Scot or an Irishman?' The intern, having received a modern education, said, 'I can't see that it makes any difference.' To me this was a serious error. In the first place, I explained, the Scot is in all likelihood a Presbyterian. In other words, his religion derives from Calvin, and it is a grim religion. An Irishman would, except in a minority of cases, be a Roman Catholic. He can confess to a sympathetic priest. He can be absolved. His mind can be relieved. The Scot cannot. And here is a fellow with duodenal ulcer. The failure of that young doctor to grasp the elementary relation between man, illness, and environment is of great significance, I thought.

"Work in the army as an intelligence officer had given me a much more detailed and extensive knowledge of foreign countries and their conditions all over the world. To that extent, I was able to serve patients better. I remember being asked to see a Peruvian on the ward. I was called because it was suspected that he had echinococcus, a cyst in the liver caused by a parasitic worm. When I talked with the man, I found that he came from a district in Russia next to Romania, where the industry is cattle raising. That is where he got his echinococcus, not in the country to which he had migrated. I was interested in relations among environment, disease, and the person, because I had worked in tropical medicine repeatedly. Later I learned more about these problems because the army had assigned me to them. At any rate, my effort was to try to see the whole person, background and all.

"Insofar as there was ever any rise in the graph of this man's life, I suppose it should be placed in the years after the war. When I was called as a consultant it was a measure of approval and was therefore encouraging and flattering. But I was not markedly conscious of a rise, or of a change in my sense of responsibility, with possibly one exception. With experience, one learns to restrain the therapeutic hand. One knows better what not to undertake. One knows that this man will remain a drunk, or that for rheumatism you could then do rather little. Like many colleagues, I always was very careful about recommending operations, but I probably was even more so as the years went by and I had seen good and bad results. Otherwise, my practice was more alike than different, from beginning to end.

"In 1961, President Kennedy appointed me a regent of the National Library of Medicine. I completed the term of four years. President Nixon later had some kind of quarrel with the National Library of Medicine, and he stopped appointing regents. Every so often a regent came to the end of his term, until there were none left. The administrators of the library have never lacked cleverness. They called back a few of us as nonregents. We met in a noncommittee, and we functioned for several years in that manner.

"A recent change in medicine [since about the 1970s] has been the increasing risk of malpractice suits and the steeply rising cost of malpractice insurance. If you have to pay high insurance rates, where can you get the money? You can get it only from your patients. The problem of malpractice is a very serious one, a very large one. The American people are so litigious. One day a new patient appeared in my office, a woman. I took her history, did the physical examination, drew the specimens and so forth. After she dressed I explained the problem to her. As far as one could tell, she was satisfied. Just as she was leaving, she tripped on the edge of the rug. I caught her so that she didn't fall. She blurted out, 'I would have sued you.' That is only one example. We pay for this attitude. We have to be insured; it is very expensive.

"On another occasion I was consulted by telephone about a young patient and said, 'It's obvious that she'd better go the hospital right away.' The family agreed. I went to the hospital and found the patient in the lobby with members of her family. They were signing the papers for her admission. One of them said to me, 'If anything goes wrong, Doc, we're going to sue you.' That was before I'd said or done anything. Because of that statement, I had to inform the medical society, write a description of the incident, and fill out forms. Nothing happened. I managed to refer her to other physicians. I got rid of the problem. The situation is much worse now. My British physician friends are astounded at what we pay for malpractice insurance and at what goes on here. The British courts wouldn't allow such things. They would punish someone for bringing a lawsuit of frivolous character.

"Regarding patients' expectations of doctors, I have the feeling that the patient's loyalty to the doctor is much less than it used to be. I don't know how we could measure this to determine the extent of it. All you know, all you learned through study and experience, is nullified if the patient dislikes you. In most practices, you need to be liked. How far one is willing to go to obtain this blissful state I don't know. I felt that I would perform my medical duties as conscientiously and thoroughly as possible, even if I lost financially, as happens when you make house calls or decline to countersign applications for drivers' licenses for people who should be at home and in bed. One can never be reimbursed properly for the amount of time that various problems require.

"I would guess that newspaper articles about sicknesses and cures may have increased public expectation about what doctors can do. Expectations are increased additionally by advertising, a mendacious activity in which the United States apparently outdoes all other countries. The term 'miracle drugs,' for example, implies supernatural powers on the part of the physician. I have been known to say to a patient occasionally, 'If you want a miracle or a prophecy, go to a rabbi.'

"If I discovered that I was twenty or thirty years younger, I wouldn't dream of reentering the practice of medicine. The reasons are as follows: First is the vexatious amount of paperwork that is now necessary. Second are the restrictions. Your fees are not determined by you or between you and the patient, even if you charge nothing. The increase in restrictions imposed by the government, accountants, and lawyers has made the practice of medicine grievous. Third is the question of what your privileges are when you are a hospital physician. Now hospitals must be notified in advance of the character of each patient's illness; they then decide how many days' stay your patient will be granted. Once the patient is admitted, a committee, which sometimes includes a physician but not always, makes the decision. This is very bad for the patient. Who wants to practice under such circumstances?

"As to the physician being his own boss, being one of the few independent characters on the American scene—that has changed. Many doctors now practice in groups, others are employed by corporations, by municipalities, or by universities. Fewer and fewer stand alone nowadays."

BEESON

Yale and Oxford—Role Model in Two Countries

DURING HIS YEARS at Emory, Beeson quickly established himself as a broadly based infectious disease expert through his publications. He investigated the transmission of hepatitis by blood transfusion, fever therapy for syphilis in the days before penicillin, and bacteremia in patients with bacterial endocarditis.

In this section he describes his chairmanship years at Yale during the period of unprecedented growth in university medical school departments. What stands out for him when he recalls those years is his relationships with students and with patients. He tried to be a role model for students, as Soma Weiss had been for him, by being interested in their work, available to them, and by passing along the traditional, humanitarian approach to caring for patients. Attempts to be empathetic, open, and caring with patients broke down, however, over the subject of disclosure of terminal illness. Beeson speaks about the practice of lying to patients, which was common during the postwar era, and how troubling that practice was for him.

He talks about his decision to leave Yale at the height of his career and accept the Nuffield chair at Oxford. He compares department chair life at the two institutions and gives his impressions of Britain's National Health Service.

"I was thrilled at the thought of becoming chairman at Yale. It was a big and prestigious department in comparison with Emory. I went up and spent a couple of days meeting people and meeting the search committee. A few days later, the dean called and said, 'We've decided to offer the job to you [1952].' I said, 'Oh, good!' There wasn't a thought in my mind of not taking it. Nowadays, a candidate for department chairman wants to think about it for six months. He wants to know how many line places are open in the budget and what the budget is. I didn't know anything about any of those things. I was delighted to be offered

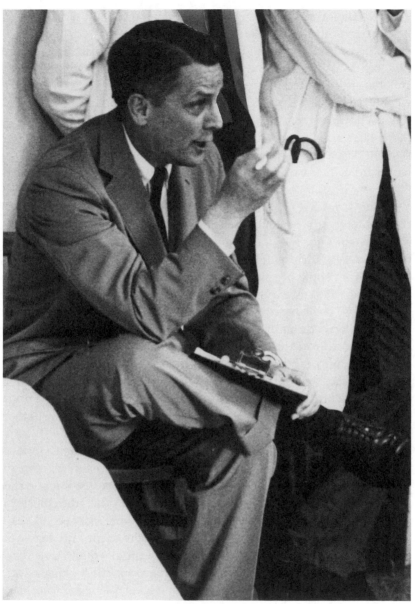

Paul Beeson, 1960.

the job. The salary was going to be eighteen thousand dollars. It had been sixteen thousand dollars at Emory.

"When I came home and told Barbara about the call, she looked a little bit dismayed. She had fashioned a happy life for herself and the children and wasn't at all excited about moving into a new community. I went up to Yale and lived in the hospital for about four months, until we found a house. Living in the hospital and having breakfasts and dinners in the cafeteria was a good way for me to get acquainted with the place. Barbara stayed in Atlanta while the children were finishing school. Then we found a house in New Haven and moved into it in August. The family got reassembled.

"I think my first years at Yale may have been where I felt there were constraints [on the career]. There were senior people in the department who thought I was too young and too ill-prepared for that job. The first two years were fairly tough years in some ways, having to win over the confidence of some people. I have often told that to other people who were going off to take a chairmanship: 'You are not going to find it too easy, because you have to wait until there are a fair number of the house staff who always thought of you as head of the department. You have to be able to convince other faculty members in the department that you are going to be fair with them and not be a difficult chief.' I was fortunate to be able to take two very good, young people up there from Emory with me—Ivan Bennett and Phil Bondy. The students liked them. The house staff liked them. They were identified with me and I could talk with them about my troubles and this helped.

"A couple of years after we were there I had to go through a series of major operations for a congenital defect of the bowel that was giving me urinary tract infections. They had to do a temporary colostomy and then go in and find this thing and obliterate it and take down the colostomy and explore the kidney on that side. For six months that second year I was really out of commission. I had a good chief resident, and there were some good people on the staff and things went all right. After that I never had any more trouble with these infections. In looking back, I think this prolonged episode of illness, involving a series of four major operations, may have been useful to me afterward. I learned how important good nursing care is. And I discovered that a seriously ill patient tends to endow physicians with special worth. The visits of my surgeons were big events of the day. I watched their expressions and recalled their exact words. I wanted them to be good, and somehow I convinced myself that they were good. Yet, a few months later, when I met the same people in the lunchroom or in a committee meeting, they had returned to their normal selves, that is, ordinary professional colleagues.

"I tried to follow in the Soma Weiss tradition of letting the students know I was interested. This is a very important thing in a medical organization. I tried to let them know that I knew where they were and what was going on. I welcomed their coming to talk to me about future jobs and so on. In running medical services, I always held the firm view that the house staff was the key to success. You've got to give time to the house staff and make them feel that you are interested in them. When we spread out our Yale house staff into the private service at New Haven Hospital and then into the VA hospital, there was some grumbling about it. They had come to work at the New Haven Hospital, not on the private service and not in the VA. I immediately set up a weekly clinical conference with the house staff in both of those places. I was seeing house staff in three separate assignments through the time I was there. I think they knew there was a familiar figure that was coming to meet with them and discuss patients with them every week.

"About three years after I had been at Yale—say, 1955—I was asked to see a private patient, a professor's wife who was dying of jaundice with carcinoma involving her liver. She was a very intelligent person. When I got there, both the doctor and the patient's husband said to me, 'We've decided that we must not tell her what the trouble is, that she has cancer. We have told her she has hepatitis.' I nodded my head and went in and examined her; there was a great big hard liver full of tumor. I told her that it looks like a severe case of hepatitis, and sometimes it takes a long time to get better. Her eyes fixed on me and she said, 'How do you know it is hepatitis?' She asked me more questions, and I just went on lying. That was an awful experience. When I left I told myself I was never going to be caught in that trap again. But I had agreed with the attending doctor and the husband that she musn't be told. The husband had read his wife wrong. She needed to be told, and she was strong enough to have coped with it. They were making her terminal illness a miserable affair.

"It took a long time to be honest with patients about death because of the perceived gulf that existed between us. We felt that it would make patients so depressed and despondent to be told the truth that it was kinder not to tell. This was the reason that was given. Indeed, patients do go through a period of anger and despondency. But they usually come out of that to live a life day by day and prepare themselves and their families. I think we didn't relate to them very well as human beings; we had the feeling that we musn't let them know. We felt, as members of a different social class, that we could make these decisions ourselves.

"I can remember that my father kept the truth from some patients, but certainly not from all. I had a little classmate, the brightest girl in our class in about fourth or fifth grade. She had juvenile diabetes and kept being sick. Insulin hadn't been discovered. My father would treat her with rest and fluids, and she would sometimes come out of it. I am positive that she did not know the prognosis before she died. It was considered ethical and noble to lie at that time. But I can remember him in Wooster, Ohio, coming out of the operating room and telling the family very promptly what he had seen. He did something that no modern surgeon would do. Sometimes he would call a member of the family into the operating room, put a mask on him and show him a malignant tumor. I was assisting him, and I saw him do that.

"The business of lying to patients is a terrible affair, and some very able physicians recognized that. They realized that the patient finds out and then feels abandoned by the doctor and the family, 'Everyone is lying to me. There is no one I can talk to about my illness.'

"Now of course, it has gone the other way around; all decisions are made in conference with the patient, and every attempt is made to bring the patient into the decision-making as early as possible. Many patients who find out they have a terminal illness say, 'You musn't tell my husband,' or 'You musn't tell my wife.' They want to keep it from members of their family. But that is the wrong thing to do. It utterly spoils that wonderful relationship that can exist toward the end of someone's life.

"I think the work of Elisabeth Kübler-Ross and the hospice movement both had a lot to do with the change in attitude. With hospice, the patient knows he is going in for terminal care, and no secret is made of it. It has worked out so well in so many parts of the world and has amply demonstrated that the patient is better off knowing. I think that often you can tell the patient in stages. Before an operation you can say, 'There may be a malignant tumor there; that is one of the reasons we have to go in.' Afterwards, you say, 'We have to have the pathologist look at it under the microscope, to be sure it is malignant.' You can prepare the patient for the bad news and then tell them a day or two later that it does look like this is a tumor. Then you can talk about chemotherapy and the possibilities of that and the course of treatment.

"Later in the decade, probably after 1965, a number of ethicists came to the medical schools, or formed liaisons with medical schools, and that changed things, as did the prospect of litigation over not telling patients the truth. I think some perceptive nurses had something to do with the change in attitude also. They realized that after the doctor had sailed gaily on, saying, 'You're all right,' the patient knew that he wasn't all right. Then very quickly medical students and house officers took this up and, almost too quickly at times, would blurt out to patients exactly what was going on. I still feel that you approach the topic of terminal illness individually, and you talk over with members of the family how you are going to tell a patient when the news is bad. Everyone has to know the same things.

"I don't think I have ever said to a patient, 'There is no hope.' I always try to hold out a little faint hope. I always say that doctors can be wrong. I also say that while we don't have a treatment that is very effective right now, there is an enormous amount of very productive research going on and that we may have something before long. We certainly will know in this medical center as soon as anything is discovered. And nowadays, there is so much therapy you can offer, not only for malignant diseases but for heart disease and chronic conditions of all kinds. You leave the patient thinking about treatment options and further diagnostic tests. Then you go back and take time with the patient.

"I think a good doctor takes time to sit down and say, 'Are there some more questions you'd like to ask as a result of what we've talked about?' I'm a nut on this business of sitting down. I just think the standing over a patient, looking down, spoils the whole interpersonal relationship. I think it is very important that your heads be on the same level and that you aren't in a hurry to get away, that you look like you have time to sit down and talk. I do try to impress this on medical students. You should never appear to be in a hurry, and you should give the patient repeated chances to ask questions and should try and answer them in the most comforting way you can. I have always made a big point of the one old thing that Trudeau said: 'to cure now and then, to help often, to comfort always.' There is always something we can do to comfort, not only the patient, but the patient's family. Talk to them on those terms.

"After I had been at Yale for six years, I felt I needed a change from the steady grind of the department. I took the year off to get a refresher. I think sabbatical years are the best thing about academic medicine. Everyone ought to go away every sixth or seventh year and break a lot of committee affiliations and personal entanglements and not have the phone ring. It is good to look at yourself from a few thousand miles away and then decide how you want to go on. I think you are worth a great deal more to the university for having been away for a year than if you had slogged away and done your regular duties.

"It was easy for me to establish in London. I knew people from when I had been there during the war. I could work at the Wright-Fleming Institute in the field of bacteriology and immunology. It was such fun. The telephone didn't ring for me all day long, and I knew what I was going to do all day. I got one nice piece of work done.[1] I went back to Yale with some ideas of what I wanted to do and tried to get a lab going, but I just could not do it.

"In 1962, when I had been chairman ten years, the members of the department at Yale were happy; we were recruiting good house staff, research fellows, and faculty and were still building space to house them. It was at Yale that this big burst of new money came in, and we could expand so rapidly. We could build labs and apply for huge grants. People were saying, 'Don't you want some more money?' It was that kind of a time. In retrospect, that time was the peak of an unnatural period of forced growth and great excitement in academic medicine, a time that will never return, I think.[2] That would be the period that I would point to now, when I seemed to have the greatest influence on other people, and as a result, the time I had the greatest responsibility.

"While I was at Yale, the regius professor at Oxford University [England] was George Pickering, a physician. A regius professor corresponds most closely to our dean. He is appointed by the monarch [queen of England]. Pickering was a very popular speaker in this country and was always being invited to be visiting professor here and there. He had been interested in some of the same problems as I had been, particularly the mechanism of fever. He had visited me at Emory and at Yale, and I had visited him on trips abroad and when I was on sabbatical in London in 1958 and 1959. We read one another's publications. I got a letter from him one day marked private and confidential. He told me that the present Nuffield professor was retiring and that he had put my name forward for the committee to consider. He wondered whether or not I was interested. The Nuffield chair was established in 1935, when the Nuffield Benefaction set up the clinical departments at Oxford. It's relatively new.

"I had been at Yale thirteen years and was becoming really fatigued by the responsibilities of this big, growing department. When you are the head of an organization that big, somebody wants to talk to you all the time. Problems come up. Sitting in my office, I had to turn my mind to a different problem every fifteen minutes. I was not seeing patients. I was not seeing medical students. I was not getting into the lab to do research. I was about fifty-seven or fifty-eight, and the thought of staying on and doing it until age sixty-five wasn't terribly attractive. A few months before Pickering's invitation arrived, I had called in some of my best friends, a half dozen of them, to come and spend an evening at my house. We talked about me and what I was doing and how I might be relieved of some of these time-consuming jobs. All of my good friends gave me no help whatever. Every time I would say something like, 'Do you think I could turn over the interviewing of intern candidates to someone else?' they would say, 'No, we think you should do that.'

"So there was this restiveness in me. I realized this might not be the way I wanted to spend the last few years of my professional life. When the offer came to go to England and work in that famous, old medieval university, and have a very small deparment and a small ward service, it was just a wonderful break for me. I got back to a department of six people. I had only forty beds in the Radcliffe Infirmary. I was able to get into the lab. I got rid of all the problems I couldn't solve at Yale. I got free of some of the people who were dependent on me for help. They kept coming to me, and I couldn't help them very much. It was a chance to get a most refreshing change in professional activity at a time when most people would like to have a change.

"When I took the post, I was moving against the tide, so to speak, because so many British scientists and clinicians had been moving to this country. But Oxford was Oxford, and a professorship there was prized. In particular, there was the historical precedent that the only other North American [a Canadian] who had moved [from Johns Hopkins in 1909] to become professor of medicine was the great William Osler. When the news of my move to Oxford got around there was a lot of gossip about it, and many letters of congratulations came in. People noted a few similarities, in that both Osler and I had attended McGill, we both had spent some time in Philadelphia, and we both had been editors of leading textbooks of medicine. Actually Osler became regius professor, like Pickering. Even now, when people introduce me to someone, they are likely to add that I was the only American to follow Osler's footsteps and take a professorship at Oxford.

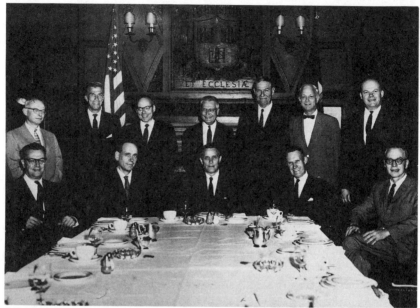

Dinner party for Paul Beeson as he was about to leave Yale for Oxford, England, June 23, 1965. All pictured were with Beeson in 1939 at the Peter Bent Brigham Hospital. Standing, from left to right: Philip Bondy, Louis H. Hempelmann, John Hickam, Jack Myers, Gustave Dammin, Max Michael, James V. Warren. Seated, left to right: John Romano, Eugene A. Stead, Paul Beeson, Charles A. Janeway, Walter Sheldon. Courtesy Edward G. Miner Library, University of Rochester Medical Center.

"Again, Barbara wasn't completely happy about picking up and leaving New Haven, where she had made a good home and some friends. She had established herself and was happy there. But as we look back on it, we now say that our nine years in England was the nicest time of our lives. The two boys had just finished at Yale, and our daughter was with us. We lived right on the outskirts of Oxford, in an area called Boars Hill. We had a horse, so we had to have land. We had a big house, not terribly beautiful, but big and comfortable. It was easy to entertain the house staff and friends there. Throughout our period in Atlanta, New Haven, and Oxford, Barbara was very good about entertaining for me. We entertained house staff and students and faculty members and had an active social life in all those places. Many Americans came through Oxford. We were always putting up visitors from home. Barbara and I used to laugh that we saw more American friends in Oxford than we saw in New Haven.

"If I had not been offered the Nuffield professorship, I probably would have stayed at Yale. I kept receiving invitations to be dean somewhere, but was not tempted. That is the sort of standard progression, from professor of medicine to dean. I left Yale in 1965, just when things were beginning to get very rocky with government subsidies; they were a little less generous than they had been. Moreover, things were rocky with the Vietnam War and the social unrest of the period. Medical students were meeting and criticizing the fact that we weren't taking care of the poor in New Haven. It wasn't going to be a very pleasant time at home. I don't think at the time I realized quite how unpleasant. My successor had a tough time dealing with all of the unrest within the department and within the medical school.

"It was again, I think, a very fortunate thing in my life, which I didn't plan, to be spared the difficulties of the academic world just when there was so much student unrest everywhere. I think that if I had stayed on, I wouldn't have been able to maintain the momentum that I had built up in those previous lush years. People would have found many things to criticize about what old Beeson was doing with the chairmanship. People would have been saying, 'Well, Beeson will have to be moved out.' I also might have asked to be moved out. I don't know. But it was a welcome change to go to England and work in that great old university and be free of all of those distractions that were getting so difficult. By the time I came back in 1974, it was all over. Everyone was remarking how our students are different people. They dress differently. They are fairly respectful. It's pleasure to work with them once again.

"Patients changed also during the nine years I was away. In that period patients had begun to ask questions. They realized they were no longer charity patients when Medicare and health insurance of all kinds came in. Then they looked around and saw that people in the medical profession are clearly very well off. They began to realize that if they were dissatisfied with something, they could sue and often recover large sums of money. Patients know very well now that they are within their rights to question a doctor's advice and ask for another opinion, and they do it. I think the disillusionment with the Vietnam War had something to do with it. Authorities can be wrong, and that was proven so amply.

"Being at Oxford was not quite like being a department chairman in the U.S. In the National Health Service, people who serve on the staffs of hospitals are appointed as consultants to the National Health Service. A consultant is always given a ward with a defined number of beds, an outpatient clinic, his own house staff, and his own nursing staff. There were five medical 'firms.' I had the firm that was the largest, with forty hospital beds. George Pickering, my great friend there, had a firm also. So there were really two university-headed firms and three National Health Service firms. Together, we totaled about 130 medical beds. There were two, three, or four physicians in each of the other firms working together. Medical students were dispersed among all those firms. We all took part in the final examinations of the students. I think that I did function as chief of a department of medicine in many ways. I inaugurated a weekly medical conference in which the five firms took turns presenting the cases and discussing them. I got them all to a meeting in one of our homes once a month, and we would talk over the problems of medicine in the Radcliffe Infirmary. We could speak with one voice and did, and we got a lot of mileage out of the fact that we were asking for the same things on the basis of these informal discussions at night.

"I thoroughly enjoyed working at Oxford as a fellow of Magdalen College. It was like belonging to a nice club. I used to go there every day for lunch and sit around in the Senior Common Room and have a glass of sherry and lunch and talk to people who had different fields of interest from mine. It was a quieter, more reflective life. And I can remember some of the formal dinners that every new professor had to go to. I remember sitting at some of those tables, listening to this talk that I could barely understand and saying to myself, 'What am I, a boy from Alaska, doing here?'

"Yet I didn't find it at all hard to become a part of medical practice or medical thinking in England. We all read the same journals on both sides of the Atlantic. We used the same drugs. We quoted the same authorities. I did get some great shocks when I realized that I was working in a government-controlled service. I didn't have the right to say, 'We'll take on a couple of more residents next year,' because that had to be approved in London, and it often wasn't approved. And of course, they kept changing the system. George Pickering complained that the National Health Service had been a marvelous system when it was first inaugurated, but that successive governments had kept tampering with it until they had made it far more bureaucratic and far less good as a patient care institution.

"I found a lot to like about it. I came back to this country and gave some unpopular talks, because socialized medicine was anathema here. In England, they can plan how many cardiologists they will have. When some revolutionary thing like coronary bypass surgery comes along, they may be left behind, because they haven't got a bunch of cardiac surgeons in training. It takes them awhile to catch up. On the other hand, it has prevented what I feel has been a very unfortunate trend to specialized practice in this country. I got awfully tired of Americans coming over to England and dropping in on a doctor's office or in a hospital for two weeks and then coming back and writing articles about how bad the National Health Service was. I think you have to work in a system for a few years to understand it, and I found an awful lot of ill-informed criticism directed to it. It has its good features and its bad features. It couldn't be transferred over to this country at all, because the expectations of our patients are very different. But it works there. The per capita cost is about half of what it is in the United States. It is very hard to show by any measure—neonatal death rate, lifespan, or anything else—that the health of Americans is any better for spending nearly twice as much money per capita on health care.

"To be able to get back to the lab and make some good hits in research after the age of fifty-eight was very rewarding. I got back to work on two problems. The first had to do with bacterial endocarditis. We stumbled onto a good way of producing bacterial endocarditis in rabbits and could produce it unfailingly every time and knew exactly when it started. This gave us a wonderful tool to study the histology of the developing lesion but also to study prophylactic chemotherapy. You know, if you have a heart murmur, when you go to the dentist you are supposed to take penicillin beforehand. We could test out various antimicrobial agents and see how effective they were. This was something we carried on over the years and enjoyed greatly.[3]

"The other study was on the mechanism of eosinophil production in parasitic infections. With trichinosis, the pork worm, you get a marked rise in eosinophils. In ordinary infections, the eosinophils disappear from the bloodsteam. We produced this in rats and inbred strains of rats to study the immunology of it. We demonstrated that the eosinophilia is mediated by T. lymphocytes.[4]

"I worked with a succession of very able young people. Marvelous people fell into my lap—Rhodes scholars and Nuffield Dominion scholars who came there for postgraduate work from all over the British

Commonwealth. We had an exceptionally bright group of young people, but not too many of them. I knew they were bright, and I could let them try out their own ideas without saying, 'You must do this and you must do that.' I had the fun of seeing things develop. It was great after having to drop out from the lab completely in my last seven years at Yale.

"I would have gladly stayed on until the retirement age of sixty-seven, but they were building a big new hospital, so I retired at sixty-five to let my successor come in and relocate the department and make the plans. It didn't seem right for me to hang onto the job; then he would have had to make do with whatever space allocations I had made.

"The nicest thing that happened was the knighthood, knight commander of the British Empire [1973]. I received a certificate signed by Queen Elizabeth and Prince Philip. It's an honorary knighthood. I can't be called Sir Paul. I didn't know anything about it until it was all arranged. It had to be cleared with the United States ambassador. There was a nice little ceremony with about thirty people. The minister of health gave me the certificate and badge. That gave me a lot of satisfaction. It was a nice symbol of being appreciated. I was pleased that it was given for services to the Oxford Clinical School."

"I still go into the VA hospital for the weekly medical conference. They discuss two cases. Sometimes the patient is brought into the room. They are all patient-oriented discussions. I occasionally ask a question or make a comment. I go simply because it's nice to be there. I just enjoy hearing medicine discussed, hearing what's going on. The only thing the audience is looking for is truth: What is the best way of doing something—making a diagnosis or treating a patient. I can make the claim for academic medicine and I think for all medicine: they all want to do the right thing for the patient. They want to make use of the best methods available. That's a great satisfaction."

OLNEY

Camp, Clinics, and Schools

OLNEY HEADED the outpatient cardiac and diabetes clinics at the University of California, San Francisco, for years while she continued her private practice. Here, she talks about how the lives of children were improved dramatically during the 1950s and 1960s because of developments in surgery, diagnosis, and treatments. Cardiac surgery corrected disabling congenital defects. Pneumonia, meningitis, and many other diseases were treatable. And diabetes was controlled more effectively. Advances in medical technology began to allow normal useful lives for children and their families who previously would have been in hopeless situations.

"I think that I enjoyed being a pediatrician most when I had my connections with the university as the head of the cardiac clinic, diabetic clinic, and luetic clinic,[1] and I was having my own private practice with families that I felt responsible for. It was very busy, but it was a happy busyness, and I think that those years were probably the best in the whole of my tenure [1960s and 1970s]. It was a nice long period. There were lots of satisfactions, and lots of input from areas that I was interested in. In cardiology there were some diagnostic things that were exciting, such as determining which congenital anomalies were operable and which ones were not. And there were the diagnostic revelations of radiopaque angiography and cardiac catheterization in order to make a precise diagnosis. Then the surgeon could correct the anomaly, and we could see a child get well and be able to carry on a normal existence. There was also satisfaction in having diabetic children under sufficient control that they weren't repeatedly hospitalized with unnecessary expense for the family. The children were holding their own with their siblings in a nondiabetic world. Those accomplishments were tremendous.

"As the head of these clinics, my colleagues who had gone into practice in far off places would write and ask me about things or ask for

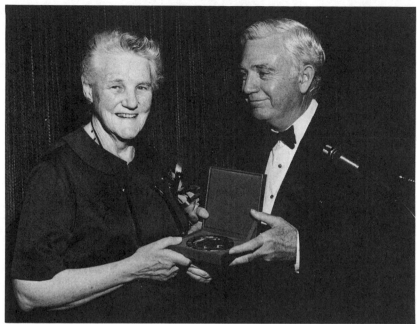

Mary B. Olney with Chancellor Francis A. Sooy, receiving the UCSF Medal Award in 1976. This most prestigious award on the UCSF campus is given to individuals who have made outstanding personal contributions to human health and well-being. Courtesy Library, Special Collections, Archives, University of California, San Francisco.

references on things that they knew I was interested in. Particularly in cardiology, I heard from people practicing who were not yet accustomed to conditions which could and could not respond to surgery. Physicians were reluctant to handle diabetics when they would see only one in maybe twenty or thirty years of practice. Diabetes has to be seen in groups in order to develop a regular procedure for handling the problem and for knowing what the difficulties are as well as knowing what new techniques are worth trying. As cardiology became more of a surgery department specialty, diabetes came more to the forefront of my work, and more referrals came through diabetes.

"I watched a boy die with bulbar polio at the university. I watched two of my patients develop polio of one extremity. They developed it approximately two months before the polio vaccine was released on the scene. That is all the polio I had in my private practice, but I saw a lot of it at Children's Hospital. It was so wonderful when they developed a vaccine. That stimulated everybody to emphasize immunization. I started talking to the parent-teacher associations at various schools, trying to interest them in having their children immunized and telling them how to protect the children from contagious diseases.

"I remember when I was a child, my mother was reluctant to let us use a pit privy at a campground, because she thought polio could be transmitted that way. People had no idea how it was transmitted. The face of medicine has changed drastically since then. What worries me now is articles that come out in the popular magazines saying that you shouldn't immunize because of the possibility of transmitting polio. Well, maybe you would have one in a colossal number of cases, but you can't stop immunization for that. How can you take that kind of responsibility for your child?

"The whole complexion of medicine changed with corrective surgery and technologies. A technique that came in and created a great change was the procedure developed by Dr. Blalock and Dr. Taussig to transplant a blood vessel so there were no longer any 'blue babies.' From there, we went to correction within the heart, closing ventricular septal defects and opening the pulmonary artery. This was a form of rehabilitation that freed a whole family. Until that surgical procedure was developed, a mother had to be almost a martyr to care for a blue baby. Later, when the child was in a wheelchair, the mother couldn't get any help. People were afraid to take care of those children. Intravenous contrast studies and cardiac catheterization made that diagnosis possible. I would say that changed the life of certain children. After surgery, some of those children went on to have families of their own. Before that, the patient might contract pneumonia or have some cerebral complication or cardiac decompensation. So what was really a hopeless situation became a useful life.

"Since we have been able to treat pharyngitis, tonsillectomies have almost become outdated and mastoid surgery rarely occurs. Pneumonias either don't happen or they can be cured. Meningitis, which carried a heavy toll, can be treated. Subacute bacterial endocarditis, which was the worry of rheumatic fever patients, can be treated. Osteomyelitis can be treated. A ruptured appendix can be treated. Great advances have been made in identifying and treating enzyme and amino acid deficiences and in immunology and genetics. Advances in the X-ray field made it possible to make diagnoses that were never possible before.

"It has been very disappointing that transplantation of the pancreas has not been very productive, perhaps because the condition which causes diabetes with the original pancreas still exists with the second. There are some youngsters who are looking forward to transplants. One little boy told me he didn't have to take care of his diabetes because he was going to get a pancreatic transplant. I asked him, 'Who is going to give you a pancreas?' He looked at me and he ceased to be cocky.

"I had so many responsibilities that I didn't participate in research until I tried in the 1950s and 1960s to create cardiac anomalies in mice. Theodore Ingalls, a Harvard physician, was among the earliest researchers to systematize the thought held at the time that all congenital anomalies in babies were a result of trauma to the mother during pregnancy. He attempted to produce a standard type of anomaly in mice subjected to low oxygen tensions. He produced septal heart defects.[2] Other research groups produced all sorts of anomalies in chickens—orthopedic and cardiac—by lowered oxygen tensions. The objective was to create a group of animals with which one could pursue research problems.

"I attempted to produce ventricular septal defects with lowered oxygen tensions, as Ingalls had done. I injected india ink into the blood vessels of newborn mice to determine the circulation throughout the heart and lungs. I was trying to duplicate his efforts to produce a standard anomaly. With a standard anomaly, you could study the effects of exercise and medication. I learned a lot about congenital heart defects and congenital anomalies from that work. Dr. Edward Shaw [chairman, Department of Pediatrics, UCSF, 1958–1966] would have liked me to continue the research, but it just didn't seem to be a very practical thing to do. It was so intricate. Trying to dissect an infant mouse's heart and identify all the structures is a lot to demand of your eyes. The length of time that it took to try to duplicate previous research didn't seem feasible. In addition, a mouse virus destroyed most of the colony at the time I was working.

"I worked with Headstart when that was set up [medical consultant, 1968–1974]. It was very interesting trying to get children from minority groups started in school and seeing how ill-prepared or disadvantaged the parents were for participating in the program. I think a big deficit of the Headstart program was that it didn't involve parents enough. Even if a man worked all day he could manage an hour in the evening for a lecture or a demonstration as part of the family. All the responsibility shouldn't have been on the mothers. Mothers could have had demonstrations on how to prepare food more easily or how to take advantage of low-cost foods to vary the menu, to make things attractive to children. This would all have been very valuable. But the program was mostly on teaching children to ride tricycles, to share, and sing together—all of which is terribly important—but more could have been done with that group.

"I was supposed to do the physical examinations to check the children for correctable defects, nutritional deficiencies, and emotional problems. I went with a social worker to inspect each site for safety. The morale was wonderful, but the people running it had too little understanding of children. In some instances the women thought that every occasion should be celebrated with chocolate cake. It required a great deal of diplomacy to teach them that that was not the best nutrition or the best way to entertain youngsters. I am afraid that sometimes I didn't have as much diplomacy as I should have. On the whole, Headstart was a very, very fine program, though it was subject to all sorts of criticism.

"A good many of the youngsters who have gone to camp go into medically related fields, in spite of the fact that they are diabetic. There have been a surprising number. I knew I had become a role model when youngsters from camp and from my private practice graduated from college and said they were going to go into medicine because they admired the way I practice medicine.

"I am impressed with the amount of team work that the practice of medicine requires now. Those who go into medicine today will need to have a much broader view, know better sources of information, learn more technology, and learn how best to apply it. How to have all those resources at one's command is a real challenge. Medicine of the future has tremendous challenges. I think some medical students must get the impression when they read about all these new developments that everything has been done. I assure them time and again that this is only the beginning, that every field of science has its contribution to make, and that they are going to see exciting times. They are going to have new problems to solve all the time, new discoveries to adapt to and many old diagnoses abandoned for better understanding of medical conditions."

RHOADS

Philanthropy and Education

WHILE CONTINUING with general surgery and nutritional research, Rhoads expanded his activities to include volunteer work with the American Cancer Society and administration and governance at the University of Pennsylvania. He felt it was extremely important to serve his community and university beyond the work he did as a surgeon, researcher, and department chairman. When he looks back over the wide range of his pursuits, he says his greatest pride is in two areas: the contributions of his research laboratory to the nutrition of surgical patients, and the successful careers of the many academic and community surgeons he trained while serving as department chair.

"I got involved in the American Cancer Society through Dr. Eugene Pendergrass, who was chairman of radiology here. He was active in the cancer society. Fairly early, he became an officer in the Philadelphia division of the American Cancer Society and was active with the national organization in New York. He asked me if I would go on the local board and said he didn't want me to say yes unless I was willing to do some work on it. So I gulped and said, 'Yes.' I was nominated as a secretary of the Philadelphia division board and from there was pushed into being president of the Philadelphia board [1955–1956]. There was a lot of friction at that time between the United Fund [now United Way] and the American Cancer Society. We did joint fund raising in industry and individual fund raising in neighborhoods. About 30 percent of the funds in Philadelphia came through the joint fund raising in industry. United Fund said that if we were going to continue to share their campaign in industry, we would have to accept their budget review and their control of how we raise money, spend money, and everything else. They wanted to use the appeal of the cancer cause to enhance the overall fund raising. Most of us didn't want to do that. We couldn't do that under our charter, which specified that we would keep 60 percent of what we raised here and send 40 percent to the national organization. I

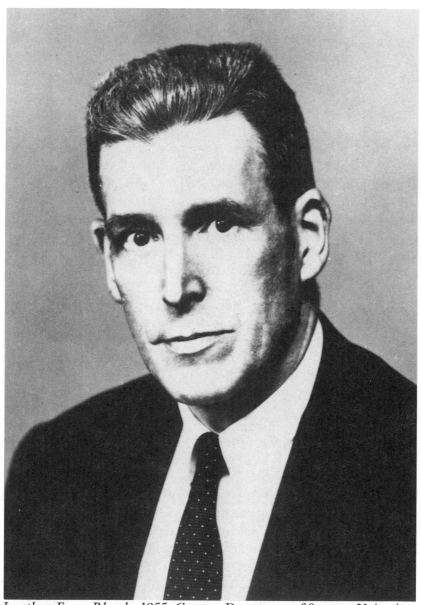

Jonathan Evans Rhoads, 1955. Courtesy Department of Surgery, University of Pennsylvania.

was in the middle of this controversy. I met with the national organization and the United Fund leadership and prominent businessmen at the Ford Motor Company headquarters. I talked about the difference between the American Cancer Society and the United Fund. I talked about why we were wiser to operate separately and said that we would like to join them in plant fund raising, which we couldn't do without the business leaders. I think from that time on I was noticed by people in the national organization. Then I got on some of the national committees and served as chairman of the professional education committee, chairman of the medical and scientific committee [1967–1968], vice-president, president elect [1968–1969], and president [1969–1970].

"That led to my being put on the scientific panel the U.S. Senate appointed when they were contemplating the new Cancer Act. After the act was passed [1971], I became a member of the new National Cancer Advisory Board. I was asked to chair it. It was a presidential appointment. I received a big certificate from President Nixon. I served three two-year appointments. I think Jimmy Carter paid so little attention to cancer that he didn't get around to appointing anyone else for more than a year, so I served a seventh year [chairman, 1972–1979]. So I had this extraordinary ringside seat on the National Cancer Research Program for seven years. Somewhere in there, I was asked to edit the journal *Cancer,* which I am still doing [1972–1991]. I don't get a chance to read too much of what goes into it. I concentrate more on what is being rejected in the hope of not rejecting something really important.

"The height of my educational career was serving as provost of the University of Pennsylvania [1956–1959]. I had been chairman of the university senate, which had been started in the mid-1950s by faculty who thought they ought to have more say in the affairs of the university. I was one of that group who believed in a higher degree of democracy in university government than we had experienced. The senate was pretty active in those days. There were numerous committees. After I had been elected chairman for a second term, the president of the university had me appointed provost. The deans of all the schools—the School of Law, the Wharton School, the College for Women, the Graduate School of Arts and Sciences, the School of Social Work, the School of Education, the library system—reported to the provost. The health schools and the engineering schools reported to the academic vice-presidents. They were supposed to report to me on educational matters. They reported to the president on fiscal matters. My aim was to increase participation of the faculty in planning and decision-making in the University of Pennsylvania and also to improve faculty remuneration. I learned a good deal about law. I learned a little about educators. I had the opportunity to participate in the appointment of new deans in the School of Education, the Wharton School (business and administration), the School of Social Work, and the Annenberg School of Communication.

"I have always been interested in educational matters. During the time I was chairman of surgery, they attempted to revamp the city schools a little. Under the charter, there was a blue-ribbon committee which included the university presidents and some representatives of community organizations who were to provide the mayor with a slate from which he might choose the members of the board of education. Someone wrote and asked if I would be willing to be nominated. I didn't like the idea very much, but I thought it was terribly important to serve. This was in the 1960s, a time when racial feelings were running high and there were riots in some other cities. We felt that anything we could do to amend things in this city would be desirable. So I said I would accept the nomination, though I didn't much want to. I was invited to come down for an interview before the blue-ribbon committee. They asked me questions I didn't really know the answers to, but I bluffed a bit. Anyhow, the mayor appointed me and I served on the board of education for four years. That was community involvement with a capital *I*. Soon after I went on the board they decided to televise their meetings. In my thinking, that was a disaster. They had always been open to the public; they had to be by law. Dr. Ravdin told me I had very bad judgment to accept. He probaby was right. In any case, it was an illuminating experience.

"The height of my surgical career was serving as chairman of the Department of Surgery at the University of Pennsylvania [1959–1972]. My primary activities were to take care of patients and to show novitiates in the art and science of surgery how I took care of patients and how they could take care of them. On top of this, I hoped to attract, by adequate remuneration and generous opportunities, men and women who would go far in their professions.

"My main conflicts as chairman of the department were with other chairmen over money and space. On the money side, the conflict was private practice versus a straight salary. This has been a conflict all over the country. For years, we had had private practice and had not depended on the university for our income to any considerable extent. We did have small stipends of fifteen hundred dollars or perhaps five thousand dollars for full professor. By and large the clinical people made their own money, and most of them put a good deal of the money they made back into their departments. We always put some money back into the operation of the department, so it was that kind of a mixture. I became the prime defender, I guess, of the private practice system way before I was chairman, when I was an assistant professor. Near the end of the war, some of the people on the university hospital board thought it would be nice to use the Mayo Clinic formula here: everybody gets a salary and then takes work assignments and makes money for the institution. I spoke out against it. Right after the war, as the men returned, they rebuilt their practices. They lost interest in the Mayo Clinic concept. They didn't want someone telling them how much money they could make. So, we've never had the Mayo Clinic type system here in surgery. But we do now have a modified system, so that some money is officially collected by the university, and that goes partly to the earner and partly to the department and partly to the dean's office. That was a source of conflict. I think it cost me a lot in relationships with other departments. They were a lot less friendly than they otherwise would have been.

"I should stress that both Dr. Ravdin and I took the position that our partnership as practitioners was separate and distinct from our relationships in the university. We felt our remuneration here should be related a good deal to what we did. So I've had no hesitancy during my chairmanship years of having other people in the department who were paid more money than I was. All the partners knew what the others were paid. So many partnerships have broken up over the fact that, as people become more senior, they earn less money, but they often want to be paid on a seniority basis. This causes the younger people who are earning the most money to want a change. We accepted the fact that you got paid more or less proportionately to what you earned. Then, if you didn't want to earn so much, you didn't have to. You could spend more time doing other things. It didn't make anybody else mad.

"I've tried not to abuse the financial aspect of the profession. I think I get that somewhat from the Quaker background. It is not peculiar to Quakers, nor universal among Quakers, but nonetheless, there were a good many people who felt that their responsibility was to do a good day's work and not haggle too much over what you got paid for it. It made it somewhat easier to stay in academic work.

"I have had particular satisfaction with the residents I worked with during the chairmanship period more than with the students, because the students come and go so rapidly. They work with so many different people that it's hard to identify with them unless they work with you on a research project. The residents are here for five, six, or seven years, and you get to know most of them pretty well. As head of the service, I had the last word on their selection and appointment, though I always spread this responsibility pretty widely among the various chiefs of service. We usually agreed on whom we liked. Many of the residents have achieved quite a degree of success. That is one reason why I always wanted to stay here. The quality of the students is so fine.

"We do a number of things for them. First, we see that they have some experience in internal medicine during their internship. We used to get them on a month of pediatrics too. Second, we find the resources so that those who want to can take a year or two to do straight research. This is an economic problem because, while they are working in the hospital, the hospital pays them from patient sources or third-party payers. Once they go over to the lab, we can't use any of those funds. We have to find outside money for them. We have gotten some from Washingtion [National Institutes of Health], some from endowments, and some from special fellowships. The research program has grown. We used to have perhaps five surgical residents assigned to research. Now, I think there are ten.

"Third, we have given them solid operating experience. By and large they have had a lot of practical experience, and they are good surgeons. They have all had a lot of independent experience, which they have handled exceedingly well. Fourth, they get a fair amount of administrative experience running a service, because a senior resident will usually have two junior residents and an intern working for him. They will cover perhaps three or four staff men, so they have to work things out to keep the peace.

"The other thing I think we've done for them is to try to bridge the gap between the time they finish their residency and the time they get an assistant professorship. We can't give them all assistant professorships here, but we have kept quite a number on by creating fellowships and so forth of a temporary sort. They don't all want to go into academic surgery. We have shied away from the idea that we are God's gift to training academic surgeons. We think it's better for everybody to train community surgeons side by side with academic surgeons, and we take a lot of pride and satifaction in many of the community surgeons we've trained. They tend to filter out at the top of their communitites just by

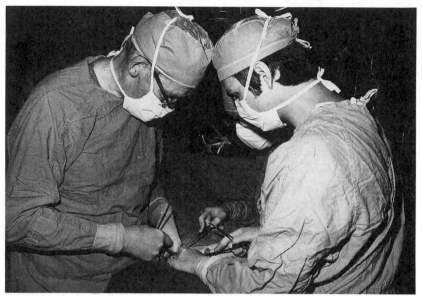

Dr. Rhoads in surgery, 1975. Courtesy Department of Surgery, University of Pennsylvania.

virture of their ability and dedication and the fact that they are reasonable, fair-minded sorts of people generally. Anyhow, I think it's wonderful that they have all done so well. I think I am more pleased with that than with anything else that I have done.

"Many of the cases I was involved with suffered from nutritional deficits. Our central research project was how to resolve these, particularly among patients who could not eat and had to be fed intravenously. In my earlier years at the university, there was no way of giving them sufficient food, and we concentrated on developing methods to do this. We were successful in finding two ways to accomplish it, one of which has been widely adopted. In retrospect, contributions to the nutrition of surgical patients, which were also applicable to many pediatric and medical patients, and the success of many doctors completing our residency program have been the most satisfying accomplishments of my time at the University of Pennsylvania."

HODGKINSON

"No Limit on What One Could Do"

AFTER HIS SERVICE in the army in Denver, Hodgkinson returned to Henry Ford Hospital in Detroit. In this section he describes some of his activities as chairman of the Department of Obstetrics and Gynecology, an appointment that began in 1952. He is extremely proud of the research laboratory he started for residents. He speaks about his years of work for the American College of Obstetricians and Gynecologists. He blossomed as a researcher during the 1950s and 1960s, and his work on urinary physiology during that period earned him a national reputation. Here he describes his creative "boot strap" research methods.

"As chairman of the Department of Obstetrics and Gynecology, I was responsible for the overall running of the department, including selection of new staff and residents, and the administrative functions of nurses, aides, and secretaries. I had little to do with budget responsibilities except in an advisory capacity. During that period, the department published many papers. We presented many medical exhibits and won many prizes. I tried, but was not always successful, to have a paper published under the name of every resident during his term of service.

"My routine was to get to the hospital early, between 4:30 and 5:00 in the morning. I worked on my papers until about 8:30. That was the only time I could do it. Then I would go make rounds and see patients, or go to the operating room, every other day. The residents always made a joke of it: 'If you want to see Dr. Hodgkinson, you better go at 5:00 in the morning.' I worked hard then.

"We had an active residency program, twelve residents. I adjusted the schedule so that a person graduated from the residency every four months. That way, no two people had the same responsibility at the same time. They rotated through the various staff people. They scrubbed with us on operations and deliveries, and teaching was largely on a one-to-one basis. They were very busy and they worked hard. I don't think a residency is any good unless the residents really have to work hard. Now

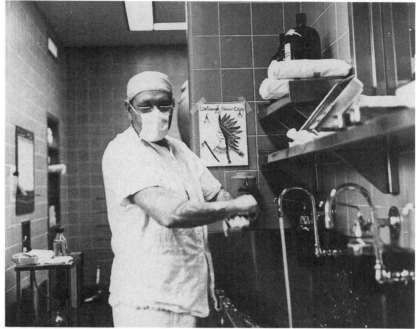

Dr. Hodgkinson scrubbing for surgery, circa 1973. Courtesy Department of Surgery, Henry Ford Hospital.

they talk about the poor residents working so hard and so long. Well, that is an opportunity. That isn't an obligation. Any resident who is worth his salt is not going to look at the clock.

"I only taught medical students in the latter part of my professional life, after the University of Michigan started to send students to Ford Hospital. When they came, we just worked them right into the residency program so that they were actually part of the team. They scrubbed with us and went to the meetings and were given assignments. Their training with us was very practical.

"Soon after I became head of the department, I started to develop the animal laboratory at Ford Hopsital. It was entirely my idea. I felt, and still feel, that resident training should include some sort of animal research. When a gynecologist makes an incision in the abdomen, he doesn't always know what he is going to get into. Sometimes there is involvement of the intestines, for instance. I think a doctor should have the knowledge and competence to do certain intestinal operations that belong in the field of general surgery. I feel deep in my heart that this is an important part of training. When the residents go out into the community, they ought to be able to take care of an emergency. You can't always find a general surgeon. When you open somebody's abdomen and find some kind of intestinal condition, you ought to be able to repair it.

"I had the advantage of having three years of general surgery before I went into OB/GYN. At first, I sent my residents over to general surgery for six months' training. But they were the tail end of the team, and they could hardly get to the operating table. The general surgical residents were there pushing them out of the way and not giving them anything to do if they could avoid it.

"So, we started a research laboratory as a way of getting around that problem. It was wonderful training. Our residents would operate on dogs and do intestinal resections and repair of ureters—that is a complication gynecologists get into not uncommonly—and other types of operations. The competence of the young surgeon grew from that kind of experience. It was invaluable and really paid off.

"I had a resident from Canada who came down and went through our program; it was a three-year residency then. He went home and got a job at a small hospital in Montreal. One summer night at about 3:00 A.M., an ambulance pulled up and brought in a man with a big towel wrapped around his neck. He had been riding in a convertible and was in an accident. The top bar of the convertible hit his neck and severed his carotid artery and both jugular veins. Blood was pouring out all over the place. Well, my former resident knew exactly what to do and knew exactly how to do it. He quickly clamped off the vessels, repaired the jugular vein, repaired the carotid artery, and performed cardiac resuscitation twice. By then his chief came in, looked over his shoulder, and said, 'It looks like you are getting along just fine.' The chief didn't even bother to scrub. The resident would never have been able to do that if it hadn't been for that experience in the dog lab. I was told that the patient comes in every month to express his appreciation to my former resident for saving his life. That dog lab paid off on just that one case. Unfortunately, after I retired from head of the department, my successor wasn't interested in that kind of thing. Gradually, it petered out, and it's gone now.

"I became interested in organizational medicine. In the 1940s, there were smaller, regional organizations of obstetricians and gynecologists. There was interest in having a national organization to represent everybody. I was an invited guest at the meeting where the American Academy of Obstetrics and Gynecology was formed [now the American College of Obstetricians and Gynecologists]. Over time, we began to form bylaws and various regional suborganizations. The organization was divided into districts. At that time there were eight districts. [Now there are ten.] District V was made up of Michigan, Ontario, Indiana, Ohio, and West Virginia. I was named chairman of District V. The organization gradually took shape, and we sent out notices of its formation. The dues were twenty-five dollars. Anybody who was a practicing obstetrician and gynecologist or who even had a major interest in obstetrics and gynecology was eligible for membership. My God! It was an avalanche. We didn't have an office, but we rented space in the office of the American Committee of Maternal Welfare in Chicago. We had wastebaskets full of applications with twenty-five dollars in each letter.

"We had our first national meeting in Cincinnati in 1951, and there I was named secretary. At that first meeting, we decided we should have a journal. We had ten thousand members. Then came the problem of qualifications for membership. We had so many applications. There were divergent opinions about who should be eligible, who shouldn't be eligible. Some were of the opinion that anybody who was interested in obstetrics and gynecology should remain eligible for membership, but the president, Woodard Beecham, disagreed. More and more people were devoting their entire professional life to obstetrics and gynecology rather than doing a little bit of everything. The only people who were going to be eligible were going to be board certified. That turned the academy around. That made it into a prestigious organization and set the stage for the specialty. It took another three years for the academy to change its name to the American College of Obstetricians and Gynecologists, comparable to the American College of Surgeons.

"As secretary, I used to work hours and hours for this organization that didn't have any protocol to go by. I was making decisions about this or that, simply because there was no precedent. After five years as secretary [1952–1956] I thought I should establish a precedent, so I refused the nomination for the next year. The college continued to grow.

"In 1960, I was elected president. That was a big responsibility. I was the tenth president. There were fifteen thousand members then. It was an extremely busy year, a wonderful year. I was away from the hospital a lot. I went to many of the district meetings, which I paid for myself. The college didn't pay me a dime. Now, they pay the president fifty thousand dollars plus expenses. It was a real thrill for me to see the college become a success, because I had put so much of myself into it, especially during the secretary years. The presidency was a challenging opportunity to bring the college together and try to make it seem worthwhile to the constituencies. Malpractice wasn't the concern then that it is now. We were interested in maternal mortality and infant mortality. We were interested in organizing the practice of obstetrics and gynecology. We formed a nurses' branch of the college, so they could have the privilege of educational programs along with the physicians. It is a big, active organization. They have meetings in conjunction with our ACOG meetings, and it's well worthwhile. I think in a lot of circumstances, the nurses feel they are not a real part of the show, and they are, especially in obstetrics. We actually made them a part of the college. It gave them a little additional dignity that they didn't have before. They knew that the doctors appreciated them. I think this is a real problem.

"In the late 1940s and early 1950s, there developed considerable gynecologic interest in stress urinary incontinence [SUI] and the anatomic relationship of the bladder and the urethra. SUI is a very common condition and occurs mostly in married women, Caucasian, usually about midlife after they have had a number of children. The incidence is extremely common. About 50 percent of women who have had children will admit that they lose some urine occasionally on coughing or sneezing. But most of the time, they can control it. But 10 percent or 15 percent of women will have uncontrollable stress incontinence. The treatment for this is surgery to change the relationship of the urethra to the bladder. It is a very, very common procedure today.

"I became interested in urinary physiology. At that time, there was a lot of interest in the subject, and there were a lot of special studies being done. Several radiographic studies showing the relationship of the bladder and urethra had been published. In those studies, a soft rubber catheter had been used to delineate the urethra. When I analyzed those studies, it was obvious that the catheter distorted the true shape of the urethra. One day, working in the operating room with one of my residents, we got to talking about how you could get a better picture of the urethra without distortion. In searching for a substitute for the soft rubber catheter, we decided that maybe we could use a metallic bead chain—a pull chain—to show the configuration of the urethra. I decided to try that.

"I had to get a chain. I didn't have anything to do in the early afternoon. I went to a few hardware stores, and they told me to try religious stores. Sometimes metallic bead chains are used to hold crosses and other things around the neck. So I went to various religious stores, and they didn't have anything either. It was getting late, and I had to get back to the office to see patients. My last stop was a large Montgomery Ward store way out on the other side of town. I went down to the hardware department, and they didn't have any. I was discouraged, but as I was walking out, I passed a table with a number of junk jewelry items, and there was a necklace. It was made out of a bunch of metallic bead chains. Well, I bought it for a dollar. I went back to the office and monkeyed around with the thing and cut the chains off. All those chains lasted me for about ten years.

"I developed the metallic bead technique for the diagnosis of stress urinary incontinence. We started to do some X-ray studies of patients with stress incontinence and some patients who didn't have stress incontinence for control, and we found that the chain did show the configuration of the urethra, so that we could diagnose SUI. After doing about four hundred or five hundred of these studies, I wrote a paper and presented it at the Central Association of Obstetricians and Gynecologists; that was in 1952. The technique was recognized nationally and internationally as showing the true urethral-vescular relationship without distorting the urethra.[1]

"We continued that study for several years. We worked up a urinary program for Ford Hospital that consisted of the metallic bead chain technique and various other tests that we were doing for bladder physiology. One of the tests for bladder physiology, called cystometry, was to measure bladder contractions in relation to bladder filling. In 1946, the test was shown to be fraught with too many dangers of error, and it was subject to emotional reactions of the patient. I thought we should be doing the test a different way. In the early 1950s, some electronic equipment came on the medical market which measured very fine, small pressures very, very accurately. It was being used for cardiac studies. It occurred to me to use this equipment for cystometry. I developed the use of electronic measuring devices for pressure changes [electronic urethrocystometry]. That was the first electronic technique that had been used for that kind of study. Electronic urethrocystometry showed several basic physiological facts not disclosed by other techniques. It became part of our routine. I published many papers on that technique.[2] Those two things occupied most of my time and my interest. One fell into the other.

"We actually discovered a new disease with this technique, because we found that some incontinent patients who didn't have stress incontinence were losing urine because their bladder contracted when it shouldn't have contracted. Sometimes a neurological condition will cause it, but these patients didn't have a neurological condition. I sent them to a neurologist, but he couldn't find anything wrong with them. So we called it detrusor dyssynergia, because the bladder was contracting when it shouldn't contract. We published a paper on that,[3] and it started a wave of enthusiasm in the people who were interested in this kind of work. Then the electronic study became widespread, and a lot of people became interested in that too. It has become a specialty all of its own now. We continued with that urinary work right up to the time I retired as head of the department [1973].

"Over the years, there has been an effort to have the gynecologist and obstetrician become the woman's physician and do the general medical care for women. Not all gynecologists believe this, but the American College of Obstetricians and and Gynecologists has taken that attitude. The idea of having routine physical examinations, gynecologic examinations, is now very well accepted, especially by obstetricians. The acceptance of the Pap smear had a lot to do with it. Women began to go for a gynecological examination and a Pap smear. Then the doctor would include a breast examination and abdominal examination and usually take the patient's blood pressure. This is generally accepted now. Most obstetrician-gynecologists I know of feel this is an obligation toward their patients. I think most women like that idea. Women often feel more free to go to an obstetrician for advice—somebody who has delivered their babies—than they would feel going to somebody they don't really know. By the time a baby is born, most women and their obstetricians know each other pretty well.

"Mammography started to come into general use in about the late 1960s. When it did, some gynecologists didn't examine the woman's breasts. A woman would come in for a routine Pap smear and gynecological examination, and the gynecologists would say, 'You had better get a mammogram.' People got the idea that mammograms are the last word. Mammography is not an absolutely accurate science, and there have been a certain number of false negative and false positive reports made. The early diagnosis of breast cancer was one of my specialties, and I put a great deal of effort into this. In my group of cases, I found a rather large percentage, up in the region of 10–12 percent, of patients with early breast cancer who had negative mammograms. Mammography is better than that now, but there are still false negatives. The breast needs a complete, careful examination done by an expert. Mammography has taken that fact out of its proper perspective.

"I fully retired from practice May 1, 1983, when the hospital made a rule that everyone had to retire at the age of of seventy-five. I was then seventy-six. Since then I've missed practicing medicine, terribly. Almost every night, I dream about something in medicine—doing an operation, seeing patients, or giving a talk."

ROMANO

Bringing Psychiatry Closer to Medicine

UNTIL THE Second World War, psychiatry was both ideologically and physically cut off from the rest of medicine, with mental hospitals being located away from acute-care hospitals and universities. The psychiatrist's primary role was neither therapeutic nor medical. In 1940, more than two-thirds of the members of the American Psychiatric Association worked in public mental institutions.[1] Romano was deeply concerned about psychiatry's outcast status. Here he talks about his objective to create more intimacy between medicine and psychiatry by training psychiatrists to be doctors in the broadest sense.

He goes on to discuss some of his activities in the community—all in terms of his own opportunity for learning. As one of the founding members of the National Institute of Mental Health, he learned to appreciate the democratic process at its best. His "political education" began when he attempted to arrange for hospital insurance for psychiatric inpatients. As consultant to a VA hospital, he was able to know medical students and residents. He learned the limitations of psychoanalysis through observing its impact on his residents and through dealing with various psychoanalytic institutes. And while chairing the faculty committee for the university trustees, he grew to appreciate the ways in which universities are governed.

"In Rochester, it took two years to build Wing R. Before it was built, we used space in other parts of the hospital. People were very kind to us. Pediatrics, especially, was friendly and gave us space and time. The dean, George Whipple, professor of pathology, supported me. He was a Nobel laureate from his work on pernicious anemia.[2]

"We put a great emphasis on undergraduate teaching, and then we began to have resident staff. I wanted to teach the first-year medical students, which I did all alone. George Engel taught the second-year students, and I did third-year teaching. Others taught with us. The first class I taught here came in 1946 and finished in 1950. They were four to

283

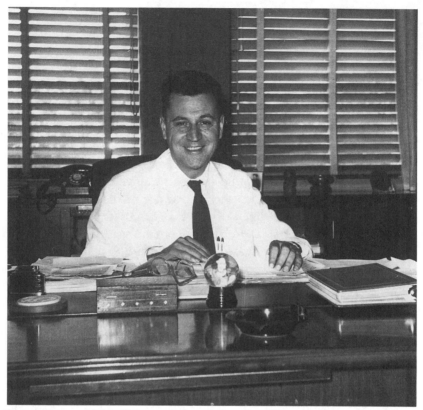

John Romano, 1954. Courtesy Edward G. Miner library, University of Rochester Medical Center.

five years older than the students who had been trained during the war years. Many were married; some had children. Many had seen combat. When it came to physics, chemistry, biology, and math, they were a bit rusty. But in terms of human affairs, they were different from the students before. They had loved and lost. I talked about grieving, sexuality, aggression. It made more sense to them than it did to ordinary first-year students. During the war years, more women were admitted to the medical school. After the war, more women came into the internships. Enrollment of women remained low until recently, with a current enrollment of about 40 percent.

"My experience with patients was broad. I saw patients young and old, black and white, rich and poor, subtly sick and blatantly disabled.

Their problems reflected a wide repertory of human distress—rebellious adolescents, drug abuse, alcoholic men and women, the aged and demented, patients with brain tumors and other organic brain disease, acute and chronic schizophrenic patients, varieties of hypomanic and manic excitements, and a great number of mildly and severely anxious and depressed persons. Our tradition here was to do clinical teaching, that is, teaching at the bedside of the patient, interviewing the patient, examining the patient. We had one-way screens, so that the patient could be interviewed without the students present. I preferred to interview without the screen, but I always allowed the patient his choice. I learned that, even with a hundred students in the room, the patient and I were so engaged with each other that it didn't matter who else was there. That has been my signature in a way—to interview patients with the students present whenever possible. In interviewing, I'd start out by saying, 'It's very good of you to come down here. What you tell us may help us understand you better, and it may help us better understand people who are sick like you.' Over more than forty years, fewer than ten patients have refused to come down and be interviewed. That was always impressive. Patients want to give too. They want to share. A lot of them say, 'Well, if it does good, I'll be happy to do that.' Young doctors, student doctors, learn from this that the dignity of the patient must be maintained.

"One of my objectives in life was to try and bring about a more intimate and effective rapport between psychiatry and medicine. I designed and then personally engaged in the educational process with all medical students, house officers from the department of psychiatry, and house officers from other clinical departments as well. We pioneered in integrating psychiatry into the medical curriculum because we did teach students in the first year, second year, third year, and fourth year. Also, we developed a liaison program. We reached out to each department. We had house officers from other departments—obstetrics and gynecology, surgery, medicine, and pediatrics—work with us. So, in addition to teaching psychiatry, psychosocial matters were dealt with in situ, within the other specialties. We had a more intimate relationship with obstetrics, because we took the person who was about to become chief resident and made him a fellow in our department for a year. I worked with the first man to do this, John Donovan, in his outpatient department. We thought it would be better for him, and not the psychiatrist, to talk about postpartum blues, or depressions, or the psychology of invasive surgery to the woman. Every year, the person who was to be chief resident in obstetrics spent a year with us. It was a very good liaison.

"I thought that a psychiatrist should be a good doctor, he should have a good medical education, a good general internship before he goes into the field of psychiatry. I wanted the psychiatrists of today and tomorrow to be well versed in the problems of medicine, surgery, pediatrics, and so on, to know what his patients are experiencing. The rotating internship that we created did that, and it strengthened relations between psychiatry and other fields too. It was a great achievement to establish that and have it continue from 1949 to 1961. It was called the Rochester two-year internship. It was six months medicine, six months psychiatry, six months pediatrics, three months obstetrics, and three months surgery. People from medicine, surgery, pediatrics, and obstetrics brought skills from psychiatry back to the those other disciplines. And they brought skills with them to psychiatry. We attracted top-drawer students from Columbia, Harvard, and other schools. We chose six interns the first year, then nine. Even the Korean War didn't trouble it. All kinds of persons came into the program. One-third went into medicine, one-sixth into pediatrics, one-sixth into psychiatry, and the remaining third into obstetrics, surgery, and other medical specialties. The idea was to offer a broad, liberal education for physicians in general medicine or for them to go on into a specialty. That was an exciting episode in my life. Over the years, the graduates of this program have written to me, those in pathology, medicine, surgery, to tell me there was no question about the value of the two-year internship in their later professional lives.

"Then a number of things happened, mostly political, which led to the decision that the internship wasn't necessary to psychiatry. People could come directly into the field without an internship, and the rotating internship was undermined. I fought this almost all alone in the country when it was abandoned. I felt alone for a long time. I thought this was a tremendous step backward, because it kept the psychiatrist from being a doctor, especially with the fourth year of medical school becoming elective and thus having less of a clinical overview. I insisted that we were physicians, not psychologists, not social workers, not clergymen. We were physicians, and we work through the role of the physician. So I fought that tooth and nail, alone. Later on the establishment capitulated. Now there are various kinds of internships for psychiatrists, four months of this, four months of that. Because of the movement towards biology, the trend is that the residents do pay more attention to medical education, to neurology, to the internship, than they had before. But I don't think the internship is as good as it used to be.

"I am truly gratified by the number of my medical students and psychiatric resident group who have achieved significant assignments and honors in academic medicine in the United States, Australia, West Germany, Canada, Lebanon, and Iceland. A number of our residents hold and have held chairman positions in departments of psychiatry, and many who emerged from our medical-psychiatric liaison program have distinguished themselves in medicine.

"For many years, many thoughtful persons have been concerned with what is the best, ideal, optimal preparation for men or women coming into medicine. Years ago [1950–1951], I took part in a national study of premedical education chaired by Harry Carmen and Aura Severinghaus, then at Columbia, and Bill Cadbury of Haverford. We made an attempt to study premedical education in America. We studied over a hundred schools, rich and poor, black and white, ivy, rural, Catholic, non-Catholic, to get some idea of how chemistry and biology, English and physics and history were taught, and what was the preparation of the student for medicine.

"I have always been in pursuit of how best to educate young men and women to become doctors in the broadest sense—not psychiatrists, psychologists, social workers, or surgeons. How can psychiatry contribute to understanding patients and families in any discipline? I'm still concerned about it.

"I don't think there was much of an intimate relationship between psychiatry and medicine during the war years. But during those years, a number of doctors became interested in coming into psychiatry because of their war experiences. Right after the war, the increase in members of the American Psychiatric Association, for example, was tremendous. And later there was a considerable change for the better, in terms of psychiatrists and medical people working with each other.

"The single most effective influence on American psychiatry in the twentieth century was the Seventy-ninth Congress passing the National Mental Health Law in 1946. I can't think of one single event which influenced modern psychiatry as much. It was due to the tremendous efforts of Claude Pepper, then senator from Florida, and Lister Hill, senator from Alabama, along with others. In order to get legislation passed, you have to have real champions supporting it. Those men did a great deal. With that one event, monies became available for the first time at the national level for research, for teaching, and for some limited aspects of clinical service. They supported all sectors of the National Institutes of Health.

"When I was leaving Cincinnati, I was appointed one of the founding members of the National Institute of Mental Health [then called the National Advisory Mental Health Council]. That was another big break in my life, another great thing that happened to me. Thomas Parran, the surgeon general, chose Robert Felix to be the first director of NIMH. It was a very good choice. Citizens were appointed to serve the government as members of committees. There was a committee for education and for service. I chaired the first research study section [1946–1948]. I chose almost all the persons for that committee: Margaret Mead and Kingsley Davis in social science; David Rappaport and Kurt Lewin in psychology; Abner Wolf and Harold Wolfe in neuropathology and neurophysiology; Houston Merritt in neurology; and Franz Alexander and Thomas French in psychoanalysis, and others. It was tops. Then we asked for the submission of grant proposals. We made recommendations to the surgeon general about what research projects should be approved, and for how much money. There was quite a bit of competition for the money, right from the beginning. In the first round, about 60 percent of the money went to neuroscience—neuroanatomy and neurophysiology. The others were in psychiatry. They were mostly clinical studies at that time. We set the standards, the guidelines, for the research. In the first year, I think we allocated about three hundred thousand dollars. Now of course, it is in the millions of dollars. Initially almost all of the money went to university-based research facilities. The NIMH intramural programs started later, in the 1950s. Later I was a member of the training section [1949–1952].

"Until 1946, there were few departments of psychiatry with more than one or two full-time members. With the creation of NIMH, there was the beginning of building psychiatry departments and developing research opportunities. The Hill-Burton Act of Congress made possible monies for the construction of psychiatric units in general hospitals. That brought psychiatry closer to medicine. It made psychiatry more involved with the medical school.

"Robert Felix was a very able fellow in many ways. He didn't want to intrude on the university. He felt that the citizens on the committees should make the decisions about which research gets approved. He felt that NIMH should support it, but not intrude. That was very good. It made me proud to be an American. It reminded me of Athens in the fifth century, the Greek democracy in which individual citizens were responsible. This was America at its best, citizens making judgments like that, trying to be fair. We examined the whole thing: Who is it who is asking for the money? What is it they wish to do with it? Where will they do it? What is the ambiance of where they will do it? What support will there be from others around them when they are doing what they want to do? These are the questions. They are very good questions. I knew how hard it was to make money in the world, but I also learned how difficult it is to spend it wisely. It's a responsibility.

"The political education of John Romano started almost as soon as I arrived in Rochester, after the building was opened up in 1948. It was stimulated by two 'gray eminences.' By the time I left Cincinnati, we had arranged for comparable and equivalent hospital insurance for psychiatric inpatients. When I came here, there was fairly good insurance for medicine, but nothing for psychiatry. Nothing in New York State. You couldn't get any insurance. Psychiatry was the last one on the totem pole for insurance. Patients could be admitted to the psychiatric floor for nine days. That's all; they were covered for nine days only. And, we had to call the patients' diseases thyrotoxicosis, irritable heart, or menopausal syndrome, instead of depression or schizophrenia. It wasn't until later that Medicare and Medicaid came and changed everything.

"I fought the battle to get psychiatric insurance all alone for about ten years, including fighting some people on the board of trustees of the university who were on the board of Blue Cross. They wouldn't accede to my wishes, and I went to all kinds of extremes. I chaired the lay board, the mental health consortium, and I met with the board of supervisors of the county. I met with insurance people. I did ten other things.

"Averell Harriman was then governor, a Democrat. So I went to a Democratic gray eminence in town. A gray eminence is somebody who runs the town but you don't hear about him; he gets things done without blowing a trombone solo about it. I explained that here are people who are sick and depressed and suicidal, and they need to be hospitalized. They can't afford to be hospitalized without being insured. We would take care of as many people as possible who couldn't pay for anything. But we couldn't afford the entire cost. So he said OK. The gray eminence called somebody in New York City, who in turn called somebody in Albany. Somebody in Albany called somebody else in

Albany, and guess what? The Rochester plan succeeded. First, we got fiften days of inpatient service for psychiatric patients once a year. Then we got thirty days. Next we got forty-five days. We got more and more things as time went on. It was a great victory, even though it took many years. It was through the gray eminence that I got the insurance provision to be changed in Albany.

"When Thomas Dewey was governor, the state passed a bill that would match state money to that spent by a county, dollar for dollar, for mental health services. Every county except Monroe was benefited. There again, I called upon the press, I called upon the Mental Health Association. One day I asked the president of the university to invite the second gray eminence to have lunch with us at a prestigious men's club downtown. I explained it all to him. He said, 'Why haven't I heard about this before?' About two weeks later, the county board of supervisors passed the bill, and Monroe County got what it should get—matching monies for whatever expenditures it made for mental health. It was somewhat shocking to me to learn that this was how things were done.

"From the very beginning in Rochester, I was also consultant and chairman of the dean's committee to the VA hospital in Canandaigua, thirty miles away, which was a hospital for chronic mental illness, mainly men. Several patients had chronic neurological disease. There were quite a few World War I veterans, and one or two Spanish-American War veterans. In 1946, World War II veterans were coming in. Since then they have had Korean War and Vietnam War veterans. For twenty-five years, I would visit every Friday morning. I took four students or four house officers with me. They would meet at my house and have a cup of coffee with my wife and son in front of the fireplace, and then we would go in my car to Canandaigua. I would have them taken on a tour of the whole place. At 10:00 A.M. they would come back and I would conduct teaching rounds. A patient would be presented to me. The nurses, social workers, nursing assistants, occupational therapists, psychologists, psychiatrists, physicians were there, as well as the dentist and clergyman. All persons relevantly concerned with the care of the patient would participate in the discussion. Then I would take these four students back with me, and we would take lunch at some little restaurant on the way home. This gave me an opportunity to know each student in the class.

"In Rochester, one constraint I've had was my relationship with psychoanalytic institutes. It is a painful story. They were so unfeeling, insensitive, and ignorant of what was going on in American academic psychiatry. I didn't belong to any analytic society. But I arranged for other members of my staff to obtain analytic training. I obtained money for people [staff members] to be analyzed, year in, year out, in Chicago, Boston, and New York. I spent thousands of dollars over the years in order to get them analyzed. I've watched them, and I didn't see many with any remarkable change in patterns of behavior. On the other hand, there are those who say that analysis brought about remarkable changes in their lives, and they feel very grateful to have had it. I continued to feel that, in some way or another, having an analytic experience would enlarge their dimensions, stretch their minds in terms of being a better psychiatrist. But I must say, that didn't always take place. In fact, analysis made some persons narrower. It made them less useful in society, I think.

"The most helpful institute was Chicago. Chicago was not a university, but it was closest to it in terms of ideas and practices. Particularly the efforts of Franz Alexander and Thomas French. Those who followed them were more rigid, more dogmatic, more doctrinaire. Franz Alexander was one of the few analysts concerned with the relationship between psychoanalysis and medicine. He began to study psychosomatic problems, and he ventured away from conventional neurosis and anxiety and hysteria and obsessive behavior. He began to study patients with thyroid disease, dermatitis, peptic ulcer, colitis. He was very much criticized by the traditional analysts for doing that. But my interest in analysis coincided with the work of Alexander.

"With psychoanalysis, it's easier to be black or white; to be gray is more troublesome. Certain analysts hated me because I supported it while I was critical of it at the same time. They insisted that I accept it all without criticism. But even though psychoanalysis is not a science, we have learned good things from it about growth and development, about transference, about the unconscious, about the life course of a person, about emotional anxiety. It should not be thrown out with the bathwater.

"My budget was reaching about six million dollars when I left the department chairmanship in 1971. We had grants from many agencies—federal, state, and local—and from private foundations—the Commonwealth Fund, Rockefeller Foundation, and the Macy Foundation. I took the chairmanship very seriously. For example, I had midyear and end-of-year interviews with every member of the faculty. We discussed what they did, what they didn't do, what they would like to do, what they would like to do but couldn't do, what their salary was, and we talked about their family. Also, I prepared annual reports, what happened in the department during the year. There haven't been any annual reports since I stepped down.

"As a department chairman, I served on the executive hospital committe, which determined hospital policy and clinical assignments. I was responsible for fund raising and for the design and implementation of research in the department. More broadly, I was chosen by the university trustees to assist them in university–wide fund drives. I enjoyed my role as professor and chairman. I learned that the skill and effectiveness in administrative matters is not due to just taking time to do something. I found that people with administrative skills were just as rare as are creative people in the arts and in science.

"I chaired the faculty committee for the university trustees that chose Allen Wallis for president of the university [1962–1963]. For nine months I spent fifteen to twenty hours a week on this assignment. I traveled with trustees all over the country searching for candidates. I learned a lot about how many fine people didn't want to be a university president. Also, about how many others who wanted to be president, but we didn't think they would be very good. I was impressed with the caliber of the trustees with whom I worked—intelligent, thoughtful, very successful men, who gave of themselves freely to the university without any recompense. They worked like hell to get money for the university. It occurred to me that it is a uniquely American phenomenon, you know, the American boards of trustees of the universities. Most universities, including professional schools, have a lay board of trustees. People forget that, that there is a lay board that is the court of final resort.

"Beyond medical school, hospital, and university, I was intimately involved in community affairs in advising city, county, and regional offices of the need for services. I tried to relate myself as intimately as I knew how to the community. I served as a consultant to the Rochester State Hospital, later called the Rochester Psychiatric Center [1946–present], to the several community hospitals, and to the Veterans Administration hospitals in Canandaigua and Batavia [1946–1973]. I tried as best I could in the years I was chairman, and since, to relate the university as intimately as possible to the various community health and welfare agencies."

"Many people think chronic mental illness is due to neglect. I want to make it clear that chronic mental illness, for the most part, is not due to neglect. It is due to the illness itself. It's part of that illness. A lot of people who grew up with psychotherapy believe that if you are with the patient long enough, are genuine enough, interested enough, committed enough, psychotherapy would win the day. No. Some kinds of psychotherapy, particularly anxiety-provoking therapy, are the worst thing you can do for a schizophrenic patient.

"Drugs are here to stay for schizophrenia. They will change; there will be better ones as time goes on. Drug therapy has led to a resurgence of interest in brain metabolism, brain biochemistry, brain physiology. All of these things are good. But none of these provide a complete answer for schizophrenia at the moment. I think major factors of cause and treatment for manic-depressive illness will be understood long before schizophrenia. Schizophrenia is more complicated. Schizophrenia is the central core of madness. It is the major problem of mental illness in terms of incidence, age of onset, length of illness, amount of money spent on those who are sick, and amount of money lost by patients not being productive.

"Depression, on the other hand, is much more common today. Maybe it has come out of the closet and people speak about it more. I think more people are depressed than anxious. Now depression is a bad term because it is so connotative. It can mean a momentary mood, something everybody feels. It can mean grief, bereavement. It can mean the black box—everything goes bad everyday: your wife is nagging you, the boss is after you, there is a bug in the car, your daughter may be pregnant. You know, ten other things. You wake up in the morning and say, 'My God, what kind of life have I got?' There is quite a bit of that. One must differentiate between the depression of everyday life and psychotic depressions.

"I think we continue to reach for a better understanding of mental illness. In some ways, psychiatry has not been good at that, because we promise too much.

"Perhaps one more word should be said about one's emotional involvement in what one is doing. Even though I have had my share of heartaches, headaches, and bellyaches, and as I told you, the good old days were never that good, still I must say that I have always remained excited about being a doctor, about caring for the sick, about sharing what little knowledge or wisdom I have with the young, and with forever being curious as to how better we could do things tomorrow. What I have done has been done *con amore.*"

AN ESSENTIAL TENSION

MEDICINE DURING the postwar years was rewarding. Trust between doctor and patient, a positive attitude toward physicians held by the public at large, drugs that cured diseases quickly and efficiently, basic scientific discoveries that both deepened understanding of human biology and paved the way for the eradication of diseases, and new technologies that enabled physicians to make more accurate and precise diagnoses, all contributed to this satisfaction. The scientific and medical optimism that was widespread in America during the late 1920s and 1930s was still prevalent in the postwar decade. Physicians were held in high esteem generally; their patients believed in them and did not mind depending on them.[1] Inequalities based on knowledge and control inherent in the doctor-patient relationship were not publicly scrutinized or condemned by consumer movements. The contemporary adversarial stance and language of patients turned health care consumers had not yet arrived.

In addition, the values of medical practice were relatively clear and generally agreed upon among physicians. Younger doctors, those who were trained in the immediate postwar period, felt they knew what it took to be a good doctor, regardless of the specialty: "to cure now and then, to help often, to comfort always," as Beeson noted. By the 1960s, when curing began to supersede caring in importance and emphasis, knowledge of what constituted a good doctor could no longer be taken for granted. We have seen that, for the most part, these doctors had mentors who were regarded by many as great clinicians. An intrinsic part of their clinical acumen lay in their abilities to empathize and communicate successfully with patients and families and to know the patient broadly and thoroughly through comprehensive history taking, detailed observations, and physical diagnosis. Those are the qualities that made a doctor good and enabled him or her to provide good care. The seven physicians learned to emulate and value those skills early in their careers. They maintained the skills and continued to value their mentors' qualities, even as they acquired scientific expertise and specialist knowledge in the years that followed. Physicians of subsequent generations would not have mentors who exhibited the qualities of Soma Weiss, I. S. Ravdin, Francis Scott Smyth, or Paul Dudley White, because the goals and emphases of medical practice changed so fundamentally after the war years. They would not be able, therefore, to emulate "good doctors" in that prewar sense.

By the mid-1960s, a fundamental tension was apparent to both physicians and health care consumers. It was a tension between traditional ideals about the physician's tasks and identity on the one hand and newer pressures to rely on technology while being financially accountable within a more demanding health care delivery system on the other. Medicine's changing priorities and values began to obscure the notion of what it took to be a good doctor. That loss of clarity was and has continued to be examined both within and outside the profession. In an address to the Harvard Medical School in 1972, psychologist Erik Erikson described the fragmentation of medical values which accompanied fragmentation in medical care delivery. He noted that both those phenomena resulted in ambiguity surrounding the doctor's identity:

> The very role of the doctor . . . is in jeopardy today because the doctor's image and self-image is linked with the conflicting images of various pursuits. There is, for example, the self-made man and the medical entrepreneur, the private practitioner, who, as a pointed complaint has it, "makes a killing." And there is the devoted teamworker. There is the gadgeteer and the computerizer, and there is the depth psychologist. There is the medical elitist in accustomed tweed and the new health populist and activist in "natural" attire. There is the specialist who must play the parts against the middle, and there is what is now called the primary physician, who in a new era insists on being as identifiable as the general practitioner of old. And there is the promising new specialty of family doctor. . . Seen in this light, the present identity crisis in medicine becomes painfully obvious.[2]

Ambiguity surrounding the physician's identity was a new development in medicine and it contributed to conflicting public views about the individual physician's responsibilities.

Medicine's dual goals in the postwar years—effective service and scientific discovery—looked to the past for moral guidance and to the future for scientific and technological direction. These broad goals remain the same today. Whether or not medical ideals forged in an earlier era can be maintained at all or successfully modified to fit current and future forms of medicine remains highly problematic. For contemporary medicine is buffeted by forces that did not exist a generation ago—the insurance industry, legal precedents and litigious patients, consumer demands, powerful technology, and a growing poor and elderly population. Problems created by these social realities have been subject to widespead professional and lay debate. But during the Golden Age, medicine's traditional ideals could still be, and were, embodied in the routine activities of many practitioners, precisely because doctors at the height of their careers lived those ideals themselves in their day-to-day work and wielded tremendous influence on others.

As we have seen, until perhaps the early or mid-1960s, the physician's work was shaped by ideals forged early in the century—duty, empathy (albeit framed by social, racial, and economic distance and a sense of superiority), care, social responsibility, and charity. Those ideals were widely retained following the Second World War. But, as time wore on, it became more and more difficult to adapt the ideals to the complex features of postwar expansion, specialization, and fragmentation. For example, as Shields points out, Medicare and Medicaid eliminated a great deal of charity work by reimbursing physicians for much of the care that they used to provide at no charge, thus fostering the decline of one of medicine's time-honored values. House calls, too, had embodied a traditional ideal—the ability to know the patient thoroughly. With greater reliance on objective diagnostic criteria located in doctors' offices, clinics, and hospitals and on effective drug treatments, house calls lost their value. Care came to be replaced largely by cure. And duty was replaced by cost effectiveness.

Pressures created by a more and more powerful scientific medicine, changing public policy, and new forms of health care delivery, all contributed to devaluing the old ideals. Yet these doctors worked to maintain those ideals in various ways. Jarcho refused to give up making house calls. Shields established a group practice "to eliminate from medicine as much of the profit element" as he could while giving the patient "the benefit of three brains." Beeson, striving to be a mentor for trainees, as Soma Weiss had been for him, established clinical conferences to let students know he was interested and available. Both Beeson and Romano stress how they worked to pass on to students the important, humanistic characteristics of the doctor: sit down rather than stand above patients, give them time, allow them to ask questions, be compassionate, and preserve their dignity. Emphasizing social responsibility, Olney, Rhoads, and Romano define their work in the broad public realm—as did their parents—as well as in the medical world. For Olney, that entailed work with public schools and the federal Headstart program for preschool children. Rhoads became provost of the University of Pennsylvania and joined the Philadelphia school board. Romano's work with NIMH committees and later with the faculty committee for the university trustees led him to view public service as an honor and a privilege.

Perhaps most important, these doctors stress the vital importance of preserving medicine's generalist identity. Shields's and Jarcho's emphasis on the priority of holistic patient care over cost effectiveness, Hodgkinson's discussion of training obstetrics and gynecology residents to be general surgeons, Romano's creation of the two-year internship to offer "a broad liberal education for the physician in general medicine," and Beeson's emphasis on training students to behave with patients in the tradition of the old-fashioned, humanitarian doctor, all speak to that goal.

Yet in this part of the volume, the doctors also speak with sadness and deep concern about the formidable power of specialization and the consequent loss of the generalist philosophy as it impacted their particular branches of medicine during the 1950s and especially during the 1960s. They have also been made uncomfortable by the transience of some features of medical knowledge and practice which they observed over the years. Jarcho was appalled to learn that, after the war, anatomical collections of slides and specimens at Columbia were being destroyed and replaced by photographs. For him, the collections represented the basis of medical knowledge, a treasure—in fact, a truth—that another generation was simply and easily ignoring and discarding.

Both Jarcho and Shields recall that they used to attend autopsies because they learned so much medicine from them. B. H. Kean, a contemporary of these doctors, commented on the meaning of the demise of the autopsy and the transience of that framework of understanding in his recent memoir:

> . . . the question arises, why then is the postmortem today facing virtual extinction? (Only 10 percent to 15 percent of all patients who die in American hospitals nowadays are autopsied, compared to four times that number four decades ago.) Fear is one great inhibitor. Recent studies have shown that, despite major improvements in diagnostic tech-

niques, as many as a quarter of all patients died following a significant error in diagnosis. While that's nothing particularly new, many doctors, who find themselves practicing in an age of escalating malpractice suits, have adopted the unfortunate attitude that what the deceased's loved ones don't know can't hurt them—the doctors.

The rapid spread of high-tech ignorance tells the rest of the story. Necropsy has long since been dropped by many medical schools as a cornerstone of a doctor's education because too few bodies are available for postmortem study. No wonder many younger physicians seem to think that autopsies have lost their relevance in an age of CAT scans and other supersophisticated methods of diagnosis. They are dead wrong. They are also missing out on one of medicine's great adventures.[3]

In other examples of how easily medical structures can be dismantled and replaced, Hodgkinson and Romano talk about programs they initiated which others later abolished. Hodgkinson created the general surgery research laboratory for his trainees in obstetrics and gynecology at Henry Ford Hospital, and Romano instituted the Rochester two-year internship. Both men's programs represented generalist ideals. They aimed to integrate specialists with other medical fields and to enable the obstetrician-gynecologist and psychiatrist, respectively, to function broadly as doctors. The continuity of generalist goals was undermined when their respective programs were discontinued after a number of years.

The doctors articulate medicine's losses. All those losses reflect the idea, suggested in Part I, that contemporary medicine does not seem to build on itself, but rather replaces one set of facts and structures with another. The transience of medical knowledge permits and sometimes even enhances the obscuring of medicine's time-honored values. The doctors respond to the impermanence of medical information, structures, and practices with a dual perspective. First, they portray the excitement over scientific discovery and the application of new techniques and treatments in the care of patients. Firmly embedded in the culture of medicine, they were committed to medicine's technological and moral imperatives. Second, with the wisdom of long experience, they express some discomfort and ambivalence in the final sections of the narratives, where they reveal that the press toward scientific discovery and specialization has antiquated an important moral stance: the need to put the good of the individual patient first.[4] Much debate about contemporary medical practice centers on how this traditional value can be actualized in the contexts of growing subspecialization, more prevalent diagnostic technology, and ever-restrictive health insurance plans.

Driven by its technological and moral imperatives, medicine grows haphazardly from the ground up, in response to both challenges that appear with the creation of new technologies and challenges of patient care, management, and life prolongation that arise within the different specialties and subspecialties. Medicine is pragmatic, applied, and action-oriented, and it is determined by the immediate need for problem-solving in particular situations. Its power and authority are derived from its day-to-day advances in patient care—such as Shields's use of pneumothoraces, Rhoads's contributions to the nutrition of surgical patients, and Hodgkinson's diagnosis of stress urinary incontinence with the metallic bead technique—and from understanding the mechanisms of disease—such as in Jarcho's studies of tropical medicine, Beeson's laboratory research on bacterial endocarditis and eosinophil production, and Olney's cardiac research with mice.

Clinical medicine's broad, applied, and practical nature is a clue to its relationship with science. While medicine depends on science for its very existence and borrows from many scientific disciplines in efforts to solve problems in patient care and to uncover mechanisms of disease, medicine itself cannot be equated with science. Rather, medicine reacts to developments in the biological, physical, and technical sciences which stand outside itself. The medical specialties use the sciences to develop in many directions at once by small, incremental innovations designed to answer only specific questions. Sick patients create the moral dimension of medicine that distinguishes it from laboratory science.

Yet with greater and greater specialization, many branches of medicine have become more scientific, ruled by the models of scientific research. Indeed, some observers have noted that many contemporary physicians view themselves as "applied scientists with the human organism as their domain and laboratory."[5] Some specialties of medicine, while becoming more and more like science, have come to define and understand medicine's moral imperative in solely operational terms: the quest for procedures, interventions, and techniques for the management of disease and prolongation of life. The development of a scientific, operational discourse and the replacement of medicine's traditional values by this new discourse have happened steadily since the postwar period. Though that gradual process of usurpation has been unplanned and accidental, its results greatly determine our notions, lay and medical alike, of medicine's purpose.

These seven narratives embody medicine's past, present, and future-oriented problem-solving nature and its embrace of science's methods and findings. The doctors' inability to specify shared values about technological intervention and the saving of lives derives from the fact that medicine has not been determined or guided by such values during the past fifty years. Instead, medicine has been constituted by its responses to particular problems and by specialization within which technological problem solving occurs. The stories of research and patient care show us how medicine actually works—by purposeful and highly particular activities. Taken together, those activities define medicine. It is the sum of the techniques, processes, methods, procedures, and treatments adapted and created in the service of patient care and life prolongation. The thousands of innovations that have occurred in the past sixty-five years, and that these doctors have been part of and witness to, have been the focus of medicine's gaze on itself, its framework for understanding itself. The always-emerging tools and practices are clinical medicine's purpose, largely taken for granted as such.

Over the past several decades, the sum of the many separate innovations has given rise to a profound qualitative change in the experience of medical practice for both physicians and patients. They, we, have been seduced by and have become servants of medicine's means (the use of and dependence on more and more sophisticated technology) and its emphasis and nearly total reliance on a *scientific approach* to its ends (the press to control disease and save lives). *We cannot imagine a medicine defined in any other way.* We now face the ethical, social, and financial ramifications of the focus on medicine's technological and *scientifically cast* moral imperatives.

MEDICINE'S MEANS AND ENDS, 1970s–1990s

Technological Superiority, Moral Confusion

THE PHYSICIAN'S life history—as subjective reflections on medicine's developments—is a largely untapped source for understanding the relationship between culture and medicine. Taken together, these seven narratives show medicine to be an agent of cultural change, a force in altering our ways of understanding fundamental truths. Through the doctors' reflective and critical voices we are able to see what has remained essential to medicine during the twentieth century and what has been transient.

Medicine's power to reconceive such matters as birth, life, and death creates the moral confusion we presently face. Medicine's overwhelming reliance on technological intervention and scientific method and its simultaneous inability to articulate shared values about those interventions and methods are the sources of that confusion. Medicine has shattered conventional ways of knowing: the body; the relationships among body, mind, and emotions; the patient and family; and communication patterns between doctor and patient, especially regarding truth-telling, responsibility, and choice. Finally, medicine has shattered its own limits as a healing practice. Here, using the seven doctors' narratives as a starting point, I wish to contrast some of medicine's traditional ways of knowing with some of its most recent practices and dilemmas. My goal is to explore the cultural effects of the latter as they heighten the state of moral confusion in which we find ourselves today.

BODY PARTS

Hodgkinson's example of the exclusion of women's breasts from the gynecologist's practice is an early illustration of how and why certain parts of the body may not be considered a specialist's responsibility. In our current age of superspecialization, a great many consumer complaints about the impersonal nature of health care delivery and lack of satisfaction in encounters with physicians stem from the fragmentation of the body among specialties. The whole patient has been dismantled and seemingly abandoned. Observations from within and outside medicine point to the need for individual doctors who have the time, training, and inclination to treat any and all ailments, or at least most of them, so that the patient may be reconstituted as a whole. Yet the tension between the perceived need to treat patients in their existential wholeness and the demand for highly knowledgeable—that is, specialized—care cannot be solved easily.

Each medical specialty has its own history, its own unique approach to constructing and understanding the body's relationship to disease processes. Patients, when moving from specialist to specialist, are in fact moving among ways of knowing (paradigms), and then treating, a particular body region and in fact the whole person. The cardiologist, oncologist, orthopedist, and psychiatrist will have different approaches to ameliorating a patient's ailments. Attempts on the part of patients to grasp paradigm shifts, as well as to cope with the medically created fragmentation of the body, have involved bewilderment in addition to frustration.

While the dismantled patient has been fostering dissatisfaction and confusion for several decades, moral dilemmas over the body emerge most dramatically today in the field of organ transplantation. The practice of transferring body parts from one being to another raises new questions about life, death, culture, and nature, obscuring traditional concepts in totally unexpected ways. Creating a class of dead patients from whom we wish to remove organs challenges cultural and religious views about treatment of the dead. Perhaps even more unsettling is the fact that organ donors represent a *new* class of dead patients. For example:

> For these are cadavers whose hearts are beating spontaneously, pumping red, oxygenated blood throughout their bodies. They may be legally dead, but their cells, tissues, and major organs continue to live and function. It is this very life that makes them such attractive donors. True, they must be aggressively maintained on ventilators with vigorous attention to blood pressure and other physiologic parameters which are extremely unstable. But this characteristic only emphasizes their similarity to other critically ill but clearly *living* patients. . . A recent study demonstrates that many health professionals are confused about their status; many do not really believe they are dead.[1]

Moreover, questions arise as to whether or not dead persons have rights which may be violated by the removal of their organs. These questions extend to anencephalic infants—those born without higher brain structure and function—as well. There is also debate about whether cells from aborted fetuses should be used for transplantation or research. The problem of inequities in the distribution of scarce organs is another dilemma. Allocation decisions are complex and charged with ethical ramifications: Should the social worth of the individual or age or gender determine eligibility, for example?[2]

Olney raised the issue of the ethics of transplantation costs when she reflected on some of today's practices. She told me:

> I don't think the costs that result from some techniques, such as transplants, are appreciated. When there were conditions that we couldn't cure, we used to say that the end of existence was nature's clearinghouse. When we try to interfere with nature's clearinghouse, we do it at great expense, and we have yet to evaluate whether or not it is ethical. There is no doubt about it in some cases. In other cases it is yet to be established. For an ordinary family to develop a seventy thousand dollar or hundred thousand dollar indebtedness or more is questionable. Kidney transplants have been so marvelous. Recent transplants of the liver and the heart and lungs have introduced fantastically expensive procedures. Whether society can continue to support that, I don't know.
>
> The most inspiring thing recently has been the discoveries of the physicist Stephen Hawking, who is unraveling questions about the universe. Despite the fact that he has amyotrophic lateral sclerosis [ALS] and can't use his arms or legs, he can use his mind. Who can say that it isn't within our means to support people like that? It leaves you in a state of complete confusion about ethics. I don't think we are in a position to make judgments, we are only in a position to make observations. And perhaps think of a way.

None of the questions posed by existing transplant practices can be answered without moral debate.

BODY-MIND-EMOTIONS

Physicians have always understood the fact that emotions and psychological states play a role in physical disease and the experience of illness. Shields's uncertainty early in his career about how to treat psychosomatic illness, Jarcho's acknowledgment that much of what he treated as an internist was psychological and emotional trouble, and Romano's struggle to define psychiatry within medicine, all exemplified medicine's lack of clarity about separation or integration of mind and brain, "psycho" and "somatic," and mind and body.

This area of confusion is not only historical. The ability to treat diseases of psychological origin and to view the experience of illness and suffering from an integrated perspective has become increasingly difficult as we rely more and more on scientific methods and sophisticated technology in order to disclose "hard" findings. Many observers of medicine today have noted that both clinicians and patients must struggle to interpret illnesses without categorizing them as either "organic" or "psychological," because we automatically assume the physical and mental to be separate and opposite.[3]

Complicating the matter is the fact that the curative power of the doctor-patient dialogue itself—a vehicle for understanding the role of emotions and psychological states in physical disease—is devalued in the press to save time and in the reliance on diagnostic technology. Much of "healing" used to reside in the doctor-patient relationship—in the doctor's ability to take time and listen, empathize, respond, and show concern for the patient and his or her problems, however they manifested themselves. Today tensions exist among the patient's need for the practitioner to view him or her as an emotional being, deserving of full attention and compassion, the patient's desire for a single pill to cure the problem quickly, and the contemporary physician's inclination to disengage the organic from the emotional so that the organic may be treated.

DOCTOR AND PATIENT

Beeson and Shields compare contemporary medical practice with earlier forms in their respective descriptions of the hospital stay and the office visit, the two settings in which doctors and patients interact most frequently. Their critique of the present situation captures the essence of their generation's ideals about the doctor-patient relationship, what remains the same and what, exactly, has been lost.

Beeson described the hospital setting today:

> I am afraid that rounds at the bedside, talking about the patient instead of to the patient, hasn't changed very much over the years. One

of the criticisms of ward round teaching now is that it isn't ward round teaching. You sit in a conference room off the ward. The student or house officer presents the case, and the rounding doctor gets up to the blackboard and talks about the latest research on this. Then he may whiz by and shake the patient's hand and go. This is too bad. This is part of the hurry of modern medicine.

In intensive care, which is really the most exciting part of modern medicine, everyone is thrilled about putting catheters in and measuring pressures here and there and measuring blood gases all the time. The talk is of "the numbers": "What are the numbers on Mrs. Jones this morning?" And you list her oxygen, CO_2, sodium, and potassium, and you talk about what you are going to do to correct those. If you go and stand in an intensive care unit, you will see a team of four or five people, usually the specialist and a fellow and the house officer and a couple of students. They come in and stand on both sides of the patient's bed, and they look across the patient and talk to one another about the numbers. No one puts a hand on the patient. No one engages in visual contact. Often the patient can't talk if he has assisted respiration. But the patient is listening, and it is so important to put a reassuring hand on the patient's arm and look him the in eye and say something. Instead of that, they talk about the numbers and then go on to the next patient.

This is one of the sad things about the technological aspects becoming so dominant in patient care. The poor patient is lying there, things attached to all four extremities, perhaps unable to speak, and never able to get off his back. The doctors come in but the patient is not able to ask those questions or get some sense of what is going on or have something explained. The doctors talk only to each other and then they leave.

We recall that during Beeson's early training years, attending physicians, interns, and student talked among themselves during ward rounds when they moved from bed to bed, and rarely communicated directly with patients. They were not taught to talk with their hospitalized patients, nor was it expected that they would. Yet, ironically, the importance of empathetic communication—though not what we would now call explanation—was stressed by the physicians who were considered "good" clinicians of the pre–Second World War era. When the consumer movement began to influence the delivery of medical care in the 1960s, patients wanted and asked for explanation of diagnoses, prognoses, and treatments and demanded participation in medical decision-making. It is those recent features of explanation and patient participation that are lost in the intensive care setting today. Beeson refers to the fact that there technology has in some sense usurped recent gains made by both doctors and patients in their desire and ability to communicate directly, honestly, and with mutual satisfaction.

Shields talked about the changed nature of the office visit:

> These days, you go into an office that has a bunch of little rooms and is often cold. You sit down in an uncomfortable place and see an assistant. That person goes down a big piece of paper and asks questions. The financial questions are all right. But when they ask the physical ones from a piece of paper, you're uncomfortable. Then they put you on the examining table, disrobed, with one of those stupid little gowns on, just about freezing to death. And the doctor comes in reading the piece of paper. You know that he doesn't have more than about five minutes. He asks you a few questions, and then he immediately puts his hands on you. He can't wait to examine you.
>
> Now how did I practice medicine? I had a consultation room. I had one consult chair. I didn't have too many, because I didn't want the family around. One consult chair for the patient. The first thing I did was to sit and talk to him, quietly. I could make each patient feel that he was the only patient I had, and that I had all the time in the world. That was just the natural way to do it, because I did feel the patient was the most important. I wouldn't remember all about him, because I can't remember people well. But I had a good record system, and I read the patient's record. If it was a return visit, I read the patient's record and knew all about him before he came into my office. I probably spent ten to fifteen minutes with the patient. Probably three times as much as doctors do now.
>
> After we talked, patients were taken into the other room by my nurse, where they disrobed and got ready for the examination. And that took more time. After I knew patients well and they were just there for a revisit, it was much shorter. I would see patients who had mainly psychosomatic difficulties in my office every time. They are a lot harder to treat.
>
> Regarding modern doctors and their problems, I was a little disturbed about my son Joe and his method of practice, because he makes absolutely no house calls and never has. I talked to him once about it, and he said, "Dad, I just can't do that. Suppose I leave my office and make a house call across town. In modern medicine, we have to have our tools. I can't do any of the things I want to do to this individual out of the office. I can't possibly spend less than ninety minutes going across town to see the patient and get back. During that time I could

not only do a much better job in the office, but I could also see at least two more patients that day. In order to do the most for my patients, I just can't afford to do house calls. I try to ascertain what the situation is and send an ambulance for them if necessary, to get them to the hospital if they are desperately sick, or get them into the office where I can see them." And he's absolutely right. That is right for all doctors now.

I have often thought that if the public could have the advantage of the physician of my father's time—the friend, the counselor who gave that sense of strength to the patients that my father did—and at the same time be able to have the things done that my son is able to do, that would be a lovely, lovely thing. But it is completely impractical. It cannot be done. There has got to be some kind of system established that will meet the needs of patients in both those ways. That is one of the great problems in medicine today.

The need for personal relationships, the need for compassion, the need for concern, for interest—all of those things haven't changed. But everything else in medicine has changed. The feelings, emotions, and intimacies of the doctor-patient relationship are different today.

PATIENT AND FAMILY

Medicine waffles, first, about the role the family plays in obtaining information about the patient and disclosing information to the patient and, second, about the role of the family in the doctor-patient relationship itself. Jarcho and Olney worked intimately with families throughout their careers. They were trained to spend time with families, to understand interpersonal dynamics that influenced the course of the patient's disease and treatment. They worked with social workers extensively in order to know families better, and they depended on social workers to act as their extensions, to provide goods and services to families, so that patient care and the family's ability to cope with illness would be enhanced. Patient and family together were the treatment unit; to disentangle them was to limit understanding of the ramifications of illness and thus to limit possibilities for treatment.

Olney notes that medical students today do not have time to pay attention to, and thus to learn the relevance of, family dynamics for patient care. She told me: "I think medical students may have a harder time now adapting to families, understanding how to appreciate what illness does in the family. You learn by sitting at the patient's bedside, seeing what happens. When the relatives came to visit, we saw what the relationships were. Now medical students are much too busy for that. They don't know what the child's absence from school does to him or the family. They don't know what it's like when the father is unemployed for a period of time with an illness that either is very threatening or very frightening to the rest of the family. Those kinds of relationships are much harder to get across to students these days." The family, a traditional aid to understanding the patient, has been replaced by technological diagnostic tools.

Shields discusses the importance of the house call as a means of enabling the doctor to know the patient in the context of family. As we just saw, he contrasts that view with the recollection of having had only one chair in the consultation room: "I didn't have too many, because I didn't want the family around." He did that to impress upon the patient the fact that he or she was the most important person in the world to him at that moment. The presence of anyone else would detract from their intimate interaction. Shields emphasized the patient, to the exclusion of family members, to promote a positive doctor-patient bond and partnership. In that context, the one-to-one relationship was more important than the family.

Recent public demands for physicians who on the one hand respect the patient's individuality and autonomy above all and who on the other hand, through their knowledge and decisions, encompass the concerns of the entire family speak to widespread cultural ambiguity about the relationship between patient and family and the role of the family during illness. One example of this ambiguity can be seen in conflicts over patient versus family "rights" to decision-making in the hospital setting. Hospitals, pressured by the need to protect legally both the welfare of patients and their own interests, currently require family permission for physicians to withdraw or withhold life-sustaining treatment from patients who lack decision-making capacity. An absence of standards about the primacy of patient or family rights is made painfully obvious when a family's decision about treatment termination or prolongation—especially cardiac resuscitation—conflicts with a physician's judgment of the patient's best interests.[4] In those conflicts, legal precedent may be sought by a patient's family or by a hospital, because *cultural* precedent, in the form of norms and clear-cut values regarding patient, family, and physician interests, does not exist.

In 1990, the U.S. Supreme Court decided that the rights of the state of Missouri to continue treatment of a comatose person (in that case, tube feeding) held sway over the rights of Nancy Beth Cruzan's family to discontinue her treatment, because "no clear and convincing evidence" about the patient's wishes for treatment termination was available. The Supreme Court's decision is one powerful illustration of the relatively small value our society currently attaches to the patient-family relationship. But deep contradictions about the role of family in health care decisions emanate from the nation's highest court; for example: "The incredible leeway the Court cedes to the states can be seen by contrasting Cruzan with another case decided on the same day. On the day the Court decided that Missouri could 'legitimately and rationally' assume that all families of incompetent patients are a danger to them, it also decided that Ohio could 'legitimately and rationally' assume that all families are loving and supportive and thus require a pregnant teenager to notify her parents before obtaining an abortion, in order to uphold 'the dignity of the family.' "[5]

The Supreme Court's double-faced stance both reflects and produces cultural unease in dealing with the patient-family relationship. And those legal mandates, while not representing the views of many citizens and not having any practical effect in many states, now become part of the cultural context in which physicians both act with patients and their families and respond to demands for patient and family rights.

TRUTH-TELLING AND DISCLOSURE

Attitudes about lying or avoiding disclosure of terminal illness have vacillated during the century, because there have been no hard and fast rules within medicine about the discussion of a bad prognosis with patients. Both Beeson and Rhoads note how their physician fathers weighed each case individually when deciding whether or not to tell a patient about a terminal illness. Beeson comments that avoiding discussion of impending death, typical of the period prior to the 1960s, was morally repugnant to him, because patients usually knew the diagnosis and prognosis anyway and felt abandoned by a physician and family who would not talk about it. Rhoads informed me that, although terminal illness was not discussed as openly with patients in the past as it is in the present, he and his colleagues did talk freely with patients about it throughout his years of practice. He claims that he has not seen a great change in patterns of communication with patients and families over the years. He told me: "We did talk to patients and we learned a great deal from what they told us. This may be because we have a substantial private patient component in the practice at the Hospital of the University of Pennsylvania as compared with some of the city hospital settings. It is true that we did not discuss fatal outcomes as much as we do now. I think perhaps this change stemmed a good deal from improvements in prognosis. As a medical student, I recall arriving at the conclusion that, if I incurred a dread disease, I would just as soon not be told about it in its early stages. As the chances for survival improve, it is easier to talk about such diagnoses."

Nevertheless, since the late 1960s and early 1970s, a change in general attitudes toward disclosure has occurred, in part because of the factors Beeson and Rhoads discussed: first, the hospice movement and an openness in some sectors of American society toward embracing the process of dying as a life cycle event to be consciously experienced; second, the federal mandate for informed consent before a patient can receive experimental treatments in cases of terminal illness; and third, the fear of litigation if a physician does not inform the patient fully of his or her condition. Telling the truth about diagnosis and prognosis can also be attributed to the consumer movement in health care, especially patient demands for greater access to all kinds of medical information and more control over treatment decisions.

Although patients are now typically told diagnoses of terminal illness and family members are usually involved in that discussion, recent research indicates that total frankness about prognosis is generally viewed by physicians as neither appropriate nor therapeutic. Studies reveal that there are styles, stages, techniques, and philosophies about disclosure and truth-telling which vary according to the physician's specialty and whether or not the physician is committed to placing patients in experimental research projects.[6]

Talking about terminal illness with patients and families is considered to be complex by physicians, and it is debated in the medical literature. The dilemma of how much information to give the patient and when represents the ongoing tension between a traditional medical morality characterized by social distance, authoritative knowledge, and protective care and the newer morality of equality between doctor and patient characterized by the patient's right to know and right to autonomy in decision-making.

PHYSICIAN RESPONSIBILITY,
PATIENT CHOICE

The American public wants medicine not only to remain powerful but to become progressively more powerful. We ask doctors to "do everything" for our terminally ill family members. We seek and demand organ transplants, artificial organs, multiple bypass surgery, and treatments for infertility. We plead for the opportunity to take experimental drugs. And we want our life spans extended. At the same time, we are frightened and angered by the possibility that our individual autonomy—perhaps our most cherished cultural value—is threatened by the applications of new medical knowledge.

Beginning in the mid-1960s, we responded to this paradox with the creation of two social movements whose goals have been to promote individual choice, opportunity, and rights in health care and to press individuals to demand some control when confronted by an increasingly technological and bureaucratic health care delivery system. These are the consumer and holistic health movements. Both had shaped physicians' and patients' knowledge of what ideal forms of health care should entail. The consumer movement, epitomized in the work of Ralph Nader, has urged people to take an active role in demanding safe, high quality, and fairly priced goods and services. The consumer movement in health care has encouraged people to seek and demand medical treatment that is competent, compassionate, honest, and relevant to their personal lives.

The holistic health movement (also termed behavioral medicine) emphasizes "wellness" rather than illness and conceives of the patient as an existential whole. It has been described as a method of potentially or partially alleviating problems of patient alienation, dissatisfaction, and loss of control brought about by a highly sophisticated, technological approach to medicine. That movement posits that the patient's psychology and behavior—as well as physiology—influence the course of illness and recovery and are directly relevant to medical care. The holistic health movement advocates patient responsibility for learning about one's condition, for making treatment decisions, and for actively participating as a member of the health care team. It also advocates physician acceptance of the patient's increased role in health care decision-making.

While most health professionals agree that well-educated and informed patients are all to the good, patient demands for information and choice upset the traditional role of physician as authority, protector, and caregiver, with unpredictable consequences for the nature of the doctor-patient relationship and for the assumption of responsibility. Both Shields and Romano echo Hodgkinson's concern about the loss of physician responsibility to patient choice. All three doctors comment that, when patients have more opportunity to participate in medical decision-making, physicians sometimes avoid or abdicate their own responsibilities, with poor health outcomes as the result. They express the view that allowing patients to make so many treatment decisions reduces or weakens physicians' responsibilities toward their patients. Shields told me: "Often the physician gives the patient choices among treatments and makes him choose without giving him the proper information. I guess I have been guilty of that. That is avoiding responsibility, and I think that is one of the things wrong with medicine today. The physician should make more decisions, rather than ask the patient to make them." Romano cited an article he had written about the extreme position of the holistic health movement: "Obviously, we have erred at both extremities. In the past, we have permitted our appropriate authority, with its commensurate responsibility and accountability, to become authoritarian. And now, in our attempt to engage the patient in his care, we have gone too far in forfeiting our time-honored responsibilities."[7]

A similar warning is given by physicians and physician advocates in recent debates about the futility of certain procedures such as cardiopulmonary resuscitation (CPR), for example. Many are asserting that the physician's integrity, ability, and responsibility both to ameliorate suffering in the individual patient and to serve the social good are jeopardized by patients and families who demand resuscitation. Those advocates argue that it is for the sake of patient autonomy and cost containment that physicians be given the opportunity (or the right) to restrict choices offered to patients and families and to override a patient's decision when a situation is deemed futile in their professional judgment.[8] Conflicts over who has the right to responsibility when treatment is considered futile are a most recent development in medicine. They arise from the regular use of highly sophisticated technologies which can prolong life.

The case of Baby L, reported in a 1990 issue of the *New England Journal of Medicine*, provides another example of the conflict over patient-family-physician control and responsibility. For over two years, a blind, deaf, quadraplegic, and severely mentally impaired infant was subjected to repeated surgical procedures and cardiopulmonary resuscitations to save her life, because the child's mother insisted that "everything possible be done to ensure the child's survival."[9] Because the child had such severe neurological deficits and could experience only pain, hospital staff finally agreed unanimously to stop medical interventions on the grounds that further procedures would be futile and inhumane. When faced with court intervention, the physicians and hospital did not alter their decision, stating that to do so would violate their ethical obligation to the patient.

Cases such as that of Baby L elicit contradictory responses about the ethics of medical decision-making. On the one hand, there is the view that a physician who merely provides a patient and family with a myriad of treatment choices, yet advocates or makes no decision himself or herself, is guilty of abdicating responsibility. Some hold that it is the physician who must exercise professional value judgments and recommend a course of action. In contrast is the belief that the physician should let the patient or family control decision-making, even when the physician believes a treatment will not benefit the patient. In that view, the goals of the patient or family, not the physician's judgment of treatment efficacy, should determine action.

A medical decision to terminate treatment because it no longer has any positive effect contradicts, and in some cases wreaks havoc with, some patients' beliefs that medicine is all-powerful in its ability to restore perfect health or normalcy. Those patients and families continue to construe medicine's powers as limitless. Their responses to catastrophic conditions or terminal illness reflect sixty years of medicine's embrace of science and technology. In that regard, some patient and family responses lag behind physicians' recent and more measured approaches to the uses of technology.

The discrepancy between those particular views has at least several effects. First, it puts the doctor-patient-family relationship in a new limbo. Second, it challenges conventional notions of medicine's authority and expertise. Third, it forces us to confront cultural expectations, born in the postwar era, that medicine can restore and, in fact, re-create normalcy.

MEDICINE AND NONMEDICINE

The consumer and holistic health movements have attempted to foster individual autonomy and control over medical decision-making and health outcomes. Yet the control they seek to create and enhance coexists with a fear about encroaching medical authority. For medicine is perceived to have *spread* into many areas of life which were not considered medical or potentially treatable a generation ago. Problems which in the past were considered social, moral, or personal concerns, or were not publicly identified at all, are now considered medical problems. These include, for example: infertility, teenage pregnancy, and menopause; obesity and anorexia; and alcohol and drug abuse. The irony surrounding the broadening of medicine's influence on these conditions is evident in our confusion toward them. We desire and demand medical treatment (and hopefully cures) for them, and we simultaneously worry about the problems of encroachment, management, and surveillance such treatments create.

Medicine's spreading perspective and power are evident also in its ability to alter our cultural and natural worlds while producing new cultural knowledge. For example, recent medical innovations have produced surrogate mothers, the technology to freeze body parts for later use and embryos for later development, and the pharmacology to end life quickly and painlessly. These and other practices are unsettling, and our unease with them is evident when we pose and confront such questions as: Should surrogacy be allowed? Should a comatose pregnant woman be allowed to have an abortion to save her life? Should a man with an inoperable brain tumor who wants to freeze his head before he dies, so that someday he can be revived and cured, have the opportunity to do so? Should the sperm of a dead man be "harvested" so that his widow may bear his child? Should physicians be allowed to practice active euthanasia? Should billions of dollars be spent on mapping human DNA? What are the ramifications for individuals and society of precise genetic knowledge of each human being? The fact that these questions are publicly aired and widely contested, both within and outside the medical profession, illustrates our concern over medicine's power to supplant old frameworks of understanding with new possibilities and thus to shatter our conceptions of what is right, wrong, appropriate, humane, and natural.

Popular concern with medicine's spread into areas of life beyond acute, serious illness did not exist before the Second World War. Recent interpretation of that spread as encroachment provides a new source of cultural anxiety. Medicine's unknown ramifications have created the desire and expressed need for experts from disciplines outside itself—

from law, philosophy, and theology, for example—to help clarify its specific responsibilities and limits, because it impinges on so many aspects of human life and human potential. Yet the problem of how medicine's ramifications can be publicly managed creates a generalized tension in society, evident in such volatile examples as the right to abortion and the right to die without the introduction of life-prolonging devices. Involvement of America's legal system in these and other issues (for example, surrogacy, cryonics), along with the media publicity which surrounds some individual cases (Karen Quinlan, Nancy Cruzan), reflects a high degree of cultural uncertainty about medicine's boundaries and responsibilities to society.

TRANSFORMING MEDICINE
AND CULTURE

THESE PHYSICIANS are members of a generation that witnessed and participated in two major upheavals in medicine's modern evolution. When they entered medicine their prime directive was to care for sick people; additionally they hoped to diagnose disease. In the vast majority of cases they could do little else. The first radical change occurred when the sulfonamides and then the antibiotics became available. For then, physicians could begin to cure life-threatening diseases; they could interrupt and halt the natural course of illness. The second upheaval arrived with the proliferation of technologies for making, reconstructing, and prolonging life. Taken together, those most recent powerful tools have enabled doctors to re-create the meaning of life, death, and human potential.

The upheavals brought about by the embrace of the scientific enterprise and the proliferation of innovative technological and pharmacological tools radically altered both physicians' and the public's notions of responsibility and possibility in medicine—from care to cure to re-creation—and that transformation happened in one lifetime. The *process of change* itself and, more important, the *ramifications of change* for the tasks of medicine and for American society were unplanned and, with few exceptions, unexamined. In fact, medicine's metamorphosis was accidental, the result of meeting countless day-to-day challenges in patient care and clinical research with the tools, models, and practices of the biomedical sciences. Both the rapidity with which that transformation occurred and the fact that it was unpredictable, unanticipated, and not subject to scrutiny or evaluation have contributed to contemporary medicine's moral quandaries.

When medicine first changed from a profession dominated by diagnosis and empathy and informed by a diffuse social responsibility to a profession dominated by cure and control and informed by values and methods of laboratory science, its traditional generalist ideals, while threatened, were able to remain viable as moral anchors because of the

316

kinds of effort exemplified by the physicians portrayed here. But later, when information, structures, and practices were made more frequently obsolete by emerging scientific and technological frameworks of understanding, medicine's long-held ideals became obscured, devalued, and in many instances abandoned.

Concentrating on day-to-day problem solving resulting in immediate, tangible payoffs, medicine's myriad activities unknowingly moved the profession beyond traditional boundaries of authority, responsibility, and care to infuse society with a great deal of confusion and ambivalence about the ultimate value of a range of practices including: genetic screening, in vitro fertilization, neonatal intensive care, the use of artificial organs, the donation and commercialization of organs for transplantation, prolonging the lives of comatose persons, euthanasia, and rationing scarce or costly resources and procedures. Developments in clinical medicine and medical science have shattered cultural definitions about the natural world of body and mind, raised countless ethical dilemmas, and made the lack of consensus about appropriate action in the face of life-threatening situations problematic for physicians, patients, and society.

The debate about whether any of the scientific disciplines, including medicine, even have the ability to conduct a conversation on morality has been lively since the use of the atomic bomb during the Second World War. Numerous observers argue that medicine, as it has assumed more scientific power, has become estranged from its ability to sustain a moral discourse, to speak with authority from a unified "moral-technical" or "samaritan" position about its ends, its limits, and its guiding principles beyond those that are scientifically determined.[1] It has been suggested that medicine, like other practices in contemporary society, has lost its notion of *shared good*.[2]

When these seven doctors entered the profession of medicine, responsibilities of the individual physician were stable and known, largely because the goals of medicine were widely shared both within and outside the profession. Practitioners of the 1920s, 1930s, and 1940s had forebears, heroes, and mentors whom they wanted to—and could—emulate, because their future tasks and limits, they thought, would remain as they had been in the past. Medicine had a relevant history—both in terms of scientific and clinical knowledge and in terms of the nature of the doctor-patient relationship—a history that could be modeled, manipulated, and built on to fashion an acceptable and predictable professional identity. Most important, medicine's time-honored end was the social good, and everyone knew it. Morality was thus inherent to the practice.

The natural course of disease controlled most outcomes. Thus "nature"—the unmanageable, uncontrollable, unknowable aspects of disease and disability—was the force that directed the conversation between doctors and patients. In doing so, it homogenized both lay and professional expectations about medicine's boundaries and ends. The vast mysteries of nature also set limits on the physician's authority.

The stories portrayed here illustrate single lifetimes in which medicine's profound changes have come about. The narratives reveal the accidental, unanticipated features of the two upheavals. They exemplify medicine's growing reliance on increasingly powerful tools in the effort to manage and control disease processes and ameliorate human suffering. They also illustrate how medicine has become imprisoned by its means and ends: its technological imperative and almost exclusively scientific approach to the management of disease and, in fact, to the management of the life cycle. And they are evidence of medicine's current fragmentation and confusion about those means and ends: its inability to work toward reclaiming, through day-to-day practices, its traditional ideals and perhaps, more important, its ambivalence about fashioning new means and ends that represent a moral as well as a scientific imperative.

These thoughtful, articulate, and distinguished physicians did not suggest ways to move beyond the current impasse. They did not talk with me about medicine's transformed identity per se over the course of their lifetimes. Nor did they propose ways in which medicine's means and ends could or should change in the future to promote a moral discourse shared with society. Those conceptions emerged in the course of my analysis and interpretation of the narratives, long after the interviews were completed. The doctors' silence regarding the future of medicine's means and ends only reflects the fact that they did not consider medicine's problems and promises in those terms. Perhaps their embeddedness in the culture of medicine—that is, their identification with medicine's tasks and limitations and their taken-for-granted knowledge of its practices—prevented them from pondering the implications of their own stories and from articulating a perspective by which to examine potential means and ends that are morally as well as scientifically grounded.

In the wake of the proliferation and dominance of ever-new technological and scientific devices and procedures and the disappearance of
broadly shared values about medicine's purposes, the moral responsibilities of the individual practitioner can only become less clear. It is well
documented that physicians in training are overwhelmed by the specific
facts and operational tasks they must remember and perform under great
stress. They look to their role models, the interns and residents, for the
perfection of discrete skills and for survival techniques in hospital settings that demand certain kinds of behavior. Medical education today is
structured so that the "leaders" are only a few years and a few steps ahead
of the trainees. Few elders, those individuals who are able to impart a
sense of vision and overall purpose to trainees, are present in a manner
sustained enough or authoritative enough to compete with the compelling, necessary, and all-pervasive procedural and technological tasks of
day-to-day hospital medicine.[3]

Doctors get their start in an overwhelmingly technologically focused, pragmatic, and action-oriented environment. They have role models, but few leave their training experiences with *culture heroes,* physicians
whose practices represent a manifestly moral set of activities and who can
serve as guiding lights. Today's physicians are thus on their own—
without explicit moral anchors inherent to the training experience or
subsequent practice—in keeping up with constantly emerging information, solving day-to-day problems, and contributing to the creation of
knowledge. They are expected to carry out these tasks within a health
care delivery system that is perceived by them to thwart, constrain, and
minimally remunerate activities that are based on time-honored values,
such as taking a lengthy history, spending time with the patient, and
making house calls.

Yet medicine, in any of its multiple facets—as an opportunity for
individual lives, an institution, a moral-technical profession, and a business enterprise—cannot be held solely responsible for either its scientifically dominated means and ends or its focus on individual (patient or
physician) rights. Nor can physicians wholly transcend the profession's
ambivalence and inability to change its own definition self-consciously.
Although medicine has had the power to shape attitudes toward its own
authority and, in fact, to influence culture, it has simultaneously been
shaped by the larger culture of which it is part.

Social scientists, philosophers, and others have observed that contemporary Western, and especially American, society holds no clear-

cut or even dominant shared values about the public or social good, because it submerges or lacks a world view and language about morals in relation to community.[4] So instead of giving medicine a morality integral to social commitment, Western culture's moral legacy to medicine in the postwar period includes, as we have seen, the following three components:

First, there is the compelling drive toward the invention and application of more powerful and pervasive technologies in all aspects of modern life. These are perceived to be *inherently good* for society. Their power to shape culture in general, and the culture of medicine specifically, is inescapable. Cultural values encourage technological development in all endeavors, and the technological imperative in medicine determines its moral force.[5]

Second, postwar individualism, as a primary value, emphasizes autonomy, individual rights, and the expression and articulation of personal preference and goals at the same time as it mutes, devalues, and renders irrelevant notions of community, compassion, duty, and social responsibility. One may well ask whether arguments over the patient's or physician's rights and the "need" to preserve the autonomy of severely disabled newborns, comatose persons, or dead organ donors, for example, have a shared moral basis or are, in fact, expressions of individual and interest group preference or attitude.[6]

Third, patients—health care consumers—though they may distrust the unknown methods, mysterious powers, and hegemonic effects of the sciences, are seduced by applications of the sciences that contribute directly to the quality of their lives, and they are usually eager to "try everything." They, we, hold a strong belief that medicine can cure, or at least help in some diffuse way, regardless of the condition. Patients usually suppose that their engagement in therapeutic efforts, their prolonged persistence with treatments, and their faith in medical expertise will ultimately be rewarded with a cure or return to normalcy. The public expects more to be better: the more interventions they seek out and receive, the closer they will be to recovery. The "more is better" attitude encapsulates one important Western cultural assumption: that the individual can acquire the ability, through training and perseverance, to reverse disease outcomes and, in fact, to overcome nature.[7] The notions of expending time, energy, and resources to conquer disease, disorder, or the unknown create the meaning that informs the behavior of health care consumers.

Thus contemporary medicine, as an integral part of Western society, has derived its meaning of social good largely, although not exclusively, from the formidable powers of technology, the primacy of individualism, and the assumption that more is better. Such a specifically informed moral stance is inadequate for confronting the difficult ethical dilemmas medicine has produced. What is needed is a moral discourse embedded in society that could be shared with medicine, that could both respond to and affect medicine, one which could pave the way toward the resolution of specific dilemmas and could work toward the construction of a set of ends relevant to today's concerns.

Appendix
Notes
Index

APPENDIX
Perspectives and Methods

THE LIFE HISTORY AS CULTURAL DOCUMENT

The life history is created through a collaboration between researcher and subject, or life historian and interviewee; it emerges in the process of dialogue. In this project, my intent was to guide the physician in talking about his or her life in the context of my concerns about medicine's relationship to culture, nature, and morality. One goal was to understand values, developments, and transitions in medicine through the unfolding of individual choices, opportunities, and constraints. This kind of account can offer us rich insights into the texture and detail of lives in medicine through time. A second goal was to look at medicine as an agent of cultural change and how it has altered our conceptions of broader cultural and moral issues.

American medicine can be conceived as a cultural system. Within that conception, my goal was to portray a variety of individual paths and voices. I wanted to represent aspects of that culture as it looked from the time these individuals were growing up in it. I sought out individuals whose work was broadly based, rather than narrowly focused or extremely specialized, in order to portray a broader picture of American medicine as it evolved through the twentieth century. I wanted enough stories that the culture of medicine could be seen from various perspectives. Yet I wanted to present few enough stories that the uniqueness and richness of the individual life could be revealed. My choices of how many life histories to collect, the branches of medicine to represent, and the amount of detail to present were all part of the problem of balancing depth and breadth to address my research questions. My broadest goal was to see if the doctors' reflections on their lives in medicine could engage us in thinking about the cultural ramifications of medicine's evolution in the twentieth century.

Because they describe both the self and culture, details of a life history add specificity and concreteness to inexact concepts such as "changing morality." By viewing social change through the lens of individual experience, we are able to move away from indefinite generalizations and abstractions into the realm of individual constructions of meaning. For it is only at the level of the individual life that larger social and cultural phenomena acquire significance and the individual-culture relationship is distinctively represented. Through the examination of several individuals' lives, we gain access both to multifaceted meanings of the self-within-culture and to a richer, more detailed portrait of the culture which contributes to and is constituted by those meanings. I elicited life histories from individuals who are in their eighties. Older people, because they are able to view their lives from a long temporal perspective, are best situated to articulate the changing relationship between the individual and culture and the meaning that membership and participation in culture has over a lifetime.

CREATING THE STORIES

These life histories stand betwixt and between biography and autobiography and yet are neither. Each one is a revelation of the self and thus is something like a confession. Yet they are only partial revelations. The personal narratives created by these individuals exist because I asked them to tell me the stories of their lives. I have influenced their content in many ways. They were collected for my purposes, not the purposes of their authors. The doctors did not tell the stories of their lives in a vacuum. They were responding to my questions, and they were responding to me—a total stranger, half their age, female, and a nonphysician. I explained that I am an anthropologist interested in the culture of medicine. There can be no question that my age, gender, and the fact that I am not a doctor all greatly influenced the manner in which they responded to my questions, chose from a storehouse of memories, and articulated their thoughts. Those basic facts about me also influenced the topics they chose to expand upon and the issues they omitted entirely, though I will never know precisely how. I do know that I am an outsider on all fronts. I was born after the Second World War and so have no personal experience of either the Depression or that war, two events which influenced each of their lives. At the time of their training and during the height of their careers, medicine was a man's world, even if there were some women in it. And, I am outside the culture of medicine: I have not been through its rigorous rites of passage; I do not know or live by its secrets, rules, and rituals. Existing outside of their history, culture, and (with one exception) gender, I asked these doctors to explain their lives to me. The features of my identity and my concerns influenced the content of their explanations. Thus, I shaped their voices. Another interviewer would have elicited another story.

I actually discerned not one but three voices in all these stories: the retrospective, the critical, and the comparative. First, these are retrospective accounts, memories of events, personalities, processes. Some memories are sharper, more vivid than others. Some aspects of the life and career are simply not remembered at all or not told in much detail. I was not interested in collecting a chronologically even reportage of facts. That would have been impossible to collect in a retrospective account at any rate. Neither did I check the accounts for accuracy. A biographer, supplementing interviews with other documents that pertain to a life, has a better opportunity for a well-rounded, if not factual, account of a life. I was interested, as in my earlier work,[1] in adult development within a particular culture. What do people remember about a life in medicine at the age of eighty? How do they characterize it? What do they choose to talk about at length, regardless of the specific questions posed? What seems unimportant now? What parts of their past animate them now? What memories, even fifty or sixty years old, make them laugh and make them cry?

The critical and comparative voices evolved from one another. From the vantage point of eighty years, approximately fifty-five of them spent in medicine, these doctors compared the way things were at any given point in time with the way things are now. Doctor-patient relations, treatments, procedures, regulations, attitudes—all are subject to historical scrutiny and the wisdom of hindsight in these accounts. Comparing their participation in past forms of medicine with their participation in more current forms allows them to judge which are better, right, and wrong.

Besides influencing the content of the material collected and the style in which the stories were told, I also edited and arranged them for presentation as a text, in a particular order and format. Each life history was told over a three-day period; they were not written. They were tape-recorded and the tapes were later fully transcribed. Working with the transcripts, I changed oral language into written language by deleting repetitions of words and phrases, altering grammatical constructions, and only occasionally substituting words for sharpening a point. Talk that seemed to be redundant or irrelevant I omitted. I made every attempt to retain the tone of the author and to let his or her personality shine through.

The original accounts were enriched over the following year or two by letters and phone conversations while the doctors reflected further on topics we had discussed and when I asked for clarification or greater detail about certain subjects. Our ongoing dialogues enabled me to know them better, and I have incorporated their additional comments by telephone or letter into the body of the texts.

The division of the life histories into particular chapters was my creation. The interviews were not structured in this way. The doctors did not answer questions or discuss topics in this order. I decided on this organization for the book after reading the transcribed interviews many times. Once I arrived at the structure of the book, I began to make some order in which to present the material. In telling the story of one's life, a narrator rambles from topic to topic, and associations between and among topics are not necessarily made explicit to the listener. Topics are discussed briefly, only to be interrupted by other ideas, which may get left behind when the original topic is again addressed in more detail. I encouraged the doctors to keep talking and to associate freely. I reordered the material later with the aim of presenting chronological, developmental, and thematic narratives that a reader can easily follow.

Finally, each doctor read and approved for publication the version of his or her story presented here. They edited the texts only slightly in order to clarify details about dates, family, teachers, colleagues, or specific research endeavors. They did not rewrite the texts. Each felt the final version was a fair representation of both the original account and his or her life in medicine.

NOTES

Introduction: Medicine, Nature, Culture

1. Leon Kass, a physician and philosopher, discusses these issues in great detail in *Toward a More Natural Science* (New York: The Free Press, 1985).

2. See Lévi-Strauss, *Structural Anthropology* (London: Allen Lane, 1963); Lévi-Strauss, *Totemism* (London: Merlin, 1964); Lévi-Strauss, *The Savage Mind* (London: Weidenfeld and Nicholson, 1966).

3. This idea is elaborated in great detail by Deborah Gordon, "Tenacious Assumptions in Western Medicine," in *Biomedicine Examined,* ed. M. Lock and D. Gordon, pp. 19–56 (Dordrecht: Kluwer Academic Publishers, 1988).

4. Sociologists and philosophers of science have demonstrated how science is socially constructed and firmly embedded in culture and how the discoveries and principles of science are constituted both by cultural values and assumptions, and by local situations, practices, interactions, and professional goals. They offer a critique of the sciences both as separate from nature and as objective, autonomous depictions of nature. See, for example, Paul T. Durbin, ed., *A Guide to the Culture of Science, Technology and Medicine* (New York: The Free Press, 1980); Thomas Kuhn, *The Structure of Scientific Revolutions* (Chicago: University of Chicago Press, 1970); Bruno Latour and Steve Woolgar, *Laboratory Life: The Social Construction of Scientific Facts* (Beverly Hills: Sage, 1979).

5. *San Francisco Chronicle,* May 1989

6. For a detailed examination of this process, see Barbara A. Koenig, "The Technological Imperative in Medical Practice: The Social Construction of a 'Routine' Treatment," in *Biomedicine Examined,* ed. M. Lock and D. Gordon, pp. 465–496. See also John B. McKinlay, "From 'Promising Report' to 'Standard Procedure': Seven Stages in the Career of a Medical Innovation," *Milbank Memorial Fund Quarterly* 59 (1981): 374–411.

7. A phrase coined by Victor R. Fuchs, "The Growing Demand for Medical Care," *New England Journal of Medicine* 279 (1968): 190–195; and Victor R. Fuchs, *Who Shall Live? Health, Economics, and Social Choice* (New York: Basic Books, 1974).

8. The technological imperative has profound economic ramifications. Many observers have noted the growing two-class system of health care delivery in the United States and the fact that poor people do not often have access to the high technology tools of medicine. Moreover, the debate over whether to spend limited health care dollars on the development and use of sophisticated technology or on prevention, prenatal care, and public health measures that would benefit greater numbers, is widely known.

9. John C. Burnham, "American Medicine's Golden Age: What Happened to It?" *Science* 215 (March 19, 1982): 1474–1479; Eliot Freidson, "Afterword, 1988" in his *Profession of Medicine,* 2d ed. (Chicago: University of Chicago Press, 1988).

Seven Doctors

1. In his review of this book, Eric Cassell, M.D., noted that I chose "great" doctors, "the best, the very best, that medicine has produced since the 1930s." My portrayal and interpretation of medicine's transformation ultimately rests on the narratives of these particular physicians. A different set of life histories in medicine would have produced, no doubt, a different interpretation. My goal, however, was to document the voices of physicians considered by their peers and successors to be outstanding practitioners of their era.

2. David E. Rogers, "The Early Years: The Medical World in Which Walsh McDermott Trained," *Daedalus* 115 (Spring, 1986): 1–18, especially p. 4. Stories of lives in medicine from other underrepresented groups have been and are being published elsewhere. It is hoped that those other stories, together with the seven portrayed here, will create a more complete picture of career opportunities and constraints on career development in twentieth-century American medicine. See, for example, Sarah Lawrence Lightfoot, *Balm in Gilead: Journey of a Healer* (Reading, Mass,: Addison-Wesley, 1988). It is known that Catholics and Italian Americans were discriminated against as well during this period. African Americans were almost completely excluded from all but their own medical institutions: Rogers, "The Early Years," p. 4. Asians, Hispanics, and other minorities in medicine were extremely uncommon until very recently.

3. Rogers, "The Early Years," p. 4.

4. Paul B. Beeson and W. McDermott, eds., *The Cecil-Loeb Textbook of Medicine:* 11th ed. (Philadelphia: W. B. Saunders, 1963); 12th ed. (1967); and 13th ed. (1971); Paul B. Beeson and W. McDermott, eds., *Textbook of Medicine:* 14th ed. (Philadelphia: W. B. Saunders, 1975); and 15th ed. (1979).

5. He has published numerous articles on these subjects as well. See, for example, Paul B. Beeson, "Clinical Medicine and the Future," *Journal of Biology and Medicine* 33 (December 1960): 235–242; Paul B. Beeson, "The Development of Clinical Knowledge," *Journal of the American Medical Association* 237,

no. 20 (May 16, 1977): 2209–2212; Paul B. Beeson, "Editorial: Training Doctors to Care for Old People," *Annals of Internal Medicine* 90, no. 2 (February 1979): 262–263; Paul B. Beeson, "Priorities in Medical Education," *Perspectives in Biology and Medicine* 25, no. 4 (Summer 1982): 673–687; Paul B. Beeson, "Making Medicine a More Attractive Profession, *Journal of Medical Education* 62, no. 2 (February 1987): 116–125.

6. For example, see John Romano, "The Elimination of the Internship—An Act of Regression," *American Journal of Psychiatry* 126, no. 11 (May 1970): 1565–1575; John Romano, "The Teaching of Psychiatry to Medical Students," *American Journal of Psychiatry* 130, no. 5 (May 1973): 559–562; John Romano, "Reflections on Informed Consent," *Archives of General Psychiatry* 30 (January 1974): 129–135; John Romano, "A Psychiatrist's View of the State of Medical Ethics," *Psychiatric Annals* 16, no. 7 (July 1986): 390–394; John Romano, "How Do We Transmit the Humanistic Factors in the Practice of Medicine?" in *Medical Education for the 21st Century,* ed. J. V. Warren and G. L. Trzebiatowski, pp. 121–139 (Ohio State University College of Medicine, 1985).

Medical Morality: Past and Present

1. This value is explored in great detail in Robert N. Bellah, Richard Madsen, William M. Sullivan, Ann Swidler, and Steven M. Tipton, *Habits of the Heart* (Berkeley: University of California Press, 1985).

2. Deborah Gordon, "Tenacious Assumptions in Western Medicine," in *Biomedicine Examined,* ed. M. Lock and D. Gordon, pp. 19–56 (Dordrecht: Kluwer Academic Publishers, 1988).

3. This list is derived largely from Edward Shorter, *Bedside Manners: The Troubled History of Doctors and Patients* (New York: Simon and Schuster, 1985), pp. 94–95.

4. Charles Rosenberg, *The Care of Strangers* (New York: Basic Books, 1987), pp. 159–160.

5. Warren I. Susman, *Culture as History* (New York: Pantheon, 1984), p. 198; and Frederick Lewis Allen, *Only Yesterday* (New York: Harper and Row, 1931), pp. 164–166.

6. For example, see David E. Rogers, "The Early Years: The Medical World in Which Walsh McDermott Trained," *Daedalus* 115 (Spring, 1986): 1–18, especially p. 5.

7. Melvin Konner, *Becoming a Doctor* (New York: Viking, 1987).

8. Lewis Thomas, *The Youngest Science* (New York: Viking, 1983).

Olney: Pediatrics—Medicine beyond Hospital Walls

1. Beginning in the 1880s, Julius Wagner-Jauregg, an Austrian psychiatrist, studied the effects of fever on mental patients by injecting them with various

bacterial substances. He eventually innoculated syphilis patients with the blood of persons infected with malaria and found that this resulted in complete remission in many cases. His "fever therapy" was received enthusiastically in Europe and the United States, and he received the Nobel Prize in 1927 for his work. See Gerald N. Grob, *Mental Illness and American Society, 1875–1940* (Princeton: Princeton University Press, 1983), p. 293. Paul Beeson also refers to fever therapy for syphilis, on p. 168.

Rhoads: Quaker Surgeon

1. I have been told by other physicians of Rhoads's age that those were the standard charges before the First World War. Dr. Karl Menninger told me in a personal interview (1986) that those were his rates through the 1920s.

Defining Medicine and the Physician's Identity

1. David E. Rogers, "The Early Years: The Medical World in Which Walsh McDermott Trained," *Daedalus* 115 (Spring, 1986): 1–18, quote appears on p. 8.

2. Margaret Clark, personal communication.

3. Paul Beeson, letter to David E. Rogers, quoted in Rogers, "The Early Years: The Medical World in Which Walsh McDermott Trained," pp. 16–17.

4. For the history of tuberculosis among American physicians and medical students, see William A. Abruzzi and Rufus J. Hummel, "Tuberculosis: Incidence among American Medical Students, Prevention and Control and the Use of BCG," *New England Journal of Medicine* 248, no. 17 (1953): 722–729; and Arthur J. Myers, Harold S. Diehl, Ruth E. Boynton, and Howard L. Horns, "Tuberculosis in Physicians," chairman's address, *Journal of the American Medical Association* 158, no. 1 (1955): 1–8.

5. That attitude may be contrasted with today's expressed fear, ambivalence, and conflict among physicians and other health care professionals about treating AIDS patients or other people known to have, or suspected of having, the HIV virus. For example, about 30 percent of American physicians surveyed by the American Medical Association in 1991 indicated that they felt no ethical responsibility to treat AIDS patients. In one recent study of AIDS and resident training, 25 percent of residents chose a training site known to be low in AIDS incidence in order to avoid treating many AIDS patients. Barbara Koenig, personal communication.

6. For example, in 1910 Salvarsan was discovered to be a treatment for syphilis. In 1922, insulin began to be used to treat diabetes. In 1926, liver extract was discovered as a cure for pernicious anemia. Surgery benefited from technical advances after 1910 as well as from new forms of anesthesia. General

research in pharmacology facilitated surgical advances, the creation of new drugs, and the refinement of existing drug treatments. The early electrocardiograph came into use during the 1920s. By 1914, new techniques in chemical analysis made laboratory work possible on a broad scale. By the early 1920s, the commercial diagnostic laboratory was established and thriving. See Richard Harrison Shryock, *The Development of Modern Medicine* (Madison: University of Wisconsin Press, 1974), pp. 438–439; and Stanley Joel Reiser, *Medicine and the Reign of Technology* (Cambridge: Cambridge University Press, 1978), especially pp. 137, 143, 184.

7. It is interesting to note that the 1920s have been referred to by one historian as medicine's "doldrum years." Physicians during that period "declared the outlook barren." Shryock, *The Development of Modern Medicine,* p. 439. Perhaps the relatively few advances in medical science during those years contributed to the sense of connection between medicine's immediate past and expected future.

8. Melvin Konner, *Becoming a Doctor* (New York: Viking, 1987), pp. 15–16.

9. Lewis Thomas, book review, "What Doctors Don't Know," *New York Review of Books,* September 24, 1988.

Combining Care and Science: The Residency

1. In 1931, only 17 percent of all doctors were full-time specialists. Rosemary Stevens, *American Medicine and the Public Interest* (New Haven: Yale University Press, 1971), p. 3. Throughout the 1930s, more than 75 percent of all physicians reported themselves to be general practitioners or specialists only on a part-time basis. Paul Starr, *The Transformation of American Medicine* (New York: Basic Books, 1982), p. 358; Stevens, *American Medicine and the Public Interest,* p. 218.

2. Regina Markell Morantz-Sanchez, *Sympathy and Science* (Oxford: Oxford University Press, 1985), pp. 334–337.

3. Ibid., pp. 323–327.

Beeson: From General Practice to Camelot

1. For a detailed description and history of work conducted at the Rockefeller Institute during the period Beeson was there, see George W. Corner, *A History of the Rockefeller Institute 1901–1953* (New York: Rockefeller Institute Press, 1964). See also A. McGehee Harvey, *Science at the Bedside* (Baltimore: Johns Hopkins University Press, 1981), chapter 5, "The Development of the Rockefeller Institute for Medical Research and Its Hospital," pp. 78–100.

2. Oswald T. Avery, C. M. MacLeod, and M. McCarty, "Transformation of

Pneumococcal Types Induced by a Desoxyribonucleic Acid Fraction Isolated from Pneumococcus Type III," *Journal of Experimental Medicine* 79 (1944): 137.

3. The five diseases chosen for study when the Rockefeller Hospital opened were: lobar pneumonia, poliomyelitis, syphilis, heart disease, and intestinal infantilism (severe intestinal disturbances in children and growth retardation). Corner, *A History of the Rockefeller Institute 1901–1953,* pp. 98–99.

4. For a personal appraisal of Soma Weiss, see Eugene A. Stead, "Soma Weiss: The Characteristics That Made Us Know He Was a Great Man," *Pharos* (Fall, 1987): 11–12.

Rhoads: Research Surgeon—From Patient to Lab and Back Again

1. As of 1991, there have been twenty-three documented cases of health-care workers infected from patients with the HIV virus. This number is assumed to be inaccurate (too low), however, because it represents only those individuals who were tested for the HIV virus before the occupational accident, and then tested again afterwards. Mary E. Chamberland, L. J. Conley, T. J. Bush, C. A. Ciesielski, T. A. Hammett, and H. W. Jaffee, "Health Care Workers with AIDS," *Journal of the American Medical Association* 266, no. 24 (1991): 3459–3462.

2. The following papers are Rhoads's scientific publications of the research described in this chapter: W. D. Thompson, I.S. Ravdin, Jonathan E. Rhoads, and I. L. Frank, "Use of Lyophile Plasma in Correction of Hypoproteinemia and Prevention of Wound Disruption," *Archives of Surgery* 36 (1938): 509–518; Jonathan E. Rhoads, A. Stengel, Jr., C. Riegel, F. A. Cajori, and W. D. Frazier, "The Absorption of Protein Split Products from Chronic Isolated Colon Loops," *American Journal of Physiology* 125 (1939): 707–712; Jonathan E. Rhoads, "Physiologic Factors Regulating the Level of the Plasma Prothrombin," *Annals of Surgery* 112 (1940): 568–574; Jonathan E. Rhoads and W. Kasinskas, "The Influence of Hypoproteinemia on the Formation of Callus in Experimental Fracture," *Surgery* 11 (1942): 38–44; Jonathan E. Rhoads, M. T. Fliegelman, and L. M. Panzer, "The Mechanism of Delayed Wound Healing in the Presence of Hypoproteinemia," *Journal of the American Medical Association* 118 (1942): 21–25; Jonathan E. Rhoads, W. A. Wolff, H. Saltonstall, and W. E. Lee, "The Use of Plasma in the Treatment of Shock Due to Burns," *Clinics* 1 (1942): 37–42; W. E. Lee, W. A. Wolff, H. Saltonstall, and Jonathan E. Rhoads, "Recent Trends in the Therapy of Burns," *Annals of Surgery* 115 (1942): 1131–1139.

Hodgkinson: Surgical Expertise and All the Emotions

1. George N. Papanicolaou and H. F. Traut, "The Diagnostic Value of Vaginal Smears in Carcinoma of the Uterus," *American Journal of Obstetrics and*

Gynecology 42, no. 2 (1941): 193–206; George N.. Papanicolaou, "A New Procedure for Staining Vaginal Smears," *Science* 95 (1943): 438–439; and George N. Papanicolaou, "The Use of Endocervical and Endometrial Smears in the Diagnosis of Cancer and Other Conditions of the Uterus," *American Journal of Obstetrics and Gynecology* 46 (1943): 421–424.

2. A 1952 editorial in the *New England Journal of Medicine* stated that it may be impractical to use the vaginal smear to screen large numbers of women for the early detection of uterine cancer: Editorial, "The Vaginal Smear," *New England Journal of Medicine* 246, no. 14 (1952): 557–558.

3. For a detailed history and analysis of the development and use of DES in American medical practice, see Susan E. Bell, "A New Model of Medical Technology Development: A Case Study of DES," in *Research in the Sociology of Health Care,* ed. J. A. Roth and S. B. Ruzek, Vol. 4, pp. 1–32 (Greenwich, Conn.: JAI Press, 1986).

4. Dr. Hodgkinson is aware of the details of the project because he was part of it. He informed me that some of the findings were not published. For results of that study, see J. P. Pratt, "A Clinical Study in Estrogenic Therapy," *Journal of Clinical Endocrinology* 1 (January 1941): 50–52.

5. When I asked him why, he told me he never had a scientific answer; it was just a feeling he had about the drug.

Romano: "Brain Spot or Mind Twist"—Attempts to Understand Psychosis

1. Romano has published a retrospective account of his training years. See, John Romano, "On Becoming a Psychiatrist: 1934–1942," *Journal of the American Medical Association* 261, no. 15 (April 21, 1989): 2240–2243.

2. John Romano and J. W. Evans, "Symptomatic Psychosis in a Case of Secondary Anemia," *Archives of Neurology and Psychiatry* 39 (June 1938): 1294–1301; John Romano and F. G. Ebaugh, "Prognosis in Schizophrenia: A Preliminary Report," *American Journal of Psychiatry* 95 (November 1938): 583–596.

3. H. H. Merritt and T. J. Putnam, "A New Series of Anticonvulsant Drugs Tested by Experiments on Animals," *Archives of Neurology and Psychiatry* 39 (1938): 1003–1015.

Becoming Agents of Change

1. Arnold Gesell, *Mental Growth of the Preschool Child* (New York: Macmillan, 1925); Arnold Gesell, "Normal Growth as a Public Health Concept," *Transactions of the American Child Health Association* 3 (1926): 48.

2. A. McGehee Harvey, *Science at the Bedside* (Baltimore: Johns Hopkins University Press, 1981), chapter 5, "The Development of the Rockefeller Institute for Medical Research and Its Hospital," pp. 86–87.

3. Harry F. Dowling, "The Impact of New Discoveries on Medical Practice: Advances in the Diagnosis and Treatment of the Infectious Diseases," in *Mainstreams of Medicine,* ed. Lester S. King (San Antonio: University of Texas Press, 1971), p. 117.

4. Harvey, *Science at the Bedside,* p. 87.

5. See his publications of that period: C. L. Hoagland, Paul B. Beeson, and W. F. Goebel, "The Capsular Polysaccharide of the Type XIV Pneumococcus and Its Relationship to the Specific Substances of Human Blood," *Science* 88 (1938): 261–263; C. M. MacLeod, C. L. Hoagland, and Paul B. Beeson, "The Use of the Skin Test with the Type Specific Polysaccharides in the Control of Serum Dosage in Pneumococcal Pneumonia," *Journal of Clinical Investigation* 17 (1938): 739–744; W. F. Goebel, Paul B. Beeson, and C. L. Hoagland, "Chemoimmunological Studies on the Soluble Specific Substance of Pneumococcus, IV," *Journal of Biological Chemistry* 129 (1939): 455–464; Paul B. Beeson and W. F. Goebel, "The Immunological Relationship of the Capsular Polysaccharide of Type XIV Pneumococcus to the Blood Group A Specific Substance," *Journal of Experimental Medicine* 70 (1939): 239–247.

6. For a comprehensive history and social analysis of the specialty of pediatrics in the United States, see Sydney A. Halpern, *American Pediatrics* (Berkeley: University of California Press, 1988).

Curing and Other Trends

1. Rosemary Stevens, *American Medicine and the Public Interest* (New Haven: Yale University Press, 1971), pp. 181, 276.

2. Paul Starr, *The Social Transformation of American Medicine* (New York: Basic Books, 1982), pp. 335–340.

3. Charles Rosenberg, *The Care of Strangers* (New York: Basic Books, 1987). Paul Starr notes that in 1930 one doctor in sixteen worked full-time in a hospital; by the 1950s one doctor in six was hospital based. Starr, *The Social Transformation of American Medicine,* p. 359.

4. Richard Harrison Shryock, *The Development of Modern Medicine* (Madison: University of Wisconsin Press, 1974), pp. 448–449.

5. Harry F. Dowling, *Fighting Infection: Conquests of the Twentieth Century* (Cambridge: Harvard University Press, 1977), chapters 8–10.

Jarcho: Independence in Internal Medicine

1. For background on these extremely influential physicians, see, for example, Harvey Cushing, *Life of Sir William Osler* (Oxford: Oxford University Press, 1925); Donald Fleming, *William H. Welch and the Rise of Modern Medicine* (Baltimore: Johns Hopkins University Press, 1987).

2. For a short autobiographical sketch by Max Wintrobe, see Allen B. Weisse, *Conversations in Medicine* (New York: New York University Press, 1984), chapter 5, "Maxwell M. Wintrobe," pp. 75–94. For a more detailed explication of antisemitism in the recent history of American medicine, see Arthur Kornberg, *For the Love of Enzymes* (Cambridge: Harvard University Press, 1989), especially chapter 10, "Reflections on My Life in Science," pp. 297–319. Also, see Jarcho's own published work on the topic of antisemitism in American medicine: Saul Jarcho, "Medical Education in the United States— 1910–1956," *Journal of the Mount Sinai Hospital* 26, no. 4 (1959): 339–385, especially pp. 357–359.

3. Saul Jarcho and D. H. Anderson, "Traumatic Autotransplantation of Splenic Tissue," *American Journal of Pathology* 15 (1938): 554–562.

4. For example, Saul Jarcho, "Giuseppe Zambeccari, a Seventeenth-Century Pioneer in Experimental Physiology and Surgery," *Bulletin of the History of Medicine* 9 (1941): 144–176; Saul Jarcho, "Experiments of Doctor Joseph Zambeccari Concerning the Excision of Various Organs from Different Living Animals," *Bulletin of the History of Medicine* 9 (1941): 311–331.

Beeson: Infectious Disease Expert

1. Paul B. Beeson, "Jaundice Occuring One to Four Months after Transfusion of Blood or Plasma. Report of Seven Cases," *Journal of the American Medical Association* 121 (1943): 1332–1334.

2. Paul B. Beeson, "Development of Tolerance to Typhoid Bacterial Pyrogen and Its Abolition by Reticulo-endothelial Blockade," *Proceedings of the Society for Experimental Biology* (N.Y.) 62 (1946): 306–307; Paul B. Beeson, "Effect of Reticulo-endothelial Blockade on Immunity to the Shwartzman Phenomenon," *Proceedings of the Society for Experimental Biology* (N.Y.) 64 (1947): 146–149; Paul B. Beeson, "Tolerance to Bacterial Pyrogens, 1. Factors Influencing Its Development," *Journal of Experimental Medicine* 86 (1947): 29–38; Paul B. Beeson, "Tolerance to Bacterial Pyrogens, 2. Role of the Reticuloendothelial System," *Journal of Experimental Medicine* 86 (1947): 39–44; Albert Heyman and Paul B. Beeson, "Influence of Various Disease States upon the Febrile Response to Intravenous Injection of Typhoid Bacterial Pyrogen; with Particular Reference to Malaria and Cirrhosis of the Liver," *Journal of Laboratory and Clinical Medicine* 34 (1949): 1400–1403.

3. Beeson's clinical observations were originally published as follows: Paul B. Beeson, Emmett S. Brannon, and James V. Warren, "Observations on the Sites of Removal of Bacteria from the Blood of Patients with Bacterial Endocarditis," *Journal of Experimental Medicine* 81 (1945): 9–23. In 1985, the article was reprinted with commentary by Beeson as: Paul B. Beeson, Emmett S. Brannon, and James V. Warren, "Classics in Infectious Disease," *Reviews of*

Infectious Diseases 7, no. 4 (July–August 1985): 565–576. I quote here at length from Beeson's retrospective commentary: "The work described in the preceding paper happened to be possible because, for a brief period, there was a 'window of opportunity' between the introduction of the technique of cardiac catheterization and the availability of penicillin for curative treatment of bacterial endocarditis. Until that time this had been a hopeless, inevitably fatal illness. This work was carried out between July 1943 and April 1944 . . . There is another compelling reason why this work could not be done now: a change in attitudes about clinical investigation of this kind. More thought and scrutiny have been given to the whole ethos of studies on humans. It should be remembered that in the early 1940s, not many people were engaged in clinical investigation. After the war, when funding of biomedical research was augmented hugely and, therefore, when many more clinical investigations were being undertaken, more thought began to be given to the propriety of doing things of this sort to people who could not possibly benefit from the procedure. Today, if I were serving on an institutional committee on human studies, I would not sanction the study we carried out so blithely in 1944. At that time the term *informed consent* had not been coined" (pp. 574–575).

4. See Charles Rosenberg, *The Care of Strangers* (New York: Basic Books, 1987), p. 302, for a brief discussion of the history of relations between African Americans and whites at Grady Hospital.

5. For the history of these developments see Daniel M. Fox, "The Politics of the NIH Extramural Program, 1937–1950," *Journal of the History of Medicine* 42 (1987): 447–466; Paul Starr, *The Social Transformation of American Medicine* (New York: Basic Books, 1982), pp. 342–347; Donald C. Swain, "The Rise of a Research Empire: NIH, 1930 to 1950," *Science* 138 (December 1962): 1233–1237.

Rhoads: Doctor, Scientist, Patient—Three Views of Illness

1. C. E. Koop, J. H. Drew, C. Riegel, and Jonathan E. Rhoads, "The Effects of Preoperative Forcefeeding on Surgical Patients," *Annals of Surgery* 124 (1946): 1165–1174.

2. For a biography of Otto Folin, professor of biological chemistry at Harvard Medical School and one of the pioneers in the development of methods for quantitative chemical analysis, see Samuel Meites, *Otto Folin: America's First Clinical Biochemist* (Washington D.C.: American Association for Clinical Chemistry, 1989).

3. For some of Rhoads's research publications during that period, see Jonathan E. Rhoads and W. Kasinskas, "The Influence of Hypoproteinemia on the Formation of Callus in Experimental Fracture," *Surgery* 11 (1942): 38–44; Jonathan E. Rhoads, M. T. Fliegelman, and L. M. Panzer, "The Mechanisms of

Delayed Wound Healing in the Presence of Hypoproteinemia," *Journal of the American Medical Association* 118 (1942): 21–25; Jonathan E. Rhoads, "Problems of Fluid Balance in the Traumatized Patient," *Annals of Internal Medicine* 18 (1943): 988–990; Jonathan E. Rhoads, C. Riegel, C. E. Koop, and I. S. Ravdin, "The Problem of Nutrition in Patients with Gastric Lesions Requiring Surgery," *Western Journal of Surgery, Gynecology and Obstetrics* 51 (1943): 229–233; C. Riegel, Jonathan E. Rhoads, C. E. Koop, R. P. Grigger, L. Bullitt, and D. Barrus, "Dietary Requirements for Nitrogen Equilibrium in the Period Immediately following Certain Major Surgical Operations," *American Journal of Medical Science* 210 (1945): 133–134; C. Riegel, C. E. Koop, J. Drew, L. W. Stevens, and Jonathan E. Rhoads, "The Nutritional Requirements for Nitrogen Balance in Surgical Patients during the Early Postoperative Period," *Journal of Clincal Investigation* 26 (1947): 18–23.

4. For a history of self-experimentation in medicine, see Lawrence K. Altman, *Who Goes First?* (New York: Random House, 1987).

Hodgkinson: Breasts, Babies, Science, and Idealism

1. C. Paul Hodgkinson and R. E. Nelson, "Penicillin, Treatment of Acute Puerperal Mastitis," *Journal of the American Medical Association* 129 (1945): 269–270; C. Paul Hodgkinson, "Penicillin and Acute Puerperal Mastitis," *American Journal of Obstetrics and Gynecology* 53 (1947): 834–838.

Romano: "One Song to Sing"—Education of the Medical Student

1. Periarteritis nodosa is a disease characterized by inflammation of small and medium-sized arteries, leading to functional impairment of tissues supplied by the affected vessels.

2. See, for example, John Romano, E. A. Stead, and Z. E. Taylor, "Clinical and Electroencephalographic Changes Produced by a Sensitive Carotid Sinus of the Cerebral Type," *New England Journal of Medicine* 223 (1940): 708–712; John Romano and M. Michael, Jr., "Partial Thenar Atrophy," *Archives of Neurology and Psychiatry* 44 (1940): 1224–1229; John Romano, M. Michael, Jr., and H. H. Merritt, "Alcohol Cerebellar Degeneration," *Archives of Neurology and Psychiatry* 44 (1940): 1230–1236; E. A. Stead, R. V. Ebert, John Romano, and J. V. Warren, "Central Autonomic Paralysis," *Archives of Neurology and Psychiatry* 48 (1942): 92–106; J. V. Warren, C. W. Walter, John Romano, and E. A. Stead, "Blood Flow in the Hand and Forearm after Paravertebral Block of the Sympathetic Ganglia," *Journal of Clinical Investigation* 21 (1942): 665–673.

3. John Romano, "Patients' Attitudes and Behavior in Ward Round Teaching," *Journal of the American Medical Association* 117 (1941): 664–667.

4. See, for example, G. L. Engel, John Romano, E. B. Ferris, J. P. Webb, C.

D. Stevens, "A Simple Method of Determining Frequency Spectrums in the Electroencephalogram," *Archives of Neurology and Psychiatry* 51 (1944): 134–146; John Romano and G. L. Engel, "Delirium. 1. Electroencephalographic Data," *Archives of Neurology and Psychiatry* 51 (1944): 356–377; G. L. Engel and John Romano, "Delirium. 2. Reversibility of Electroencephalogram with Experimental Procedures," *Archives of Neurology and Psychiatry* 51 (1944): 378–392; G. L. Engel, John Romano, and T. R. McLin, "Vasodepressor and Carotid Sinus Syncope," *Archives of Internal Medicine* 74 (1944): 100–119; John Romano and G. L. Engel, "Studies of Syncope," *Psychosomatic Medicine* 7 (1945): 3–15; G. L. Engel, John Romano, and E. B. Ferris, "Variations in the Normal Electroencephalogram during a Five-year Period," *Science* 105 (1947): 600–601.

5. The Office of Scientific Research and Development was created by President Roosevelt in 1941. One of its committes, the Committee on Medical Research, began a comprehensive research program to deal with the range of medical problems created by the war. Paul Starr, *The Social Transformation of American Medicine* (New York: Basic Books, 1982), pp. 340–341.

6. For example, John Romano, G. L. Engel, J. P. Ferris, H. W. Ryder, and M. A. Blankenhorn, "Syncopal Reactions during Simulated Exposure to High Altitude in the Decompression Chamber," *War Medicine* 4 (1943): 475–489; John Romano, G. L. Engel, E. B. Ferris, H. W. Ryder, J. P. Webb, and M. A. Blankenhorn, "Problems of Fatigue as Illustrated by Experiences in the Decompression Chamber," *War Medicine* 6 (1944): 102–105; J. P. Webb, G. L. Engel, John Romano, H. W. Ryder, C. D. Stevens, M. A. Blankenhorn, and E. B. Ferris, "The Mechanism of Pain in Aviators' Bends," *Journal of Clinical Investigation* 23 (1944): 934.

7. For results of that research, see G. L. Engel, John Romano, and E. B. Ferris, "Effect of Quinacrine (Atabrine) on the Central Nervous System," *Archives of Neurology and Psychiatry* 58 (1947): 337–350.

8. See L. H. Bartemeier, L. S. Kubie, K. A. Menninger, John Romano, and J. C. Whitehorn, "Combat Exhaustion," *Journal of Nervous and Mental Disorders* 104 (1946): 358–389.

A Moral-Technical Profession

1. Eric J. Cassell, *The Healer's Art* (New York: Penguin Books, 1976).

2. For an examination of research on humans conducted prior to and during the Second World War, see David J. Rothman, *Strangers at the Bedside* (New York: Basic Books, 1991).

3. Henry Beecher, "Ethics and Clinical Research," *New England Journal of Medicine* 274 (1966): 1354–1360. See also, Henry Beecher, "Experimentation on Man," *New England Journal of Medicine* 274 (1966): 1382–1383.

4. For a thorough discussion of the development of federal policy on informed consent and the nature and ramifications of Henry Beecher's analysis, see Rothman, *Strangers at the Bedside.*

5. Andrea Sankar, "Patients, Physicians and Context: Medical Care in the Home," in *Biomedicine Examined,* ed. M. Lock and D. Gordon, pp. 155–178 (Dordrecht: Kluwer Academic Publishers, 1988).

6. Romano and Olney defined the patient very broadly and their conceptions of responsibility to the patient were drawn broadly as a result. Their work—as psychiatrist and pediatrician, respectively—extended the boundaries of clinical interest beyond the strictly biomedical. It can be argued that psychiatry and pediatrics continue to draw boundaries of care, treatment, and authority more widely than other medical specialties. This situation both reflects and contributes to their relatively low status (and in the case of psychiatry, marginal status as well) among the medical specialties.

7. For an excellent discussion of both sides of the debate in historical perspective, see William Ray Arney, *Power and the Profession of Obstetrics* (Chicago: University of Chicago Press, 1982).

Idealism and Conflict in the Golden Age

1. Eliot Freidson, *Profession of Medicine* (Chicago: University of Chicago Press, 1988), p. 384.

2. Paul B. Beeson, "One Hundred Years of American Internal Medicine," *Annals of Internal Medicine* 105 (1986): 436–444; Paul B. Beeson, "Too Many Specialists, Too Few Generalists," *Pharos* (Spring, 1991): 2–6.

Beeson: Yale and Oxford—Role Model in Two Countries

1. Paul B. Beeson and D. Rowley, "The Anticomplementary Effect of Kidney Tissue. Its Association with Ammonia Production," *Journal of Experimental Medicine* 110 (1959): 685–697.

2. Beeson's years at Yale coincided with the period of greatest growth in academic medicine and medical research. Paul Starr writes, "Between 1955 and 1960, unswerving congressional support pushed up the NIH budget from $81 million to $400 million." Paul Starr, *The Social Transformation of American Medicine* (New York: Basic Books, 1982), p. 347.

3. David T. Durack and Paul B. Beeson, "Experimental Bacterial Endocarditis, 1. Colonization of a Sterile Vegetation," *British Journal of Biology and Medicine* 43 (1971): 351–357; David T. Durack and Paul B. Beeson, "Experimental Bacterial Endocarditis, 2. Survival of Bacteria in Endocardial Vegetations," *British Journal of Experimental Pathology* 53 (1972): 50–53; D. T. Durack, Paul B. Beeson, and R. G. Petersdorf, "Experimental Bacterial Endo-

carditis, 3. Production and Progress of the Disease in Rabbits," *British Journal of Experimental Pathology* 54 (1973): 142–151.

4. A. Basten, M. H. Boyer, and Paul B. Beeson, "Mechanism of Eosinophilia, 1. Factors Affecting the Eosinophil Response of Rats to *Trichinella spiralis*," *Journal of Experimental Medicine* 131 (1970): 1271–1287; A. Basten and Paul B. Beeson, "Mechanism of Eosinophilia, 2. Role of the Lymphocyte," *Journal of Experimental Medicine* 131 (1970): 1288–1305; M. H. Boyer, A. Basten, and Paul B. Beeson, "Mechanism of Eosinophilia, 3. Suppression of Eosinophilia by Agents Known to Modify Immune Responses," *Blood* 36, no. 4 (1970): 458–469.

Olney: Camp, Clinics, and Schools

1. For a concise history of pediatric clinics and pediatric subspecialization, see Sydney Halpern, *American Pediatrics* (Berkeley: University of California Press, 1988).

2. Theodore H. Ingalls, "The Study of Congenital Anomalies by the Epidemiologic Method," *New England Journal of Medicine* 243, no. 3 (1950): 67–73; and Theodore H. Ingalls, F. J. Curley, and R. A. Prindle, "Experimental Production of Congenital Anomalies," *New England Journal of Medicine* 247, no. 20 (1952): 758–768.

Hodgkinson: "No Limit on What One Could Do"

1. C. Paul Hodgkinson, "Relationships of the Female Urethra and Bladder in Urinary Stress Incontinence," *American Journal of Obstetrics and Gynecology* 65 (1953): 560–573; and C. Paul Hodgkinson and H. P. Doub, "Roentgen Study of Urethrovesical Relationships in Female Urinary Stress Incontinence," *Radiology* 61 (1953): 335–345.

2. C. Paul Hodgkinson, H. P. Doub, and W. T. Kelly, "Urethrocystograms," *Clinical Obstetrics and Gynecology* 1, no. 3 (September 1958); and C. Paul Hodgkinson and N. Cobert, "Direct Urethrocystometry," *American Journal of Obstetrics and Gynecology* 79 (1960): 648–664.

3. C. Paul Hodgkinson, M. A. Ayers, and B. H. Drukker, "Dyssynergic Detrusor Dysfunctions in the Apparently Normal Female," *American Journal of Obstetrics and Gynecology* 87 (1963): 717–730.

Romano: Bringing Psychiatry Closer to Medicine

1. Gerald N. Grob, *Mental Illness and American Society, 1875–1940* (Princeton: Princton University Press, 1983); and Gerald N. Grob, "The Forging of

Mental Health Policy in America: World War II to New Frontier," *Journal of the History of Medicine* 42 (1987): 410–446.

2. In 1934 George Whipple shared the Nobel Prize with George Minot and William Murphy for demonstrating the effects of diet on pernicious anemia.

An Essential Tension

1. Paul B. Beeson and Russell C. Maulitz, "The Inner History of Internal Medicine," in *Grand Rounds: One Hundred Years of Internal Medicine*, ed. R. C. Maulitz and D. E. Long, pp. 15–54 (Philadelphia: University of Pennsylvania Press, 1986).

2. Erik Erikson, "On Protest and Affirmation," *Harvard Medical Alumni Bulletin* 46, no. 6 (July–August 1972): 30–32.

3. B. H. Kean, *M.D.* (New York: Ballantine Books, 1990), p. 75.

4. A great deal has been written about the threat to and need for a stronger moral stance in medicine. For example, see Eric J. Cassell, *The Healer's Art* (New York: Penguin Books, 1976); Eric J. Cassell and M. Siegler, eds., *Changing Values in Medicine* (Frederick, Maryland: University Publications of America, 1985); Arthur Kleinman, *The Illness Narratives* (New York: Basic Books, 1988); Edmund D. Pellegrino, *Humanism and the Physician* (Knoxville: University of Tennessee Press, 1979); Edmund D. Pellegrino and David C. Thomasma, *A Philosophical Basis of Medical Practice* (New York: Oxford University Press, 1981); David C. Thomasma, "Establishing the Moral Basis of Medicine," *Journal of Medicine and Philosophy* 15 (1990): 245–267.

5. Richard M. Zaner, "Medicine and Dialogue," *Journal of Medicine and Philosophy* 15 (1990): 305.

Medicine's Means and Ends, 1970s–1990s: Technological Superiority, Moral Confusion

1. S. J. Youngner, "Organ Retrieval: Can We Ignore the Dark Side?" *Transplantation Proceedings* 22, no. 3 (1990): 1014–1015.

2. Joel Feinberg, "The Mistreatment of Dead Bodies," *Hastings Center Report* 15 (1985): 1; Raymond A. Belliotti, "Do Dead Human Beings Have Rights?" *Personalist* 60 (1979): 201–210; A. Lynch, "Respect for the Dead Human Body: A Question of Body, Mind, Spirit, Psyche," *Transplantation Proceedings* 22, no. 3 (1990): 1016–1018; Norman Fost, "Removing Organs from Anencephalic Infants: Ethical and Legal Considerations," *Clinics in Perinatology* 16, no. 2 (1989): 331–337; J. A. Robertson, "The Ethical Acceptability of Fetal Tissue Transplants," *Transplantation Proceedings* 22, no. 3 (1990): 1025–1027; Arthur L. Caplan, "Equity in the Selection of Recipients

for Cardiac Transplants," *Circulation* 75, no. 1 (1987): 10–19; A. P. Monaco, "Transplantation: The State of the Art," *Transplantation Proceedings* 22, no. 3 (1990): 896–901.

3. For example, see Nancy Scheper-Hughes and Margaret Lock, "The Mindful Body: A Prolegomenon to Future Work in Medical Anthropology," *Medical Anthropology Quarterly,* n.s., 1 (1987): 6–41; Laurence J. Kirmayer, "Mind and Body as Metaphors: Hidden Values in Biomedicine," in *Biomedicine Examined,* ed. M. Lock and D. Gordon, pp. 57–94 (Dordrecht: Kluwer Academic Publishers, 1988); Howard Stein, *American Medicine as Culture* (Boulder, Colo.: Westview Press, 1990).

4. J. Chris Hackler and F. Charles Hiller, "Family Consent to Orders Not to Resuscitate: Reconsidering Hospital Policy," *Journal of the American Medical Association* 264, no. 10 (1990): 1281–1283; Elisabeth Rosenthal, "Rules on Reviving the Dying Bring Undue Suffering, Doctors Contend," *New York Times,* October 4, 1990. See also, Mark Siegler, "A Physician's Perspective on a Right to Health Care," *Journal of the American Medical Association* 244, no. 4 (1980): 1591–1596.

5. George J. Annas, Sounding Board, "Nancy Cruzan and the Right to Die," *New England Journal of Medicine* 323, no. 10 (1990): 670–673.

6. Mary-Jo Del Vecchio Good, Byron J. Good, Cynthia Schaffer, and Stuart E. Lind, "American Oncology and the Discourse on Hope," *Culture, Medicine and Psychiatry* 14 (1990): 59–79; Kathryn M. Taylor, "Physicians and the Disclosure of Undesirable Information," in *Biomedicine Examined,* ed. Lock and Gordon, pp. 441–464.

7. John Romano, "The Future Is Not What It Used to Be," *Medical Review* (University of Rochester Medical Center) (Fall, 1984).

8. Tom Tomlinson and Howard Brody, "Futility and the Ethics of Resuscitation," *Journal of the American Medical Association* 264, no. 10 (1990): 1276–1280; and Rosenthal, "Rules on Reviving the Dying Bring Undue Suffering, Doctors Contend."

9. John J. Paris, Robert K. Crone, and Frank Reardon, Occasional Notes, "Physicians' Refusal of Requested Treatment: The Case of Baby L," *New England Journal of Medicine* 322 (1990): 1012–1014.

Transforming Medicine and Culture

1. See, for example, America's Doctors, Medical Science, Medical Care, special issue of *Daedalus* 115 (Spring, 1986); Heyward Brock, ed., *The Culture of Biomedicine: Studies in Science and Culture,* Vol. 1 (London and Toronto: Associated University Presses, 1984); Howard Brody, *The Healer's Power* (New Haven: Yale University Press, 1992); Eric J. Cassell, *The Nature of Suffering* (New York: Oxford University Press, 1991); Ronald J. Christie and C. Barry

Hoffmaster, *Ethical Issues in Family Medicine* (New York: Oxford University Press, 1986); Renee C. Fox, "Ethical and Existential Developments in Contemporaneous American Medicine: Their Implications for Culture and Society," *Milbank Memorial Fund Quarterly* 52 (1974): 445–483; Renee C. Fox and Judith P. Swazey, "Medical Morality Is Not Bioethics—Medical Ethics in China and the United States," *Perspectives in Biology and Medicine* 27 (1984): 336–360; Edmund Pellegrino, *Humanism and the Physician* (Knoxville: University of Tennessee Press, 1979); Charles E. Rosenberg, "Disease and Social Order in America: Perceptions and Expectations," *Milbank Quarterly* 64, Suppl. 1 (1986): 34–55; Harmon L. Smith and Larry R. Churchill, *Professional Ethics and Primary Care Medicine* (Durham: Duke University Press, 1986); David C. Thomasma, "Establishing the Moral Basis of Medicine," *Journal of Medicine and Philosophy* 15 (1970): 245–267; Kerr L. White, *The Task of Medicine* (Menlo Park, Calif.: The Henry J. Kaiser Family Foundation, 1988).

2. Robert N. Bellah, Richard Madsen, William M. Sullivan, Ann Swidler, and Steven M. Tipton, *Habits of the Heart* (Berkeley: University of California Press, 1985); Robert N. Bellah, Richard Madsen, William M. Sullivan, Ann Swidler, and Steven M. Tipton, *The Good Society* (New York: Alfred A. Knopf, 1991); Alasdair MacIntyre, *After Virtue,* 2d ed. (South Bend, Ind.: University of Notre Dame Press, 1984); Charles Taylor, *Sources of the Self* (Cambridge: Harvard University Press, 1989).

3. Perri Klass, *A Not Entirely Benign Procedure* (New York: New American Library, 1987); Melvin Konner, *Becoming a Doctor* (New York: Viking, 1987); Lewis Thomas, book review, "What Doctors Don't Know," *New York Review of Books,* September 24, 1988.

4. Bellah, Madsen, Sullivan, Swidler, and Tipton, *Habits of the Heart;* MacIntyre, *After Virtue.*

5. Barbara A. Koenig, "The Technological Imperative in Medical Practice: The Social Construction of a 'Routine' Treatment," in *Biomedicine Examined,* ed. M. Lock and D. Gordon, pp. 465–496 (Dordrecht: Kluwer Academic Publishers, 1988).

6. MacIntyre, *After Virtue.*

7. Deborah Gordon, "Tenacious Assumptions in Western Medicine," in *Biomedicine Examined,* ed. M. Lock and D. Gordon, pp. 19–56.

Appendix: Perspectives and Methods

1. Sharon R. Kaufman, *The Ageless Self: Sources of Meaning in Late Life* (Madison: University of Wisconsin Press, 1986).

INDEX

347

Life Course Studies

David L. Featherman
David I. Kertzer
  General Editors

Nancy W. Denney
Thomas J. Espenshade
Dennis P. Hogan
Jennie Keith
Maris A. Vinovskis
  Associate General Editors

Family, Political Economy, and Demographic Change:
The Transformation of Life in Casalecchio, Italy, 1861–1921
David I. Kertzer and Dennis P. Hogan

Dolor y Alegría: Women and Social Change in Urban Mexico
Sarah LeVine,
in collaboration with
Clara Sunderland Correa

Family, Class, and Ideology in Early Industrial France:
Social Policy and the Working-Class Family, 1825–1848
Katherine A. Lynch

Event History Analysis in Life Course Research
Karl Ulrich Mayer and Nancy B. Tuma, eds.

Family Dynamics in China: A Life Table Analysis
Zeng Yi